Emergency General Surgery

Editors

PAUL J. SCHENARTS
RONALD F. MARTIN

SURGICAL CLINICS OF NORTH AMERICA

www.surgical.theclinics.com

Consulting Editor
RONALD F. MARTIN

October 2018 • Volume 98 • Number 5

ELSEVIER

1600 John F. Kennedy Boulevard • Suite 1800 • Philadelphia, Pennsylvania, 19103-2899

http://www.surgical.theclinics.com

SURGICAL CLINICS OF NORTH AMERICA Volume 98, Number 5
October 2018 ISSN 0039-6109, ISBN-13: 978-0-323-64099-2

Editor: John Vassallo, j.vassallo@elsevier.com
Developmental Editor: Meredith Madeira

Surgical Clinics of North America (ISSN 0039–6109) is published bimonthly by Elsevier Inc., 360 Park Avenue South, New York, NY 10010-1710. Months of publication are February, April, June, August, October, and December. Business and Editorial Offices: 1600 John F. Kennedy Blvd., Suite 1800, Philadelphia, PA 19103-2899. Periodicals postage paid at New York, NY and additional mailing offices. Subscription prices are $350.00 per year for US individuals, $802.00 per year for US institutions, $100.00 per year for US students and residents, $420.00 per year for Canadian individuals, $1015.00 per year for Canadian institutions, $475.00 for international individuals, $1015.00 per year for international institutions and $225.00 per year for Canadian and foreign students/residents. To receive student/resident rate, orders must be accompanied by name of affiliated institution, date of term, and the *signature* of program/residency coordinator on institution letterhead. Orders will be billed at individual rate until proof of status is received. Foreign air speed delivery is included in all *Clinics* subscription prices. All prices are subject to change without notice. POSTMASTER: Send address changes to *Surgical Clinics*, Elsevier Health Sciences Division, Subscription Customer Service, 3251 Riverport Lane, Maryland Heights, MO 63043. **Customer Service (orders, claims, online, change of address): Telephone: 1-800-654-2452 (U.S. and Canada); 314-447-8871 (outside U.S. and Canada). Fax: 314-447-8029. E-mail: journalscustomerservice-usa@elsevier.com (for print support); journalsonline support-usa@elsevier.com (for online support).**

Reprints. For copies of 100 or more, of articles in this publication, please contact the Commercial Reprints Department, Elsevier Inc., 360 Park Avenue South, New York, New York 10010-1710. Tel. 212-633-3874, Fax: 212-633-3820, E-mail: reprints@elsevier.com.

The Surgical Clinics of North America is also published in Spanish by McGraw-Hill Interamericana Editores S.A., P.O. Box 5-237 06500 Mexico D.F. Mexico; and in Portuguese by Interlivros Edicoes Ltda., Rua Comandante Coelho 1085, CEP 21250, Rio de Janeiro, Brazil; and in Greek by Paschalidis Medical Publications, Athens Greece.

The Surgical Clinics of North America is covered in *MEDLINE/PubMed (Index Medicus), EMBASE/Excerpta Medica, Current Contents/Clinical Medicine, Current Contents/Life Sciences, Science Citation Index*, and *ISI/BIOMED*.

Contributors

CONSULTING EDITOR

RONALD F. MARTIN, MD, FACS
Colonel (retired), United States Army Reserve, Chief, Department of Surgery, York Hospital, York, Maine

EDITORS

PAUL J. SCHENARTS, MD, FACS
Professor and Vice Chairman, Department of Surgery, Section of Trauma, Surgical Critical Care and Emergency General Surgery, University of Nebraska, College of Medicine, Omaha, Nebraska

RONALD F. MARTIN, MD, FACS
Colonel (retired), United States Army Reserve, Chief, Department of Surgery, York Hospital, York, Maine

AUTHORS

FARRELL C. ADKINS, MD
Assistant Professor of Surgery, Carilion Clinic and Virginia Tech Carilion School of Medicine, Roanoke, Virginia

COLLEEN M. ALEXANDER, MD
Clinical Instructor, Fellow, Division of General and Gastrointestinal Surgery, The Ohio State University, Columbus, Ohio

JUAN A. ASENSIO, MD, FACS, FCCM, FRCS (England), KM
Vice Chairman of Surgery, Chief, Division of Trauma Surgery and Surgical Critical Care, Director of Trauma Center and Trauma Program, Professor, Department of Surgery, Professor of Clinical and Translational Science, Department of Translational Science, Creighton University School of Medicine, Omaha, Nebraska; Adjunct Professor of Surgery, Uniformed Services University of the Health Sciences, F. Edward Hébert School of Medicine, Walter Reed National Military Medical Center, Bethesda, Maryland

ZACHARY M. BAUMAN, DO, MHA, FACOS
Assistant Professor, Department of General Surgery, Division of Trauma, Emergency General Surgery and Critical Care Surgery, University of Nebraska Medical Center, Omaha, Nebraska

CURTIS E. BOWER, MD
Carilion Clinic and Virginia Tech Carilion School of Medicine, Roanoke, Virginia

KATIE LOVE BOWER, MD, MSc
Assistant Professor of Surgery, Carilion Clinic and Virginia Tech Carilion School of Medicine, Roanoke, Virginia

JENNY CAI, MD
Department of Surgery, Division of Trauma and Acute Care Surgery, East Carolina University, Brody School of Medicine, Greenville, North Carolina

LOURDES CASTANON, MD
Staff Surgeon, Department of Surgery, Allegheny General Hospital, Pittsburgh, Pennsylvania

ANN YIH-ANN CHUNG, MD
Clinical Instructor, Department of Surgery, University of North Carolina at Chapel Hill, Chapel Hill, North Carolina

MICHAEL DITILLO, DO
Department of Surgery, Allegheny General Hospital, Pittsburgh, Pennsylvania

MEREDITH COLLEEN DUKE, MD, MBA, FACS
Assistant Professor, Department of Surgery, University of North Carolina at Chapel Hill, Chapel Hill, North Carolina

BRYAN A. EHLERT, MD
Assistant Professor, Department of Cardiovascular Sciences, East Carolina University, Brody School of Medicine, Greenville, North Carolina

CHARITY H. EVANS, MD, MHCM, FACS
Assistant Professor, Department of General Surgery, Division of Trauma, Emergency General Surgery and Critical Care Surgery, University of Nebraska Medical Center, Omaha, Nebraska

NICOLE M. GARCIA, MD
Department of Surgery, Division of Trauma and Acute Care Surgery, East Carolina University, Brody School of Medicine, Greenville, North Carolina

BRADLEY ROUNSBORG HALL, MD
Department of General Surgery, University of Nebraska Medical Center, Omaha, Nebraska

ABDULRAHMAN Y. HAMMAD, MD
Department of Surgery, Allegheny General Hospital, Pittsburgh, Pennsylvania

JASON W. KEMPENICH, MD
Assistant Professor, Department of Surgery, The University of Texas Health Science Center at San Antonio, San Antonio, Texas

DANIEL I. LOLLAR, MD
Assistant Professor of Surgery, Carilion Clinic and Virginia Tech Carilion School of Medicine, Roanoke, Virginia

DAVID T. LUYIMBAZI, MD
Assistant Professor of Surgery, Carilion Clinic and Virginia Tech Carilion School of Medicine, Roanoke, Virginia

MICHAEL M. McNALLY, MD, FACS
Assistant Professor, Department of Surgery, Division of Vascular Surgery, University of Tennessee, Knoxville, Tennessee

MICHAEL P. MEARA, MD, FACS
Assistant Professor, Division of General and Gastrointestinal Surgery, The Ohio State University, Columbus, Ohio

DAVID W. NELMS, MD
General Surgery Residency Program, UnityPoint Health, Des Moines, Iowa

JACOB ORAN, MD
Department of General Surgery, University of Nebraska Medical Center, Omaha, Nebraska

CARLOS A. PELAEZ, MD
General Surgery, Trauma and Critical Care, The Iowa Clinic, Trauma Services, General Surgery Residency Program, UnityPoint Health, Des Moines, Iowa

PAUL J. SCHENARTS, MD, FACS
Professor and Vice Chairman, Department of Surgery, Section of Trauma, Surgical Critical Care and Emergency General Surgery, University of Nebraska, College of Medicine, Omaha, Nebraska

LISA L. SCHLITZKUS, MD, FACS
Assistant Professor, Department of Surgery, Section of Trauma, Surgical Critical Care and Emergency General Surgery, University of Nebraska, College of Medicine, Omaha, Nebraska

KENNETH R. SIRINEK, MD, PhD
Professor, Department of Surgery, The University of Texas Health Science Center at San Antonio, San Antonio, Texas

JESSICA I. SUMMERS, MD, FACS
Assistant Professor, Department of Surgery, Section of Trauma, Surgical Critical Care and Emergency General Surgery, University of Nebraska, College of Medicine, Omaha, Nebraska

TIFFANY NICOLE TANNER, MD, FACS
Associate Program Director, Assistant Professor of Surgery, Department of General Surgery, Minimally Invasive and Bariatric Surgery, University of Nebraska Medical Center, Omaha, Nebraska

DUSTIN JOHN TUBRE, MD
Resident, General Surgery, Creighton University School of Medicine, Omaha, Nebraska

JUNIOR UNIVERS, MD
Fellow, Department of Surgery, Division of Vascular Surgery, University of Tennessee, Knoxville, Tennessee

MICHEL WAGNER, MD, FACS
Assistant Professor, Department of Surgery, Division of Trauma Surgery and Surgical Critical Care, Assistant Professor of Clinical and Translational Sciences, Department of Translational Science, Creighton University School of Medicine, Creighton University Medical Center, Omaha, Nebraska

BRANDT D. WHITEHURST, MD, MS
Clinical Assistant Professor, Department of Surgery, Southern Illinois University School of Medicine, Springfield, Illinois

SHARON L. WILLIAMS, MD
Assistant Professor of Surgery, Carilion Clinic and Virginia Tech Carilion School of Medicine, Roanoke, Virginia

Contents

Foreword: Emergency General Surgery xiii

Ronald F. Martin

Preface: Emergency General Surgery xvii

Paul J. Schenarts and Ronald F. Martin

Acute Biliary Disease 877

Ann Yih-Ann Chung and Meredith Colleen Duke

Acute biliary disease is a ubiquitous acute surgical complaint. General surgeons managing emergency surgical patients must be knowledgeable and capable of identifying and caring for common presentations. This article discusses the workup, diagnosis, and management of the varying pathologies that make up biliary disease, including cholelithiasis, cholecystitis, biliary dyskinesia, choledocholithiasis, cholangitis, gallstone pancreatitis, and gallstone ileus. Also addressed are more challenging and rare presentations, including pregnancy and bariatric anatomy.

Pancreatitis 895

Abdulrahman Y. Hammad, Michael Ditillo, and Lourdes Castanon

Acute pancreatitis is an inflammation of the glandular parenchyma of the retroperitoneal organ that leads to injury with or without subsequent destruction of the pancreatic acini. This inflammatory process can either result in a self-limited disease or involve life-threatening multiorgan complications. Chronic pancreatitis consists of endocrine and exocrine gland dysfunction that develops secondary to progressive inflammation and chronic fibrosis of the pancreatic acini with permanent structural damage. Recurrent attacks of acute pancreatitis can result in chronic pancreatitis; acute and chronic pancreatitis are different diseases with separate morphologic patterns. Acute pancreatitis has an increasing incidence but a decreasing mortality.

Pneumoperitoneum 915

Tiffany Nicole Tanner, Bradley Rounsborg Hall, and Jacob Oran

Pneumoperitoneum has a wide differential diagnosis and presents with varying degrees of severity; however, not all causes require operative intervention. It is imperative that all patients with this diagnosis are evaluated by a surgeon. A thorough history, physical examination, and workup, aimed at localization of the source of pneumoperitoneum, will ultimately determine the necessary treatments, including the need for operative intervention. The authors provide the reader with a working knowledge regarding the evaluation and treatment of patients with pneumoperitoneum.

Acid Peptic Disease 933

Jason W. Kempenich and Kenneth R. Sirinek

The management of peptic ulcer disease has radically changed over the last 40 years from primarily surgical treatment to medical therapy nearly eliminating the need for elective surgery in these patients. Although there has been a decline in patients requiring acute surgical intervention for complications of peptic ulcer disease (perforation, bleeding, and obstruction), these patients still make up a significant proportion of hospital admissions every year. The modern acute care surgeon must have significant knowledge of the multiple treatment modalities used to appropriately care for these patients.

Small Bowel Obstruction 945

Katie Love Bower, Daniel I. Lollar, Sharon L. Williams, Farrell C. Adkins, David T. Luyimbazi, and Curtis E. Bower

Identifying patients with small bowel obstruction who need operative intervention and those who will fail nonoperative management is a challenge. Without indications for urgent intervention, a computed tomography scan with/without intravenous contrast should be obtained to identify the location, grade, and cause of the obstruction. Most small bowel obstructions resolve with nonoperative management. Open and laparoscopic operative management are acceptable approaches. Malnutrition needs to be identified early and managed, especially if the patient is to undergo operative management. Confounding conditions include age greater than 65 years, post Roux-en-Y gastric bypass, inflammatory bowel disease, malignancy, virgin abdomen, pregnancy, hernia, and early postoperative state.

Volvulus 973

Zachary M. Bauman and Charity H. Evans

Intestinal volvulus, regardless of location, is a rare disease process but one that requires high suspicion and timely diagnosis given the increased incidence of intestinal necrosis and potential mortality. Most patients with intestinal volvulus require some form of surgical intervention. However, over the last few decades, the workup and management of intestinal volvulus has changed given constant advancements in technology and patient care. Most important, however, is recognizing the need for emergent versus more elective surgery because this influences the morbidity and mortality for the individual patient.

Acute Gut Ischemia 995

Bryan A. Ehlert

Acute mesenteric ischemia is a surgical emergency commonly caused by embolic or thrombotic occlusion of the superior mesenteric artery. Prompt diagnosis, fluid resuscitation, systemic anticoagulation, and mesenteric revascularization are key tenets to the treatment of this lethal condition. Revascularization can be performed via open thromboembolectomy or surgical bypass, endovascular techniques, or a hybrid approach of the

two. Despite technologic advancements, mortalities remain high, and the plan of care and revascularization should be based on the patient's clinical status and available medical center resources.

Evolution and Current Trends in the Management of Acute Appendicitis **1005**

Michel Wagner, Dustin John Tubre, and Juan A. Asensio

The treatment of appendicitis has evolved since the first appendectomy in the eighteenth century. It seems to have come full circle with nonoperative management in the era before frequent surgical interventions, to open surgical interventions, minimally invasive interventions, and now back to a renewed interest in nonoperative management of acute appendicitis. Scoring systems to help refine the diagnosis of acute appendicitis and advances in medical imaging have also changed the management of this condition. Scientific investigations into the effects the microbiome of the appendix play in this disease process are also being considered.

Emergency Presentations of Diverticulitis **1025**

Michael P. Meara and Colleen M. Alexander

Acute diverticulitis is a common condition that has been increasing in incidence in the United States. It is associated with increasing age, but the pathophysiology of acute diverticulitis is still being elucidated. It is now believed to have a significant contribution from inflammatory processes rather than being a strictly infectious process. There are still many questions to be answered regarding the optimal management of acute diverticulitis because recent studies have challenged traditional practices, such as the routine use of antibiotics, surgical technique, and dietary restrictions for prevention of recurrence.

The Acute Upper Gastrointestinal Bleed **1047**

David W. Nelms and Carlos A. Pelaez

Upper gastrointestinal bleeding (UGIB), defined as intraluminal hemorrhage proximal to the ligament of Treitz, can range from mild and asymptomatic to massive life-threatening hemorrhage. For the purposes of this article, the authors define an acute UGIB to be one that results in new acute symptoms and is, therefore, potentially life-threatening. UGIB requires a systematic approach to evaluation and treatment, similar to the management of a trauma patient. Surgeon involvement in UGIBs remains integral despite the rare need for operative management. Endoscopy is the primary tool for diagnosis and treatment.

Lower Gastrointestinal Bleeding **1059**

Brandt D. Whitehurst

Lower gastrointestinal bleeding entails a range of severity and a multitude of options for localization and control of bleeding. With experience in trauma, critical care, endoscopy, and definitive surgical interventions, general surgeons are equipped to manage this condition in various clinical settings. This article examines traditional and emerging options for bleeding localization and control available to general surgeons.

SURGICAL CLINICS OF NORTH AMERICA

FORTHCOMING ISSUES

December 2018
Enhanced Recovery After Surgery: Past, Present and Future
Daniel I. Chu, *Editor*

February 2019
Issues in Transplant Surgery
Juan Palma-Vargas, *Editor*

April 2019
Diseases of the Biliary Tract
J. Bart Rose, *Editor*

RECENT ISSUES

August 2018
Management of Breast Cancer
Catherine C. Parker, *Editor*

June 2018
Current Concepts in Hernia Surgery
Ajita S. Prabhu, *Editor*

April 2018
Vascular Surgery: Current Concepts and Treatments for Venous Disease
Marc A. Passman, *Editor*

ISSUE OF RELATED INTEREST

Thoracic Surgery Clinics, February 2018 (Vol. 28, Issue 1)
Thoracic Surgery in the Special Care Patient
Sharon Ben-Or, *Editor*
Available at: www.thoracic.theclinics.com

Foreword
Emergency General Surgery

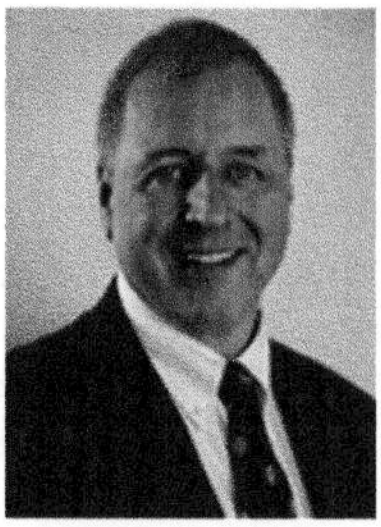

Ronald F. Martin, MD, FACS
Consulting Editor

As it has been said, change is the one constant you can count on. Our discipline of surgery is no exception to this rule. Sometimes changes come via gradual evolutionary processes, and sometimes events alter more rapidly. And sometimes it is hard to tell the difference even when you are right in the middle of the changes.

The discipline of general surgery continues to morph along many lines. Each change seems to usher in further division within our group. Historically, the evolution of specialty training and development was designed to add capability and to expand practice. At a certain point, hard to say when exactly, the effort and ability required to maintain the highest standards on the specialty focus became incompatible with also maintaining the requirements for highest standards on the broader base discipline. So, it followed that specialists in many cases abandoned their primary source of training in favor of full-time focus on their specialty efforts. For the most part, this was probably a good thing. Of course, one not-necessarily-intended consequence of this collection of choices was that it further raised the bar of competition for the generalist—being now compared to the specialist—in many areas that were traditionally in the purview of the generalist.

As medicine itself and the business of medicine writ large have evolved on a separate but possibly related path, we find ourselves encountering a number of new forces at play. Perhaps chief among them is the desire of some of our colleagues to pursue career paths that limit their responsibility or place limits on the amount of time the profession can demand of them. "Specialty" training can be sometimes used as a way to compartmentalize one's responsibility or to avoid either some undesired clinical activity or some time responsibility, such as call.

As with all such changing landscapes, things don't always go as planned. The discipline of trauma surgery might be a prime example. Many decades ago, trauma care was poorly organized, haphazard, and highly variable in quality. This was, of course, recognized, and extraordinary efforts were put in place to not just improve the

Surg Clin N Am 98 (2018) xiii–xv
https://doi.org/10.1016/j.suc.2018.07.018
0039-6109/18/© 2018 Published by Elsevier Inc.

operative aspect of care for the traumatized patient but also look systematically at all the other in-hospital as well as out-of-hospital elements of the trauma care system. As you undoubtedly are aware, amazing progress has been made for this discipline. The system's successes as well as the improvement in personnel training provided an excellent platform for discipline development. As our imaging technology also improved—in particular the image processing technology—we surgeons found ourselves in an interesting position: as a group, we were rapidly converting what had been a technically demanding operative specialty into a specialty that was to become largely nonoperative (at least for the general surgery component).

The success of nonoperative strategies for the management of traumatized patients, particularly patients who suffered blunt trauma but increasingly those with some forms of penetrating trauma as well, gradually eroded the operative opportunities for a substantial fraction of trauma surgeons and trauma centers. This continued to such a degree that some surgeons, even at Level 1 trauma centers, were performing very few operations per year. The American College of Surgeons Committee on Trauma recognized this as a concern and started to place some operative volume requirements as part of its certification process. Perhaps by serendipity, this happened at an interesting time as it coincided with a growing number of surgeons who were "less than enthusiastic" about operating at all hours of the day and night. We had a growing number of surgeons (trauma surgeons) who needed more opportunity to go to the operating room coupled with a growing number of surgeons (general and specialty surgeons) who would prefer to not operate at night or on weekends. It would seem like a match made in heaven.

Or possibly not so fast.

We may have solved the problem of who would work at what time, but we had not solved the issues created by the generalist/specialist divided in terms of experience or depth of training that we had been brewing for more than half a century. To make it worse in some regards, we were asking those with the least amount of recent operative experience to tackle some of the most challenging operative problems across a very wide spectrum of concerns, sometimes with the least amount of collegial support.

The difficulty inherent in this transition was fairly obvious to just about everybody, so we did what we usually do: we created a new fellowship model and called it Acute Care Surgery. The training for this acute care paradigm combines training for emergent problems for both trauma and non-trauma-related maladies. In theory, this should work, but it may depend somewhat upon who is the trainee and who are the trainers in order to generate a group of surgeons who work comfortably in both worlds. Despites claims by many, the final results of this experiment are not completely in yet.

Regardless of the historical arc that ushered in the era of Acute Care Surgery, we now seem to once again be dividing the group of patients who arrive unexpectedly into the trauma population and those who require "emergency general surgery." It probably makes sense to do so, as while some would still like to conflate the two topics, they are in many respects distinct. Part of the original separation of trauma surgery as a specialty from general surgery was an understanding of the benefit of detailed knowledge of critical care principles and the nuanced care required for complex resuscitation in the physiologically deranged patient. The operative demands of that discipline lessened, and perhaps we could have left it at that. Perhaps we could have solved the shortage of operative experience on some trauma teams by other means. We added general surgery emergencies to the trauma team plate in large part for the matched unexpected workload with available personnel without regard to the observation that there is a lot less skill set requirement in common, for instance, between caring for the patient with free intraperitoneal perforation from diverticulitis or one with hepatic hemorrhage secondary to blunt trauma than there would be comparing the care of the patient with diverticulitis to caring of the patient with sigmoid colon cancer.

For the last century, much, though certainly not all, of the increase in our collective surgical knowledge was a product of the specialization into organ-based care (as opposed to etiology-based or technique-based care). In order to maintain a round-the-clock level of excellence in operative as well as surgical care, our future emergency general surgeons will need to acquire their operative skill sets in much the same way that their counterparts provide "scheduled care." In the past we tackled this problem within the general surgery residency programs, but perhaps we are not doing that as well as we thought given the number of people who seek additional training to feel comfortable treating emergently ill patients.

There are many more factors that contribute to our current state of affairs in this matter than I have discussed. Surgeons converting from being largely self-employed to hospital-based employees, shifting demographics of patient bases as well as surgeon distribution, increasing competition between hospital systems, ever changing reimbursement models, and even the changes or uncertainties inherent to the larger national debates on health care all have been forces at play in creating our new models of care delivery. In some respects, how we got here isn't that important: what is important is that we realize that we have new challenges to how we collectively provide surgical care for those members of our communities who need our help—day or night. Whatever solutions we devise should be designed to solve the problem for the patients first and foremost.

As with every topic we bring forward in the *Surgical Clinics of North America* series, we do so with the hope of providing a collection of articles that is helpful on the individual basis but even more helpful when collected as a complete issue. I am deeply grateful to our collaborators on this issue, in particular, my longtime friend and colleague, Dr Paul (P.J.) Schenarts, for their excellent effort. We hope that if you find yourself getting hammered on call some night that this issue may provide you an easy place to turn should you need help.

Ronald F. Martin, MD, FACS
Department of Surgery
York Hospital
15 Hospital Drive
York, ME 03909, USA

E-mail address:
rmartin@yorkhospital.com

Preface
Emergency General Surgery

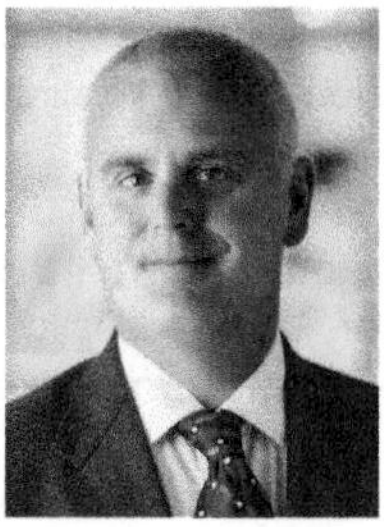
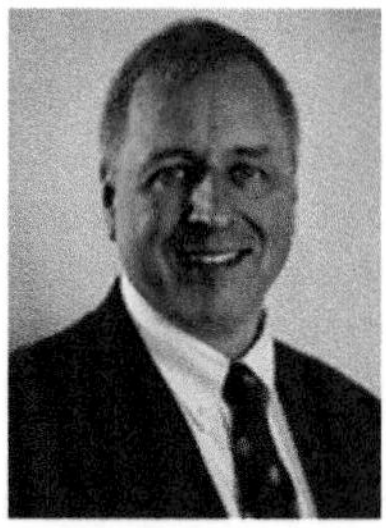

Paul J. Schenarts, MD, FACS   Ronald F. Martin, MD, FACS
Editors

The care of the patient who presents with surgical concerns on an unexpected basis was once solely in the domain of the general surgeon who also practiced in the scheduled realm. While that remains the case in many hospital systems, it is increasing being replaced by care delivered by surgeons who primarily, if not only, encounter these patients on an urgent basis. This evolving paradigm has caused us to transition from pairing the patient who has a certain clinical problem with a surgeon who has a certain clinical skill set to pairing the patient with the person who happens to be at the facility at that time.

This new arrangement has some benefits for patients and providers alike in that it may de-conflict schedules as well as provide some assurance of timely availability of both professional and facility resources. However, it may create areas of mismatching of patient needs with availability of clinical expertise. Sometimes that mismatch is recognized early and mitigated; sometimes not.

As we have evolved from general surgery to acute care surgery to emergency general surgery models, our paths to skill and experience acquisition (spelled residency and fellowship training) have struggled to keep pace. We find ourselves now with a group of surgeons who are being asked to cover a broader waterfront of problems with sometimes considerably less preparation than in days passed. Furthermore, some of these encounters happen at odd hours or times when other specialty assistance may be difficult to find.

When we first imagined this issue, we thought of titling something like, "Guidebook to night on call from Hell." Of course, even momentary reflection made us think we needed a more appropriate title. Still, the notion that we would try to colocate in one issue a broad spectrum of topics that any surgeon might encounter covering *any* hospital emergency department was the paramount driver. We considered producing an issue on "Acute Care Surgery," but as mentioned above, we felt that trauma was a broad enough topic of its own that has been peeling away from acute care in the broad

Surg Clin N Am 98 (2018) xvii–xviii
https://doi.org/10.1016/j.suc.2018.07.017

sense. Also, the need for trauma expertise and the requirement for that knowledge may be far more variable between institutions than what we perceive as the more universal need to provide Emergency General Surgery no matter where one is.

To that end, we reached out to those who we felt could bring a depth and breadth of knowledge from both our civilian and military environments that would allow us to compile an easy-to-find and easy-to-use issue to get one through the difficult night of call and perhaps beyond. We did not design this to be the definitive guide to every clinical endpoint but rather as a tool to help anyone play "zone defense" until definitive strategies could be operationalized.

We are deeply indebted to our colleagues, who have shared their expertise on these matters. The generosity of their time and effort as well as their insights is of great value to all of us as a community. We are also indebted to our publisher, John Vassallo, for his tireless efforts on this series as well as all of our production staff from Elsevier, especially Meredith Madeira.

We hope that no one ever has to deal with all these topics in one day or even over a couple of days, but if one did, we hope this issue could be of some use.

Paul J. Schenarts, MD, FACS
University of Nebraska
Omaha, NE, 68182, USA

Ronald F. Martin, MD, FACS
Department of Surgery
York Hospital
15 Hospital Drive
York, ME 03909, USA

E-mail address:
rmartin@yorkhospital.com

Acute Biliary Disease

Ann Yih-Ann Chung, MD*, Meredith Colleen Duke, MD, MBA

KEYWORDS

• Emergency surgery • Acute care surgery • Biliary • Cholelithiasis • Cholecystitis • Choledocholithiasis • Gallstone pancreatitis • Cholecystectomy

KEY POINTS

- This article will discuss the work-up and diagnosis of biliary diseases including cholelithiasis, cholecystitis, biliary dyskinesia, choledocholithiasis, gallstone pancreatitis, and gallstone ileus.
- This article will review the management of acute presentations of biliary disease for the emergency general surgeon.
- This article will describe the management of biliary disease in unique populations, such as pregnant women, and post bariatric surgery individuals.

INTRODUCTION

Approximately 700,000 to 800,000 cholecystectomies are performed in the United States annually making it the most common elective abdominal operation at present.[1] Given the prevalence of biliary disease, it is important for the general surgeon to be able to recognize its many manifestations and how to manage them. Acute biliary-related presentations are typically secondary to the presence of gallstones and can range from simple symptomatic cholelithiasis to cholangitis causing septic shock. In addition, surgeons often encounter gallbladder disease in complicated populations, such as pregnant women or patients who have had bariatric surgery. This article discusses the work-up, diagnosis, and management of the varying pathologies that make up biliary disease including cholelithiasis, cholecystitis, biliary dyskinesia, choledocholithiasis, cholangitis, gallstone pancreatitis, gallstone ileus.

CHOLELITHIASIS

In the United States, 10% to 15% of the population have gallstones. Of this group, about 10% to 25% develop symptoms related to their gallstones with the risk of asymptomatic gallstones becoming symptomatic at 1% to 2% per year. Incidental gallstones are commonly noted on routine imaging. In patients who are otherwise asymptomatic, it is not recommended to proceed with an elective prophylactic

---

Disclosure Statement: The authors have nothing to disclose.
Department of Surgery, University of North Carolina-Chapel Hill, 4035 Burnett-Womack, Campus Box 7081, Chapel Hill, NC 27599-7081, USA
* Corresponding author.
E-mail address: Ann_Chung@med.unc.edu

Surg Clin N Am 98 (2018) 877–894
https://doi.org/10.1016/j.suc.2018.05.003
surgical.theclinics.com

cholecystectomy. Multiple studies have been performed to identify prognostic factors to predict the need for cholecystectomy in patients with gallstones, but they have all been inconclusive. Currently, the only relative indications for prophylactic cholecystectomies for asymptomatic cholelithiasis are in post heart transplant patients, or patients with sickle cell anemia or hereditary spherocytosis who need a splenectomy, and patients who are found to have a single gallstone that is greater than 1 cm, which has been shown to be a risk factor for malignancy.[2]

Diagnosis

Symptomatic cholelithiasis typically presents with right upper quadrant abdominal pain that occurs after eating, usually fatty foods, and lasts for about 30 minutes. It is also associated with nausea and emesis. This disease is also known as biliary colic. It is caused by intermittent obstruction of the cystic duct or neck of the gallbladder by a gallstone. Symptoms can be mistaken for other gastrointestinal processes, such as gastroesophageal reflux disease or irritable bowel disease. Transabdominal ultrasound remains the best initial diagnostic imaging study for biliary pathology and has been proven to have the best sensitivity and specificity for evaluating gallstones.[3] Gallstones are often seen on computed tomography (CT) scans but although CT scans are helpful in evaluating for other biliary pathology, it is less sensitive than ultrasound for identifying gallstones. MRI is equivalent to ultrasound for visualizing gallstones; however, because of the increased cost and timeliness of this study, it is of low benefit as an initial diagnostic modality. Both CT scans and MRIs are more often used to evaluate for complex biliary disease.[4]

Management

Unlike asymptomatic cholelithiasis, the indication for surgery for biliary colic is clear. Laparoscopic cholecystectomy is recommended for symptomatic cholelithiasis in appropriate surgical candidates, because these patients can go on to develop further complications of cholelithiasis, such as choledocholithiasis or cholecystitis. It is important to rule out concurrent choledocholithiasis because this changes the treatment plan. This is typically done by obtaining a hepatic function panel, specifically concerning the total bilirubin and alkaline phosphatase, and evaluating the diameter of the common bile duct on ultrasound. Any indication of possible biliary obstruction, including enzyme elevation or a dilated common bile duct, should prompt further work-up for choledocholithiasis. Although cholecystectomy for symptomatic cholelithiasis is typically an elective procedure, patients do often present to the emergency department with severe pain from biliary colic and it is not unreasonable to proceed with a semiurgent cholecystectomy in that situation.

ACUTE CALCULOUS CHOLECYSTITIS

Acute calculous cholecystitis occurs when a gallstone obstructs the cystic duct leading to inflammation, gallbladder distention, and eventual ischemia. Symptoms typically include right upper quadrant abdominal pain, nausea, vomiting, and fever. A common finding on physical examination is Murphy sign, which is defined as inspiratory arrest caused by pain during deep palpation in the right upper quadrant of the abdomen. Its sensitivity and specificity for acute cholecystitis has been reported as 62% and 96%, respectively.[5] It is important to consider other diagnoses when confronted with this clinical presentation, which is somewhat generalized. Peptic ulcer disease, acute pancreatitis, gastroenteritis, nephrolithiasis, and even myocardial ischemia can present in a similar fashion.

Diagnosis

The Tokyo Guidelines, which were most recently updated in 2013, are often used to diagnose and guide management of acute cholecystitis. Diagnostic criteria include local signs of inflammation, such as the presence of a Murphy sign, systemic signs of inflammation including fever or leukocytosis, and imaging findings of cholecystitis. When all three are present, the Tokyo Guidelines report a 91% sensitivity and 97% specificity for acute cholecystitis.[6]

A right upper quadrant ultrasound remains the initial diagnostic imaging of choice to evaluate biliary pathology. Ultrasound findings show gallstones, gallbladder wall thickening (4 mm or greater), and pericholecystic fluid. Similar to the evaluation for cholelithiasis, CT and MRI can also be used. If the diagnosis of cholecystitis is equivocal based on imaging, but clinical suspicion remains high, a hepatobiliary iminodiacetic acid (HIDA) scan can be used. It has a higher sensitivity and specificity for acute cholecystitis compared with ultrasound, but it is costlier and more time-consuming to obtain limiting its use.[3]

Laboratory tests should also be obtained including a complete blood count and hepatic functional panel. Patients may demonstrate leukocytosis. It is not uncommon to have elevation of alkaline phosphatase. Elevated bilirubin levels should raise suspicion for biliary obstruction, which would require further evaluation to rule out choledocholithiasis.

It is important to remember that acute calculous cholecystitis remains a largely clinical diagnosis. Patient factors, such as congestive heart failure or primary liver disease, can also demonstrate similar findings to cholecystitis on imaging (eg, pericholecystic fluid) and laboratory values. Thus, the patient's symptoms and physical examination are just as critical in making the accurate diagnosis of acute calculous cholecystitis as is the interpretation of tests.

Management

The Tokyo Guidelines categorizes acute calculous cholecystitis into three stages: mild (grade I), moderate (grade II), and severe (grade III). For all three categories of cholecystitis, early laparoscopic cholecystectomy is recommended if the patient can tolerate the procedure. For severe (grade III) cholecystitis where the patient shows organ dysfunction and/or severe local inflammation, other options are suggested if the patient is not clinically stable to undergo a surgery.[7] Proceeding initially with open cholecystectomy, even in severe cases of cholecystitis, is no longer suggested although conversion from laparoscopic to open surgery does occur in 10% to 30% of cases typically secondary to complications or difficult anatomy. In the era of early laparoscopic surgery, acute cholecystitis was actually considered a relative contraindication to a laparoscopic approach because of the concern for higher rates of complication. However, with improvement in laparoscopic technique, laparoscopic cholecystectomy has shown to have improved mortality and morbidity as compared with open surgery with benefits of decreased length of hospital stay, decreased hospital costs, and shorter overall recovery time.[8]

It is in part because of the advent of laparoscopy that the timing of surgery for cholecystitis remains controversial. During the early adoption of laparoscopic cholecystectomy, surgical treatment of acute cholecystitis was believed to be of higher risk. Common practice was to administer a course of antibiotics to allow the gallbladder to "cool down" and to then perform a delayed laparoscopic cholecystectomy. This was typically performed 4 to 6 weeks following initial presentation, once the acute inflammation had resolved, which presumably would decrease risks of complications, such as bile duct injury. Once laparoscopic cholecystectomy was adopted as the procedure of choice for acute cholecystitis, numerous retrospective and prospective studies were performed to look at early versus delayed cholecystectomy resulting in the current consensus favoring early cholecystectomy within 24 hours of presentation. This recommendation is somewhat muddled by the duration of symptoms before presentation, which was widely variable among the studies (1–7 days). The 2013 Tokyo Guidelines recommend cholecystectomy within 24 hours of presentation for those patients whose symptoms have been present for no longer than 72 hours.[7] This is in the absence of complicating pathology including gallstone pancreatitis and choledocholithiasis (discussed later). Despite the contested timing of symptoms, the studies evaluating the outcomes of early versus delayed laparoscopic cholecystectomy agree that the morbidity and specifically the rate of bile duct injury is no different in early versus delayed surgery. With early operative intervention, the rates of conversion to open surgery, readmission, and other biliary complications, such as gallstone pancreatitis and choledocholithiasis, are equivalent, if not lower.[4,9]

Antibiotics should be initiated immediately before surgery and should target enteric pathogens, such as gram-negative aerobes, *Escherichia coli*, *Klebsiella pneumonia*, and anaerobes. Duration of antibiotic therapy varies on the presentation and severity of the infection and inflammation and there is no true consensus. For uncomplicated acute cholecystitis, antibiotics are not continued following cholecystectomy.[4] In cases in which early cholecystectomy is not performed, typically patients are treated with a full course of antibiotics (10–14 days) before a delayed cholecystectomy.

In circumstances where patients are not candidates for general anesthesia, typically secondary to severe medical comorbidities, or are critically ill and cannot tolerate a surgery, cholecystectomy is not recommended. In these patients, a tube cholecystostomy is the suggested treatment in addition to antibiotics.[10] This is a procedure often performed by interventional radiology and is a tube that is directed percutaneously into the gallbladder either transhepatic or transperitoneal. This method allows drainage of the gallbladder without the risk of an operation and has an 85% to 90% success rate in clinical improvement. The cholecystostomy tube can then be removed in 4 to 6 weeks after tube cholangiography confirms patency of the cystic duct. The tube should remain in place if the cystic duct remains obstructed. Elective laparoscopic cholecystectomy should then be offered in these patients because there is a high rate of recurrence of biliary disease in this population even if the cystic duct opens following biliary drainage. In patients who continue to be poor surgical candidates, the tube is removed once the cystic duct is proven to be patent or their biliary disease is managed with the tube.[11]

ACALCULOUS CHOLECYSTITIS

Acute acalculous cholecystitis is a phenomenon that occurs in the critically ill population, associated with severe trauma, burns, sepsis, recent complex surgery, and patients requiring prolonged total parenteral nutrition. The exact pathophysiology of acalculous cholecystitis is still somewhat elusive but results from bile stasis and gallbladder ischemia likely as a response to systemic inflammation and illness. It is difficult to diagnose and there must be a high index of suspicion. It has been associated with high morbidity and mortality, in part secondary to the critically ill status of these patients, but also because there is often a delay in diagnosis. Presentation is nonspecific and is similar to the symptoms of calculous cholecystitis, such as right upper quadrant pain, fevers, leukocytosis, and elevated liver function enzymes (alkaline phosphatase, bilirubin).[12]

Diagnosis

Once acalculous cholecystitis is suspected, work-up should begin with an ultrasound. Although the sensitivity and specificity of ultrasound for acalculous cholecystitis is lower compared with that for calculous cholecystitis, it is performed rapidly and at bedside. Many of these patients are critically ill with mechanical ventilation and transport to the radiology suite is risky and cumbersome. Ultrasound findings suggestive of acalculous cholecystitis include gallbladder wall thickening (the most sensitive finding), pericholecystic fluid, hydrops, and intramural gas. A HIDA scan is the next most useful modality in diagnosing acalculous cholecystitis with sensitivity and specificity ranging from 67% to 100% and 38% to 100%, respectively. Some would argue that it is the best radiographic tool to help diagnose acalculous cholecystitis; however, because the test can take 1 to 6 hours and requires transport, it is often not a feasible option in a critically ill patient. It is often used in settings where ultrasound is indeterminate. A positive HIDA scan would demonstrate lack of filling of the gallbladder after 1 hour of injection of technetium or 30 minutes after injection of morphine. Finally, CT scan can also be used with findings similar to that of ultrasound.[12] Some patients are incorrectly given the diagnosis of acalculous cholecystitis, because stones were not visualized on imaging. This is caused by stone passage, or lack of visualization, more common in the setting of obesity.

Management

Prompt diagnosis and intervention is key in the management of acute acalculous cholecystitis because this diagnosis carries a high morbidity and mortality. The suggested treatment depends on the stability of the patient. If they can tolerate general anesthesia, immediate laparoscopic cholecystectomy is recommended. Should the patient not tolerate the procedure, a drainage tube is left in the gallbladder during laparoscopy. Most patients with acute acalculous cholecystitis are not candidates for surgery, thus tube cholecystostomy is typically the more common treatment. Tube management is similar to that of calculous cholecystitis. Tube removal follows confirmation of cystic duct patency. Oftentimes patients do not require a cholecystectomy following tube removal, because the inciting factors for the development of acute acalculous cholecystitis have resolved by that time.[12]

BILIARY DYSKINESIA/SPHINCTER OF ODDI DYSFUNCTION

Functional gallbladder disorders are a controversial group of disease entities that general surgeons face, frequently in the acute setting. The diagnosis and determination of need for surgery is complicated, so it may be more prudent to manage on an elective basis. Biliary dyskinesia and sphincter of Oddi dysfunction make up functional gallbladder disorders in which patients have biliary colic, right upper quadrant and/or epigastric pain following eating, in the absence of gallstones or evidence of gallbladder inflammation. The cause and pathophysiology of these entities is unclear but biliary dyskinesia is typically defined as gallbladder dysmotility, whereas sphincter of Oddi dysfunction suggests elevated pressures of the sphincter of Oddi also causing emptying issues. Both of these then lead to biliary colic similar to that experienced by patients with symptomatic cholelithiasis. The incidence of functional gallbladder disorders is almost three-fold higher in the female population.[13]

Diagnosis

Because the primary symptom of both biliary dyskinesia and sphincter of Oddi dysfunction is pain, the diagnosis of these disorders is perplexing. It is often a diagnosis of exclusion, so it is important to rule out other more common causes of right upper quadrant abdominal pain, such as gastroesophageal reflux disease, dyspepsia, irritable bowel syndrome, and pancreatitis. The Rome III Criteria has been cited to help in the diagnosis of these disorders.[14] Laboratory values are typically normal with no leukocytosis/leukopenia and no abnormalities in liver function enzymes. Imaging should be obtained to rule out cholelithiasis, and any other cause for abdominal pain, but note that ultrasound has a low sensitivity for detecting very small stones (<3 mm) or sludge so it is not uncommon to find sludge or microcholelithiasis when operating on these patients. Endoscopic ultrasound (EUS) does have a higher sensitivity and specificity for the detection of very small gallstones and is used as an adjunct to rule out cholelithiasis.[15]

Once all other potential causes have been evaluated for and ruled out, HIDA scan with cholecystokinin stimulation should be obtained to evaluate for biliary dyskinesia and endoscopic retrograde cholangiopancreatography (ERCP) with sphincter of Oddi manometry should be performed for sphincter of Oddi dysfunction. Reduced ejection fraction of the gallbladder less than 35% is considered to be consistent with biliary dyskinesia, whereas sphincter of Oddi basal pressures in excess of 40 mm Hg is consistent with sphincter of Oddi dysfunction.[14]

Management

Laparoscopic cholecystectomy should be considered in patients who have undergone a thorough work-up and have been concluded to have biliary dyskinesia. Studies have shown that patients with reproducible pain after cholecystokinin injection do have clinical improvement following cholecystectomy. It is important to discuss with the patient that their symptoms may not completely resolve following surgery. The studies regarding cholecystectomy as the treatment of biliary dyskinesia are limited and the results range widely from 38% to 90% symptom resolution depending on the study.[16]

The management of sphincter of Oddi dysfunction is sphincterotomy without cholecystectomy. This has traditionally been performed via an open transabdominal approach through the duodenum, but more recently endoscopic management has been feasible and much more common. Studies have shown that the endoscopic approach is as effective and safe as the open approach.[14] There are limited studies available looking at the rate of symptom resolution following this procedure. Again, it is important to discuss with the patients preoperatively that their symptoms may not resolve or even improve with these interventions.

CHOLEDOCHOLITHIASIS

The exact incidence of choledocholithiasis is unknown but has been estimated as 5% to 20% in patients with cholelithiasis.[17] Choledocholithiasis is seen more commonly in its secondary form because of the existence of cholelithiasis. Primary choledocholithiasis is less common and these stones form de novo secondary to biliary strictures or certain bacterial infections. Secondary choledocholithiasis can present in varying forms: concurrently with cholelithiasis, acute gallstone pancreatitis, or acute cholangitis.[1] In the setting of pancreatitis and cholangitis, choledocholithiasis is presumed to be present as the cause of biliary obstruction leading to these conditions. In the case of cholelithiasis, the presence of choledocholithiasis is more difficult to elucidate.

Diagnosis

Clinical symptoms of choledocholithiasis are similar to those of symptomatic cholelithiasis with right upper quadrant/epigastric abdominal pain and nausea. Jaundice can also be found on physical examination. Oftentimes, patients do not demonstrate any symptoms and the diagnosis is only suspected based on findings from laboratory values and imaging studies.

All patients being evaluated for symptomatic cholelithiasis should also be worked up for choledocholithiasis. The patient's history should be noted for any previous episodes of jaundice or pancreatitis. The initial diagnostic work-up for cholelithiasis should prompt suspicion for choledocholithiasis and determine the need for further work-up or intervention. White blood cell (WBC) is often normal in cases of choledocholithiasis; liver function enzymes (bilirubin, alkaline phosphatase, and even transaminases) can be elevated and ultrasound may demonstrate a dilated common bile duct (>6 mm) (**Table 1**). These are established risk factors for choledocholithiasis; however, there has not been a consensus in the surgical or gastrointestinal medicine communities regarding how to proceed once the diagnosis has been confirmed.

Ultrasound remains the primary imaging modality to screen for biliary pathology, although its accuracy for detecting choledocholithiasis is low. ERCP and intraoperative cholangiogram (IOC) are both considered the gold standards for diagnosing choledocholithiasis. However, because of invasiveness, they are rarely used as purely diagnostic studies. EUS and magnetic resonance cholangiopancreatography (MRCP) have higher sensitivity and specificity than ultrasound for identifying common bile duct stones and are often used as confirmatory diagnostic tests for choledocholithiasis.[18]

No single algorithm has been adopted to guide confirmation of the diagnosis of choledocholithiasis and then subsequent management. A well-studied guideline was published by the American Society of Gastrointestinal Endoscopy in 2010 that classified risks factors as "very strong," "strong," and "moderate," then categorized patients into "high risk," "intermediate risk," and "low risk" for choledocholithiasis. Based on their risk profile, recommendations were made for high-risk patients to proceed to ERCP before cholecystectomy. Intermediate-risk patients should obtain further imaging, such as EUS or MRCP, to confirm choledocholithiasis before undergoing ERCP if needed. Low-risk patients are safe to undergo laparoscopic cholecystectomy with no further interrogation of the common bile duct.[19]

Table 1
American Society for Gastrointestinal Endoscopy categorized risk factors for choledocholithiasis

	Very Strong	Strong	Moderate
Risk factors for choledocholithiasis	CBD stone on transabdominal ultrasound	Dilated CBD on ultrasound (>6 mm with existing gallbladder)	Abnormal liver function test other than bilirubin
	Clinical ascending cholangitis	Bilirubin 1.8–4 mg/dL	Age >55 y
	Bilirubin >4 mg/dL		Clinical gallstone pancreatitis

	High	Low	Intermediate
Likelihood of choledocholithiasis	Presence of any very strong risk factors	No risk factors present	All other patients

Abbreviation: CBD, common bile duct.

Adapted from American Society for Gastrointestinal Endoscopy. The role of endoscopy in the evaluation of suspected choledocholithiasis. Gastrointest Endosc 2010;71(1):2; with permission.

Management

The timing and method of removal of common bile duct stones continues to be debated with no universally accepted course. A variety of options are available to the surgeon for management of choledocholithiasis, which include laparoscopic versus open common bile duct exploration and preoperative, postoperative, or intraoperative ERCP (**Table 2**). Multiple studies have attempted to define the optimal approach to management of common bile duct stones. No one technique has emerged as the most effective. Data have demonstrated that ERCP and IOC have equivalent outcomes with no significant differences in ductal clearance rate, mortality, morbidity, and need for additional interventions. Proponents of a "one-stage approach" argue that laparoscopic cholecystectomy with IOC is more cost effective with equal efficacy to preoperative or postoperative ERCP. Unfortunately, treatment is often dictated by the resources available to surgeons and surgical expertise. With the availability and safety of ERCP, the most widely used strategy in contemporary times includes preoperative ERCP for clearance of common bile duct stones with a sphincterotomy, followed by laparoscopic cholecystectomy within the same hospitalization.[20]

CHOLANGITIS

Cholangitis refers to biliary duct inflammation and infection secondary to obstruction. Choledocholithiasis is the most common cause of biliary obstruction. Frequently isolated bacteria include *E coli*, *Klebsiella*, *Enterobacter*, and *Enterococcus*. Cholangitis is a life-threatening condition that can rapidly escalate into septic shock.[21] Identification and emergent management is critical.

Diagnosis

The classic symptoms associated with cholangitis are summarized in Charcot triad: fever, jaundice, and right upper quadrant abdominal pain. In practice, approximately 50% of patients demonstrate all three findings. Jaundice is most commonly present. Reynolds pentad includes Charcot triad with the addition of altered mental status and hypotension, denoting severe disease with sepsis. This is present in only about 5% of patients.[19] Because these symptoms are nonspecific the diagnosis of cholangitis is

Table 2
American Society for Gastrointestinal Endoscopy recommendations for management of choledocholithiasis based on risk factors

Likelihood of Choledocholithiasis	Management
High	Preoperative ERCP
Intermediate	1. Laparoscopic IOC a. Positive → laparoscopic CBDE or postoperative ERCP b. Negative → laparoscopic cholecystectomy 2. Preoperative EUS or MRCP a. Positive → preoperative ERCP b. Negative → laparoscopic cholecystectomy
Low	Laparoscopic cholecystectomy, no cholangiography

Abbreviation: CBDE, common bile duct exploration.

Adapted from American Society for Gastrointestinal Endoscopy. The role of endoscopy in the evaluation of suspected choledocholithiasis. Gastrointest Endosc 2010;71(1):2; and Tse F, Barkun JS, Barkun AN. The elective evaluation of patients with suspected choledocholithiasis undergoing laparoscopic cholecystectomy. Gastrointest Endosc 2004;60(3):443; with permission.

made in combination with laboratory values and imaging studies. WBC and bilirubin can be elevated. The initial imaging study to obtain should be a transabdominal ultrasound, which may show a dilated common bile duct suggesting biliary obstruction. Further imaging is usually unnecessary. Signs of infection with biliary obstruction should prompt high suspicion for cholangitis.

Management

There are three key features to the treatment of cholangitis: resuscitation, antibiotics, and biliary drainage. Antibiotics should target biliary and enteric organisms. The 2013 Tokyo Guidelines categorizes cholangitis into mild, moderate, or severe forms and suggests timing of biliary decompression depending on the severity of the disease process. ERCP should be urgently performed for biliary decompression, allowing infection effervescence. Should ERCP not be available, a percutaneous transhepatic catheter is placed to decompress the biliary system proximally with definitive clearance of the biliary obstruction at a later date. If these interventional options are both unavailable, a laparoscopic choledochotomy with T-tube drainage is performed, although this should be done as a last resort. For patients with cholangitis secondary to choledocholithiasis, definitive management includes a laparoscopic cholecystectomy to remove the risk of recurrent biliary complications. This is typically done during the same hospitalization once the patient has stabilized.[18]

GALLSTONE PANCREATITIS

Gallstones are the most common cause of acute pancreatitis in the Western world and account for 50% of all pancreatitis cases.[22] Inflammation of the pancreas occurs because of blockage of the pancreatic duct and/or common bile duct by gallstones. Other common causes of pancreatitis include alcohol, hypertriglyceridemia, hypercalcemia, certain medications and antibiotics, and anatomic variations of the pancreas. The severity of the disease process can vary widely from a mild, self-limited course to a severe presentation requiring intensive critical care. Scoring systems, such as Ranson criteria, which uses specific laboratory values and vital signs, are often used to help risk-stratify patients.[23] It is important to categorize the severity of the disease and initiate adequate and appropriate care immediately.

Diagnosis

The most common symptom of pancreatitis is severe epigastric abdominal pain radiating to the back. Nausea and vomiting can be present in addition to low-grade fevers. It is important to clinically monitor for jaundice. Laboratory values including a complete blood count and comprehensive metabolic panel (CMP) with amylase and lipase should be obtained. Elevated levels of amylase and lipase are diagnostic for pancreatitis. White blood cell count (WBC) and liver function enzymes may be mildly elevated. If liver function enzymes, such as bilirubin, are elevated, it is important to trend the levels to help determine if there is persistent biliary obstruction. Triglyceride and calcium levels should also be obtained to evaluate alternate sources of the disease.

Pancreatitis is often diagnosed based on amylase and lipase levels. Imaging studies are used as adjuncts to elucidate the cause of the process and help determine the severity of the disease. An abdominal ultrasound with findings of cholelithiasis can support a biliary cause. CT is often used to evaluate the level of pancreas inflammation. It can also demonstrate complications of pancreatitis, such as necrosis, infection, or pseudocysts. MRCP also has high sensitivity and specificity for pancreatitis but is more often used in settings where the biliary anatomy must be further elucidated.[24]

Management

This discussion focuses on treatment of mild episodes of biliary pancreatitis that resolve shortly with supportive care. All cases of pancreatitis should initially be managed with intravenous fluid resuscitation and bowel rest. There is no role for prophylactic antibiotics in the absence of infection. Resolution of pancreatitis is hallmarked by improvement of abdominal pain. The recommended definitive management of gallstone pancreatitis is a laparoscopic cholecystectomy once the episode of pancreatitis has resolved and the patient is appropriate for surgery. Because of the high rate of early recurrent biliary complications (up to 30%), studies suggest that surgery should occur during the same hospitalization and/or as soon as possible. There have been no studies that have demonstrated any benefit in performing a delayed cholecystectomy.[18]

The need to evaluate the common bile duct for choledocholithiasis in the setting of gallstone pancreatitis with ERCP or IOC remains controversial. Routine preoperative ERCP or IOC for gallstone pancreatitis is no longer recommended because it has been demonstrated that only about 25% of patients with gallstone pancreatitis have common bile duct stones.[25] In patients who display evidence of biliary obstruction, such as persistently elevated bilirubin levels, preoperative ERCP or IOC should be used. The current trend favors preoperative ERCP but both methods have been shown to be equivalent in detecting choledocholithiasis and ductal clearance. For the category of patients who show normalizing bilirubin levels, the question to interrogate the common bile duct is unclear. Risks and increased hospital costs associated with ERCP and IOC have pushed the debate away from their use in this patient population with the presumption that a downtrending bilirubin level indicates the passage of stones. A recent 2016 retrospective study argued that in the setting of mild gallstone pancreatitis with normalizing bilirubin levels, routine IOC and/or ERCP is not required because most common bile duct stones are clinically silent and additional interventions result in overtreatment.[26]

GALLSTONE ILEUS

Gallstone ileus is an uncommon manifestation of biliary disorders and a rare cause of small bowel obstruction, with an estimated range of 1% to 3%. It occurs in 0.3% to 0.5% of patients with cholelithiasis and is often preceded by an episode of acute cholecystitis. It is defined as a mechanical intestinal obstruction caused by an impacted gallstone within the gastrointestinal tract. Inflammation from an episode of cholecystitis leads to adhesions adhering a portion of the gastrointestinal tract to the gallbladder. Then pressure effect from an offending gallstone causes formation of a fistula between the gallbladder and the gastrointestinal tract leading to passage of the gallstone into the intestines where it ultimately becomes impacted leading to an intestinal obstruction. The duodenum is the most commonly affected portion of the gastrointestinal tract because of its natural proximity to the gallbladder but the stomach, small bowel, and transverse colon have all been reported as involved. Typically stones smaller than 2 cm pass to the rectum without obstruction. The rate of impaction increases with stones larger than 2 cm. The most common site of obstruction is at the terminal ileum and the ileocecal valve because of their small intraluminal diameter. An uncommon site of obstruction is the stomach where the stone has migrated proximally causing a gastric outlet obstruction. This phenomenon is also known as Bouveret syndrome. The incidence of gallstone ileus occurs highest in elderly, female patients.[27]

Diagnosis

The symptoms of gallstone ileus correlate to those of a small bowel obstruction, such as nausea, emesis, abdominal pain and distention, and obstipation. Biliary symptoms are rarely present, but patients can demonstrate jaundice on examination. Laboratory values are similarly nonspecific. WBC may be normal or mildly elevated; liver function enzymes are typically normal unless there is an associated common bile duct obstruction. Classically, an abdominal plain film may show pneumobilia, complete or partial bowel obstruction, and a calcified gallstone outside of the area of the gallbladder. These findings are only present in about 20% to 50% of cases. In contrast to most biliary pathology, gallstone ileus is more commonly diagnosed via CT scan rather than ultrasound. Ultrasound can demonstrate pneumobilia and ectopic gallstones; however, CT scan is superior with a sensitivity of up to 93% in diagnosing gallstone ileus. Findings of obstruction, pneumobilia, and ectopic gallstones is higher in CT scans relative to plain films and ultrasound. Other imaging modalities, such as upper gastrointestinal studies or MRCPs, are rarely used except in cases where CT scan is still indeterminate.[25]

Management

The primary goal in treating gallstone ileus is to relieve the obstruction by removing the impacted gallstone. Patients often present severely dehydrated with electrolyte and metabolic derangements secondary to the obstruction and these should be addressed before surgical intervention. Once patients are stable for surgery, operative intervention should be pursued. Surgical approach is typically via laparotomy because this disease process is uncommonly encountered; however, there are an increasing number of reports of successful laparoscopic extraction of impacted gallstones via small incision extension. No head-to-head studies have been performed to date comparing laparotomy with laparoscopy for gallstone ileus. It is at the discretion of the surgeon depending on their comfort and expertise in complex laparoscopy. A crucial part of the surgical procedure is to thoroughly explore the entire bowel to ensure there are not multiple stones present throughout the gastrointestinal tract. Thus, laparotomy may be the preferred and recommended approach for most surgeons.

The recommend surgical technique for impacted stone extraction includes longitudinal enterotomy on the antimesenteric border of the bowel proximal to the site of obstruction, then gently milk the gallstone proximally and remove it via the enterotomy. An important aspect of the surgery should include palpation of the entire intestine to remove any other ectopic gallstones. The enterotomy should then be closed transversely to avoid narrowing the lumen. In rare cases, a bowel resection may need to be performed. Numerous studies have been conducted to look at whether a concurrent chole-enteric fistula takedown and cholecystectomy should be performed at the initial operation versus in a delayed fashion versus no further surgery. Based on the results, current data recommend against performing a one-stage operation except in the rare cases where patients are stable and can tolerate the longer procedure. Controversy remains over whether patients should undergo a delayed fistula takedown and cholecystectomy at all, because of the potential risk of duodenal fistula formation versus the benefit of preventing recurrent gallstone ileus. The data are sparse, and the results are highly heterogenous. This is a disease of elderly, frail patients, and a complex prolonged initial operation and reoperation carry significant morbidity and mortality. The risk of gallstone ileus recurrence has been reported up to 8% with reoperation for biliary symptoms, such as cholecystitis and cholangitis, and up to 10% following enterolithotomy alone. Given these findings, it is reasonable to perform a delayed fistula takedown and cholecystectomy only in patients with recurrent symptoms; however, the surgeon should exercise their clinical judgment in making this decision because the data remain unclear.[28]

BILIARY DISEASE IN POST BARIATRIC SURGERY PATIENTS

Rapid weight loss following bariatric surgery has been well documented to be associated with the development of gallstones or sludge.[29] Routine cholecystectomy at the time of bariatric surgery has been suggested[30] although other studies have shown the efficacy of prophylactic ursodiol to decrease gallstone formation following weight loss.[31] The incidence of biliary disease seems to be low following bariatric surgery; however, it remains important for acute care surgeons to be comfortable caring for these patients.

Management of symptomatic cholelithiasis and acute cholecystitis should follow that of the general population. In patients who have undergone a Roux-en-Y gastric bypass and present with choledocholithiasis, cholangitis, or gallstone pancreatitis, how to interrogate the common bile duct becomes a conundrum. A variety of techniques have been studied and introduced to tackle this problem. One key is to accurately define the patient's bariatric anatomy. The most common bariatric procedure performed today is the sleeve gastrectomy, which maintains direct access to the ampulla of Vater. Many patients and consulting physicians falsely assume or report bariatric anatomy, which can significantly alter treatment plans. Review of operative notes, and radiologic studies including CT scans, and barium swallow studies can help define the anatomy.

The difficulty arises in how to gain access to the ampulla of Vater when the remnant stomach is excluded from the proximal gastric pouch. A surgical approach is undertaken with a laparoscopic or open common bile duct exploration. This is not frequently used likely because of the ready availability of skilled gastroenterologists and discomfort of surgeons with performing a laparoscopic common bile duct exploration while not wanting to subject the patient to an open surgery. One of the earliest methods described is the laparoscopic (or open) assisted transgastric ERCP combining the joint efforts of the surgeon and the gastroenterologist. Typically, a gastrostomy is created, a 15-mm port is placed directly into the remnant stomach, and the sterilized duodenoscope is introduced through the port and gastrostomy to perform the ERCP and stone retrieval as is done with normal anatomy. The gastrostomy site can then be closed or a temporary tube is left in place if future access is necessary. Sometimes the gastrostomy is created with interventional radiology guidance, although this procedure is limited by difficulty in distending the remnant stomach with air. The efficacy and safety of this method is well established.[32] Access to the common bile duct via transhepatic cholangiography has also been described.[33]

Other entirely endoscopic techniques are currently being used and investigated. Standard peroral ERCP is often unsuccessful because of the long length of the Roux limb. The emergence of balloon-assisted enteroscopy has allowed deeper enteroscopy with the ability to reduce small bowel loops to facilitate further advancement of the scope through the Roux limb. This method is limited in patients with long Roux limbs and in these situations, a laparoscopic- assisted transgastric ERCP may be necessary.[34] A novel approach referred to as EUS-directed transgastric ERCP is currently under investigation. The procedure includes creation of an internal gastrogastric or gastrojejunal fistula directed by EUS guidance. A stent is placed from the gastric pouch or Roux limb to the remnant stomach to create a direct passage to the duodenum to perform ERCP.[35] Another innovative approach to addressing choledocholithiasis in altered foregut anatomy is an endoscopic transhepatic approach. A passage is created from the gastric pouch through the left lobe of the liver to access the intrahepatic left hepatic duct. A tract is formed and dilated, then a stent is placed. Antegrade stone manipulation can take place including stent placement, lithotripsy, balloon dilation, and sweeping. This procedure has been described in 17 patients, which is currently the largest experience in the United States. These complex endoscopic techniques are currently experimental and should only be undertaken by advanced endoscopists.

This specific patient population is difficult to manage because of their anatomy and limited resources available to the acute care surgeon. It is prudent to involve a surgeon comfortable with bariatric anatomy and a skilled endoscopist to help determine treatment options and manage potential complications.

BILIARY DISEASE IN PREGNANT PATIENTS

Acute biliary disease and appendicitis make up the most common nonobstetric surgical emergencies complicating pregnancy, affecting approximately 1 in 500 women.[36] The goal in acute management is to accurately and rapidly diagnose the cause of acute abdominal pain while minimizing risks of diagnostic modalities. The best way to protect the fetus is to treat the mother appropriately. Ultrasound is the initial imaging modality of choice for abdominal pain, particularly with concern for biliary pathology. In the past, conservative or nonoperative management of benign biliary disease was recommended at all stages of pregnancy. Laparoscopy was then applied more liberally during the second trimester of pregnancy to treat benign biliary disease. In uncomplicated biliary disease, the rates of preterm labor and spontaneous abortion are similar for operative and nonoperative management. Delaying cholecystectomy until after delivery leads to high rates of recurrent symptoms, emergency department visits, and recurrent hospitalizations. Given the low risk of laparoscopic cholecystectomy to the pregnancy woman and fetus, the Society of American Gastrointestinal and Endoscopic Surgeons guidelines for the use of laparoscopy during pregnancy now defines laparoscopic cholecystectomy as the treatment of choice in the pregnant patient with symptomatic gallbladder disease, regardless of trimester. Treatment of choledocholithiasis should be managed in the systematic method routinely used including ERCP, IOC, laparoscopic cholecystectomy, and laparoscopic common bile duct exploration.[37]

Technical Considerations

Certain technical considerations should be addressed while performing laparoscopic biliary procedures on pregnant patients. Patients should be placed in modified left lateral decubitus position to minimize compression of the vena cava. The surgeon should use the abdominal access method in which they have the most comfort. There are no data to support superiority of open or Hasson access to Veress needle, or optical trocar techniques.[38] Location of initial port placement should be adjusted according to fundal height. Routine insufflation pressure of 10 to 15 mm Hg can be safely used, with adjustments for individual patient physiology.[34] Deep venous thrombosis chemoprophylaxis is not required if pneumatic compression devices and early postoperative ambulation are used. In patients with significant risk factors (recognizing that pregnancy is a hypercoagulable state) deep venous thrombosis chemoprophylaxis including low-molecular-weight heparin (or lovenox) or unfractionated heparin is recommended.[39]

INTERVENTIONS

Laparoscopic Cholecystectomy

Laparoscopic cholecystectomy is one of the most commonly performed surgeries in the United States and is now the favored surgical approach to managing gallbladder pathology. The mortality rate of the operation is low at 0.1% to 0.5% with morbidity ranging from 2% to 6%.[40] There are a plethora of variations to this common procedure. Laparoscopic cholecystectomy is performed using a single-port platform, but is more commonly performed with multiple ports, typically four total. Usually one larger port is used as the specimen extraction site. The smaller ports are 5 mm, or even smaller needlescopic instruments. Sometimes one of the working ports necessitates size increase to provide additional manipulation options, either larger clips, sutures, or staples. Steps of the procedure include elevation of the fundus over the liver with lateral retraction of the infundibulum. The lateral and medial peritoneal attachments from the gallbladder to the liver are scored, allowing further retraction of the infundibulum. This facilitates performance of the key step, which is adequately identifying the "critical view of safety." This critical view is achieved by exposing the hepatocystic triangle: the area bordered by the cystic duct, common hepatic duct, and the visceral surface of the liver. Once the space is exposed, the cystic duct and artery should be skeletonized and isolated as the only two structures entering the gallbladder. Once this has been confirmed, they can safely be clipped and divided.[41] The structures are secured with metal or locking clips. Alternative options include ties, loops, or sutures. A stapler is used, particularly in the setting of partial cholecystectomy. The artery is divided with sharp, monopolar, ultrasonic, or bipolar methods. There is a wide array of routine approaches to cholecystectomy, and complex maneuvers to address complicated anatomy. Approximately 25% of all cholecystectomies are performed open. Of the remaining cases that are undertaken laparoscopically, conversion to open occurs 5% to 10% of the time. The most common reasons for conversion are adhesions, severe inflammation, and difficult anatomy.[42] Elective laparoscopic cholecystectomy is most often performed on an outpatient basis, whereas many acute presentations typically require hospital admission and monitoring. Bile leaks are managed expectantly if the drainage is low, typically less than 500 mL over 24 hours. Minor leaks often resolve spontaneously with percutaneous drainage. In leaks that are greater than 500 mL over 24 hours, ERCP with sphincterotomy and stent placement should be performed to assist in resolution of the leak. Retained common bile duct stones often present later and should be suspected in patients who have new acute-onset of right upper quadrant abdominal pain and jaundice. Similar to the management of choledocholithiasis, retained common bile ducts stones are treated with ERCP and sphincterotomy.[43]

Common bile duct injury is the most dreaded complication of cholecystectomy with an incidence less than 1%. It typically occurs secondary to difficulty in identifying the accurate anatomy. Common bile duct injuries need to be definitively repaired with a Roux-en-Y hepaticojejunostomy. Timing of diagnosis affects overall management. When identified intraoperatively, definitive management with reconstruction is performed immediately. However, this should only be undertaken by surgeons with skills capable of performing advanced hepatobiliary surgery. If such a surgeon is unavailable, drains should be placed, and the patient transferred to a center with experience in management of biliary complications. Oftentimes, the injury is diagnosed postoperatively. Patients present with symptoms of a biliary leak or biliary obstruction. In these cases, the initial management is directed at control of the leak and biliary decompression, which is performed percutaneously and/or via ERCP. Definitive reconstruction of the biliary tract with a Roux-en-Y hepaticojejunostomy is delayed until intra-abdominal contamination is resolved.[44]

Tube Cholecystostomy

Percutaneous cholecystostomy tube placement has become the recommended initial approach for patients with acute cholecystitis who are too high risk for general anesthesia and surgery. It is a procedure that is performed with intravenous sedation and local anesthetic. The tube is placed transperitoneally or transhepatically into the gallbladder under ultrasound or fluoroscopic guidance. It achieves drainage of the infected gallbladder and allows time for inflammation to resolve and the patient to recover from severe illness. Cholecystostomies can also be placed laparoscopically. This typically takes place in the setting where cholecystectomy was attempted; however, because of severe inflammation, the surgeon alternatively places a cholecystostomy tube. Interval cholecystectomy can then be performed if necessary.[11]

Intraoperative Cholangiogram

The role of IOC during laparoscopic cholecystectomy has evolved. It was once recommended that IOC be routinely performed to delineate biliary tract anatomy and evaluate for choledocholithiasis. Multiple studies have demonstrated that routine IOC does not prevent bile duct injury but rather only assists in earlier identification of injuries thus most surgeons have abandoned performing routine IOC during all cholecystectomies. More commonly, IOC is selectively undertaken during cases where difficult anatomy is encountered. IOC can also be performed to diagnose common bile duct stones, although with the increasing availability of ERCP, which is diagnostic and therapeutic, it is now often favored over IOC in cases of choledocholithiasis.[45]

Table 3
Overview of biliary disease

Disorder	Symptoms	Laboratory Studies	Imaging	Management
Cholelithiasis (biliary colic)	RUQ abdominal pain following eating fatty foods	LFTs	Transabdominal US	Laparoscopic cholecystectomy
Cholecystitis	RUQ abdominal pain, fevers	LFTs, CBC	Transabdominal US	Laparoscopic cholecystectomy, antibiotics
Choledocholithiasis	RUQ abdominal pain, jaundice	LFTs	Transabdominal US, ± EUS or MRCP	Laparoscopic cholecystectomy with IOC or ERCP
Cholangitis	RUQ abdominal pain, jaundice, fevers	LFTs, CBC	Transabdominal US	Resuscitation, antibiotics, biliary decompression, laparoscopic cholecystectomy
Gallstone pancreatitis	Epigastric abdominal pain, jaundice	LFTs, CBC	Transabdominal US, CT scan	Resuscitation, laparoscopic cholecystectomy
Gallstone ileus	Abdominal pain, N/V, obstipation	CBC, BMP	CT scan	Resuscitation, bowel rest, enterolithotomy, ± interval laparoscopic cholecystectomy
Functional gallbladder disorders	RUQ abdominal pain	LFTs	Transabdominal US, HIDA scan	Laparoscopic cholecystectomy

Abbreviations: BMP, basic metabolic panel; CBC, complete blood count; LFT, liver function test; N/V, nausea/vomiting; RUQ, right upper quadrant; US, ultrasound.

Endoscopic Retrograde Cholangiopancreatography

ERCP has emerged as an important diagnostic and therapeutic tool for biliary pathology. Because of its less invasive nature and fairly low risk profile, it has overtaken IOC and common bile duct exploration as the current most commonly used tool to diagnose and manage choledocholithiasis, gallstone pancreatitis, and bile leaks. The morbidity associated with ERCP is low at 1% to 10% with complications including cholangitis, pancreatitis, hemorrhage, and perforation.[46] These typically are managed conservatively and rarely need operative intervention. ERCP has proven to be safe and efficacious in addressing biliary pathology.

SUMMARY

Biliary pathologies are one of the most common disorders encountered by general surgeons. The spectrum of diseases often presents in an acute fashion and it is important for emergency general surgeons to be able to quickly identify and diagnose the correct syndrome and implement a plan of care (**Table 3**). Surgeons should be comfortable with laparoscopic cholecystectomy and open surgery should the need for conversion arise. Emerging technologies, such as ERCP, has made more traditional techniques, such as IOC and common bile duct exploration, less familiar to young surgeons; however, these are important tools in the armament for managing biliary disease and should not be neglected.

REFERENCES

1. Stinton LM, Shaffer EA. Epidemiology of gallbladder disease: cholelithiasis and cancer. Gut Liver 2012;6(2):172–87.
2. Khashab M, Giday SA. Gallbladder and biliary tree. Current surgical therapy. 10th edition. Philadelphia: Elsevier; 2011. p. 335.
3. Pinto A, Reginelli A, Cagini L, et al. Accuracy of ultrasonography in the diagnosis of acute calculous cholecystitis: review of the literature. Crit Ultrasound J 2013; 5(Suppl 1):S11.
4. Ansaloni L, Pisano M, Coccolini F, et al. 2016 WSES guidelines on acute calculous cholecystitis. World J Emerg Surg 2016;11:25.
5. Jain A, Mehta N, Secko M, et al. History, physical examination, laboratory testing, and emergency department ultrasonography for the diagnosis of acute cholecystitis. Acad Emerg Med 2017;24(3):281–97.
6. Takada T, Strasberg S, Solomkin J, et al. TG13: updated Tokyo guidelines for the management of acute cholangitis and cholecystitis. J Hepatobiliary Pancreat Surg 2013;20:1–7.
7. Miura F, Takada T, Kawarada Y, et al. Flowcharts for the diagnosis and treatment of acute cholangitis and cholecystitis: Tokyo guidelines. J Hepatobiliary Pancreat Surg 2007;14:27–34.
8. Lu N, Biffl W. Acute biliary disease. In: Moore LJ, Todd SR, editors. Common problems in acute care surgery. 2nd edition; 2017. p. 243–52.
9. Peitzmann AB, Watson GA, Marsh JW. Acute cholecystitis: when to operate and how to do it safely. J Trauma Acute Care Surg 2014;78(1):1–12.
10. Abi-Haidar Y, Sanchez V, Williams SA, et al. Revisiting percutaneous cholecystostomy for acute cholecystitis based on a 10-year experience. Arch Surg 2012; 147(5):416–22.
11. Berber W, Engle KL, String AS, et al. Selective use of tube cholecystostomy with interval laparoscopic cholecystectomy in acute cholecystitis. Arch Surg 2000;135:341–6.

12. Huffman JL, Schenker S. Acute acalculous cholecystitis: a review. Clin Gastroenterol Hepatol 2010;8:15–22.
13. Goussous N, Kowdley GC, Sardana N, et al. Gallbladder dysfunction: how much longer will it be controversial? Digestion 2014;90:147–54.
14. Drossman DA. The functional gastrointestinal disorders and the Rome III process. Gastroenterology 2006;130:1377–90.
15. Behar J, Corazziari E, Guelrud M, et al. Functional gallbladder and sphincter of Oddi disorders. Gastroenterology 2006;130:1498–509.
16. Rastogi A, Slivka A, Moser AJ, et al. Controversies concerning pathophysiology and management of acalculous biliary-type abdominal pain. Dig Dis Sci 2005; 50:1397–401.
17. Collins C, Maguire D, Ireland A, et al. A prospective study of common bile duct calculi in patients undergoing laparoscopic cholecystectomy: natural history of choledocholithiasis revisited. Ann Surg 2004;239(1):28.
18. O'Connor O, O'Neill S, Maher MM. Imaging of biliary tract disease. AJR Am J Roentgenol 2011;197:W551–8.
19. ASGE Standards of Practice Committee, Maple JT, Ben-Menachem T, Anderson MA, et al. The role of endoscopy in the evaluation of suspected choledocholithiasis. Gastrointest Endosc 2010;71(1):1–9.
20. Demehri FR, Alam HB. Evidence-based management of common gallstone-related emergencies. J Intensive Care Med 2016;31(1):3–13.
21. Jonnalagadda S, Strasberg S. Acute cholangitis. Current surgical therapy. 10th edition. Philadelphia: Elsevier; 2011. p. 345.
22. Fogel EL, Sherman S. ERCP for gallstone pancreatitis. N Engl J Med 2014;370: 150–7.
23. Ranson JH, Rifkind KM, Roses DF, et al. Prognostic signs and the role of operative management in acute pancreatitis. Surg Gynecol Obstet 1974;139:69–81.
24. O'Connor O, McWilliams S, Maher MM. Imaging of acute pancreatitis. AJR Am J Roentgenology 2011;197:W221–5.
25. Chang L, Lo S, Stabile BE, et al. Preoperative versus postoperative endoscopic retrograde cholangiopancreatography in mild to moderate gallstone pancreatitis: a prospective randomized trial. Ann Surg 2000;231:82–7.
26. Pham XD, de Virgilio C, Al-Khouja L, et al. Routine intraoperative cholangiography is unnecessary in patients with mild gallstone pancreatitis and normalizing bilirubin levels. Am J Surg 2016;212:1047–53.
27. Nuno-Guzman C, Marin-Contreras ME, Figueroa-Sanchez M, et al. Gallstone ileus, clinical presentation, diagnostic and treatment approach. World J Gastrointest Surg 2016;8(1):65–76.
28. Ravijumar R, Williams JG. The operative management of gallstone ileus. Ann R Coll Surg Engl 2010;92:279–81.
29. Caruana JA, McCabe MN, Smith AD, et al. Incidence of symptomatic gallstones after gastric bypass: is prophylactic treatment really necessary? Surg Obes Relat Dis 2005;1(6):564–7.
30. Fobi M, Lee H, Igwe D, et al. Prophylactic cholecystectomy with gastric bypass operation: incidence of gallbladder disease. Obes Surg 2002;12(3):350–3.
31. Sugerman HJ, Brewer WH, Shiffman ML, et al. A multicenter, placebo-controlled, randomized, double blind, prospective trial of prophylactic ursodiol for the prevention of gallstone formation following gastric-bypass-induced rapid weight loss. Am J Surg 1995;169(1):91–7.

32. Falcão M, Campos JM, Galvar NM, et al. Transgastric endoscopic retrograde cholangiopancreatography for the management of biliary tract disease after Roux-en-Y gastric bypass treatment for obesity. Obes Surg 2012;22(6):872–6.
33. Ahmed AR, Husain S, Saad N, et al. Accessing the common bile duct after Roux-en-Y gastric bypass. Surg Obes Relat Dis 2007;3(6):640–3.
34. Schreiner MA, Chang L, Gluck M, et al. Laparoscopic-assisted versus balloon enteroscopy-assisted ERCP in bariatric post-Roux-en-Y gastric bypass patients. Gastrointest Endosc 2012;75(4):748–56.
35. Kedia P, Tyberg A, Kumta NA, et al. EUS-directed transgastric ERCP for Roux-en-Y gastric bypass anatomy: a minimally invasive approach. Gastrointest Endosc 2015;82(3):560–5.
36. Pearl JP, Price RR, Tonkin AE, et al. SAGES guidelines for the use of laparoscopic during pregnancy. Surg Endosc 2017;31(10):3767–82.
37. Nasioudis D. Laparoscopic cholecystectomy during pregnancy: a systematic review of 590 patients. Int J Surg 2016;27:165–75.
38. Overby DW, Apelgren KN, Richardson W, et al. SAGES guidelines for the clinical application of laparoscopic biliary tract surgery. Surg Endosc 2010;24(10):2368–86.
39. Richardson WS, Hamad GG, Stefanidis D, et al. SAGES VTE prophylaxis for laparoscopic surgery guidelines: an update. Surg Endosc 2017;31(2):501–3.
40. Agresta F, Campanile FC, Vettoretto N, et al. Laparoscopic cholecystectomy: consensus conference-based guidelines. Langenbecks Arch Surg 2015;400:429–53.
41. Van Arendonk KJ, Duncan MD. Acute cholecystitis. Current surgical therapy. 10th edition. Philadelphia: Elsevier; 2011. p. 338.
42. Livingston EH, Rege RV. A nationwide study of conversion from laparoscopic to open cholecystectomy. Am J Surg 2004;188:205–11.
43. Duca S, Bala O, Al-Hajjar N, et al. Laparoscopic cholecystectomy: incidents and complications. A retrospective analysis of 9542 consecutive laparoscopic operations. HPB (Oxford) 2003;5(3):152–8.
44. Sicklick JK, Camp MS, Lillemoe KD, et al. Surgical management of bile duct injuries sustained during laparoscopic cholecystectomy: perioperative results in 200 patients. Ann Surg 2005;241(5):786–95.
45. Tabone LE. To 'gram or not'? Indications for intraoperative cholangiogram. Surgery 2011;150:810–9.
46. Szary NM, Al-Kawas FH. Complications of endoscopic retrograde cholangiopancreatography: how to avoid and manage them. Gastroenterol Hepatol 2013;9(8):496–504.

Pancreatitis

Abdulrahman Y. Hammad, MD, Michael Ditillo, DO,
Lourdes Castanon, MD*

KEYWORDS

• Pancreatitis • Epidemiology • Management

KEY POINTS

- Acute pancreatitis is an inflammation of the glandular parenchyma of the retroperitoneal organ that leads to injury with or without subsequent destruction of the pancreatic acini. This inflammatory process can either result in a self-limited disease or involve life-threatening multiorgan complications.
- In contrast, chronic pancreatitis is a syndrome that consists of endocrine and exocrine gland dysfunction that develops secondary to progressive inflammation and chronic fibrosis of the pancreatic acini with permanent structural damage.
- Recurrent attacks of acute pancreatitis can result in chronic pancreatitis; it is thought that acute and chronic pancreatitis are 2 different diseases with 2 separate morphologic patterns.
- Acute pancreatitis has an estimated annual incidence of 4.9 to 40 cases per year per 100,000, which has been increasing over the last several decades, albeit with a decreasing mortality.

INTRODUCTION

Acute pancreatitis (AP) is an inflammation of the glandular parenchyma of the retroperitoneal organ that leads to injury with or without subsequent destruction of the pancreatic acini. This inflammatory process can either result in a self-limited disease or involve life-threatening multiorgan complications. In contrast, chronic pancreatitis (CP) is a syndrome that consists of endocrine and exocrine gland dysfunction that develop secondary to progressive inflammation and chronic fibrosis of the pancreatic acini with permanent structural damage. Recurrent attacks of AP can result in CP; it is thought that AP and CP are 2 different diseases with 2 separate morphologic patterns.[1–4] AP has an estimated annual incidence of 4.9 to 40 cases per year per 100,000, which has been increasing over the last several decades, albeit with a

Disclosure: The authors have nothing to disclose.

Department of Surgery, Allegheny General Hospital, 320 East North Avenue, Pittsburgh, PA 15212, USA
* Corresponding author.
E-mail address: lourdes.castanon@ahn.org

Surg Clin N Am 98 (2018) 895–913
https://doi.org/10.1016/j.suc.2018.06.001 surgical.theclinics.com
0039-6109/18/

decreasing mortality.[5,6] The incidence of CP ranges from 5 to 12 cases per year per 100,000, with an estimated prevalence of 50 per 100,000.[6,7]

Peery and colleagues[8] reported in 2012 that AP was the most common gastrointestinal admission diagnosis, with an inpatient cost estimate of $2.6 billion per year. AP is reported to carry a mortality risk of approximately 1%; however, a subset of patients can have a more severe form of the disease with a mortality approaching 30%.[8,9] CP was reported to have a mortality as high as 20% to 25%.[10,11] Hence, proper management of those diseases requires a multidisciplinary team approach with the involvement of gastroenterologists, endocrinologists, pain specialists, psychiatrists, surgeons, and support groups.

Cause

Acute pancreatitis

The cause of AP can be readily identified in most patients, with gallstones and alcohol being the leading causes (40%–70% and 25%–35% respectively).[12,13]

Gallstone size negatively correlates with an increased risk of pancreatitis. Smaller stones are more likely to migrate down the bile or pancreatic duct and cause an obstruction, which in return increases ductal pressure and unregulated digestive enzymatic activity.[14] Because gallstones have a high prevalence, the best way to evaluate for cholelithiasis is by performing abdominal ultrasonography on all patients with AP. However, only 3% to 7% of patients who have gallstones develop AP.[15] Moreover, men with gallstones have a higher risk of developing AP, whereas women have a higher incidence of gallstone pancreatitis because of a higher prevalence of gallstones.

AP associated with alcohol consumption is usually considered in patients with AP who have a history of 5 years or more of heavy drinking. Because clinically identified AP is only prevalent in 5% of heavy drinkers, there may be additional genetic and environmental factors that contribute to a person's sensitivity to the negative effects of alcohol (eg, failure to inhibit trypsin activity, tobacco use).[12,14,16]

Other infrequent causes of AP include hypercalcemia secondary to hyperparathyroidism, hypertriglyceridemia, endoscopic retrograde cholangiopancreatography (ERCP), drugs, and infections. Primary or secondary hypercalcemia can lead to calcium deposition in the pancreatic duct or activation of trypsinogen in the pancreas.[17] However, this only occurs inconsistently in 1% to 4% of AP cases.[12,14,18] Similarly, hypertriglyceridemia accounts for 1% to 4% of AP cases, potentially resulting in AP attacks following a serum triglyceride concentration more than 1000 mg/dL.[12] Hypertriglyceridemia can be acquired by many factors (eg, obesity, diabetes mellitus, hypothyroidism) or caused by inherited lipoprotein metabolism disorders.

ERCP can potentially cause AP because of various associated risks. After the procedure, 35% to 70% of the patients develop asymptomatic hyperamylasemia.[14,19] If the hyperamylasemia presents with persistent severe abdominal pain, nausea, and vomiting, it is generally diagnosed as post-ERCP pancreatitis.[14,20] The risk for AP associated with ERCP is higher when it is used to treat sphincter of Oddi dysfunction (25%) but is much lower if used for removal of gallstones (5%). In addition, diagnostic ERCP is only associated with AP in 3% of the patients.[14,21] Further ERCP-induced AP-associated risks include young age, female sex, and poor emptying of the pancreatic duct after the procedure.[14] To prevent post-ERCP pancreatitis in patients at higher risk, a temporary pancreatic stent may be placed during the procedure.[22] In addition, prophylactic nonsteroidal antiinflammatory drugs were also reported to be effective in preventing post-ERCP pancreatitis.[23]

Several reported cases show that various medications (eg, 6-mercaptopurine, aminosalicylates, sulfonamides, diuretics, valproic acid) are associated with inducing pancreatitis through various mechanisms, such as immunologic reactions, direct toxic effects, accumulation of toxic metabolite, ischemia, and increased pancreatic juice viscosity.[14,24,25] However, drug-induced pancreatitis has a good prognosis with a low mortality.[26]

AP has been linked with various viral and bacterial infections (eg, mumps, hepatitis B, human immunodeficiency virus [HIV], *Mycoplasma*, and *Salmonella*) but none have been identified as a direct cause.[14] AP specifically was shown to have occurred in some patients with HIV because of the opportunistic infection itself or complications raised by infection, medication, or the antiretroviral therapy.[27,28]

Idiopathic AP describes patients who present with the disease but without obvious cause after considering history, laboratory tests, and imaging results. About 10% to 15% of patients with AP are in this category. This diagnosis becomes one of exclusion after pursuing the appropriate diagnostic imaging modalities.[12]

Chronic pancreatitis

Alcohol consumption is currently thought to be the most common cause of CP.[29–31] The risk seems to be related to the duration of intake and amount consumed rather than the type (beer, wine, or spirits) or the manner of consumption (daily vs binge).[29] Alcohol consumption more than 40 g/d has been shown to be associated with increasing risk of AP and/or CP.[32] However, recent evidence indicates that alcohol is a significant contributor to the pathogenesis, although it is not the main cause of the disease for most patients.[30] This can be extrapolated from the fact that CP can progress even after cessation of alcohol intake. Another risk factor that has been reported is cigarette smoking. A multicenter study by Yadav and colleagues[31] examining more than 1000 patients showed that cigarette smoking is an independent risk factor for CP.

Pancreatic ductal obstruction secondary to strictures, tumors, or pancreatic divisum can lead to CP. Sphincter of Oddi dysfunction was also reported to be associated with CP in patients with unexplained pancreaticobiliary pain.[33] A subsequent study reported an improvement of clinical symptoms, cholestasis, and improvement of exocrine pancreatic function following endoscopic sphincterotomy.[34] Pancreatic divisum, a failure of the 2 pancreatic buds from the primitive foregut to fuse together, is currently debated as a cause of CP. A minority of patients affected with pancreatic divisum present with CP.[29] At present, the literature supports investigating other sources of abdominal pain in patients with known pancreatic divisum and no evidence of pancreatitis because their symptoms are most likely secondary to another cause. Surgical drainage procedures might provide symptomatic relief in patients with pancreatic divisum who present with CP.[35]

Tropical pancreatitis has been the most common cause of CP in tropical Africa and Asia.[36] Children are most commonly affected and often die in early adulthood secondary to endocrine and exocrine dysfunction. Although the underlying pathogenesis is not fully understood, certain genetic mutations have been identified in some patients.[37,38]

Idiopathic cause of CP is another distinct entity with bimodal distribution of age (juvenile type at 10–20 years and senile type at 50–60 years) and an equal male to female ratio.

Hereditary pancreatitis accounts for a minor proportion of patients with CP. CP is inherited in an autosomal dominant fashion with a point mutation on chromosome 7. Most individuals develop clinical symptoms before the age of 20 years and a strong family history is often elicited.[29] There is an increased risk of pancreatic adenocarcinoma in patients with hereditary CP and, hence, early surgical resection or complete pancreatectomy with autotransplant of the islet are recommended.[39]

Other genetic causes include mutations in the cystic fibrosis transmembrane conductor regulator (CFTR) gene.[40] Most patients with cystic fibrosis can present as acute recurrent pancreatitis but ultimately progress into CP. Mutations in other genes, such as the SPINK1 and chymotrypsin-C genes, have also been associated with CP.[30,41] Alpha1-antitrypsin deficiency was previously described in patients with CP, although its rule remains unclear and is currently considered not be associated with CP.[42–44] Other less commonly reported causes for CP include hyperparathyroidism, hypertriglyceridemia, systemic lupus erythematosus, and blunt and penetrating trauma to a pancreatic injury.[45–48]

Diagnosis

Signs and symptoms

Acute pancreatitis The most common symptom for patients with AP is acute onset of severe abdominal pain. Pain is typically pronounced in the epigastric region or the left upper quadrant. Fifty percent of patients may complain of pain radiating to their back, whereas others may complain of pain radiating to their chests or flanks, although nonspecific.[49] Other complaints include persistent nausea or vomiting.[49] On physical examination, epigastric tenderness is usually present. Severe epigastric pain or even a more diffuse abdominal pain that can be associated with severe pancreatitis is typically present. Systemic manifestations such as fever, hypotension, hypoxia, tachypnea, and tachycardia may also be present in patients with severe pancreatitis. Abdominal distention and hypoactive bowel sounds secondary to an ileus may also be present. In patients presenting with AP secondary to choledocholithiasis, scleral icterus may be seen.

Chronic pancreatitis Pain is the most common presenting symptom for CP. This pain is typically in the epigastric area and may radiate to the back. This pain can be associated with nausea and vomiting. The pain typically presents after meals, although it can be independent of oral intake. The pain in CP is multifactorial and involves inflammatory and neuropathic components. The pain is typically discordant with the imaging findings.[50,51] As the disease progresses, the pain can be present in a more continuous fashion.[52] In contrast, pain might decrease over the course of years in patients who abstain from alcohol intake.[29] Although abdominal pain is the most common finding in patients with CP, some patients remain asymptomatic. A minority of patients present with other symptoms related to pancreatic exocrine dysfunction.[52] Loss of pancreatic exocrine function can lead to fat malabsorption with subsequent diarrhea, steatorrhea, fat-soluble vitamin deficiency, and weight loss. Glucose intolerance and diabetes mellitus may occur later in the course of the disease. Less common presentations include pleural effusion, splenic vein thrombosis, bile duct or duodenal obstruction, and pancreatic cancer.[7,11]

Laboratory Investigations

Acute pancreatitis

Serum amylase and serum lipase levels increase within the first few hours of the onset of symptoms and are used for diagnostic purposes. These increased levels occur because of a blockade of digestive enzyme secretion causing them to leak out of the acinar cells into the interstitial space and, subsequently, the systemic circulation. Serum lipase level increase is more sensitive compared with serum amylase in diagnosing AP.[53] Other laboratory findings may include leukocytosis, increased hematocrit secondary to hemoconcentration caused by third spacing, increased blood urea nitrogen (BUN) level, hypocalcemia, and hyperglycemia. Other markers that can be used to adjunct the diagnosis of AP include C-reactive protein, interleukin-6, interleukin-8, interleukin-10, tumor necrosis factor, and polymorphonuclear elastase.[54] At present, CRP level at 48 hours correlates with the severity of AP.[53] Trypsinogen activation peptide is another marker that might be useful in the detection of early pancreatitis.[55]

Chronic pancreatitis

Although serum amylase and lipase levels may be increased in CP, their levels are often normal. Complete blood count, electrolyte levels, and liver function tests are typically normal as well. Sudan red stain of stool samples is currently obsolete and a 72-hour measurement of fecal fat, which was previously considered the gold standard in the diagnosis of CP, is now done less commonly. At present, measurement of fecal elastase is considered the most appropriate test.[56] Direct pancreatic function testing using secretin is considered the most sensitive test for the early diagnosis of CP, although it is only performed at a few centers in the United States.[51] Other laboratory tests that have been used include stool chymotrypsin level, immunoglobulin G4, rheumatoid factor, antinuclear antibody, erythrocyte sedimentation rate, and anti–smooth muscle antibody titers are all considered markers of immune activation. In patients with exocrine dysfunction, fasting glucose levels and hemoglobin A1c levels should be checked.

Imaging

Acute pancreatitis

Abdominal ultrasonography is a simple and readily available tool that can aid in the investigation of AP. In the acute phase, the pancreas appears hypoechoic and diffusely enlarged on ultrasonography. In patients presenting with AP secondary to gallstones, ultrasonography can uncover gallstones in the common bile duct (CBD) or in the gallbladder. Although ultrasonography is highly accurate in detecting gallstones, its accuracy is generally lower in patients presenting with gallstone-induced pancreatitis. This reduced accuracy is partly caused by excessive gas accumulation in AP, and is also partly caused by the association of pancreatitis with smaller gallstones.[57,58] Other abnormalities on ultrasonography include hypoechoic peripancreatic areas of inflammation, heterogeneous echo patterns, and decreased pancreatic echogenicity compared with the liver.[59]

Abdominal computed tomography (CT) with contrast remains the gold standard in the initial staging as well as in predicting the severity of the disease. The severity of AP can be determined using a CT severity index (CTSI) that was developed by Balthazar and colleagues.[60] Repeat CT is typically not indicated unless there is an acute change in clinical status suggesting that there might be an evolving complication. MRI is an alternative to CT that offers less radiation exposure. In addition, MRI is more sensitive than CT scan in diagnosing early AP and in characterizing pancreatic, bile duct, and vascular complications (eg, pseudoaneurysms and venous thromboses).[61,62] In addition, MRI can play a major role in determining the cause of the AP attack, particularly for calculi and pancreatic divisum.[63] Other common diagnostic modalities that can aid in the diagnosis but are not necessarily needed include endoscopic ultrasonography (EUS) and ERCP.

Chronic pancreatitis

In patients presenting with CP, a wider variety of imaging modalities, including abdominal radiographs, ultrasonography, CT, and MRI scans, as well as endoscopic modalities can be used to facilitate the diagnosis. Although plain radiographs play a small role in diagnosing CP, calcifications of the pancreatic duct and calcium deposition in the pancreas might be seen in approximately 30% of the cases.[64] Ultrasonography, CT scan, and MRI may show calcifications, ductal dilatation, fluid collections, or glandular atrophy or enlargement with varying degrees of sensitivity and specificity.[30] At present, magnetic resonance cholangiopancreatography (MRCP) is gaining favor as the most accurate and noninvasive imaging modality in diagnosing CP because it can show calcifications and biliary/pancreatic duct microlithiasis. It is also specifically helpful in recognizing altered ductal anatomy such as dilatation, strictures, or leaks. Secretin-enhanced MRCP is becoming more popular in studying the exocrine function of the pancreas and in further visualizing the pancreatic duct abnormalities.[30]

ERCP has been considered the test of choice for the diagnosis of CP. In addition to its ability to show changes in the pancreatic duct with dilatations and/or strictures with the characteristic beading sign, ERCP is therapeutic and can be used for dilatation, stone extraction, and stent placement. With the wide spread of alternative noninvasive imaging modalities, the use of ERCP is becoming limited to cases with a potential need for therapeutic intervention.[65] EUS is another highly sensitive modality that can be used to aid in the diagnosis of CP. It can be used for identifying pancreatic anatomic abnormalities and/or confirming choledocholithiasis.[66] However, this modality is limited by being user dependent and requiring an advanced level of training, making it unpopular in diagnosing the disease. CT, MRI, and EUS can be used to exclude other conditions that can mimic symptoms of CP, such as intraductal papillary mucinous neoplasms or pancreatic adenocarcinoma.[30]

Scoring AP cases can range from mild to severe. Hence, it is vital to rate the severity of the disease in its earlier stages, identify patients who are at risk, and initiate the appropriate treatment.[67] Many scoring systems have been used to predict the severity of AP. Although superior to clinical judgment for assigning critical care and aggressive therapy to patients, these systems have varying accuracy in predicting the severity of AP at the beside.[68] In addition, many are not used routinely because they may be time consuming, cumbersome, invasive, too specific to certain complications, or inadequately specific or sensitive. Those severity scores include the Ranson criteria, the acute physiology and chronic health evaluation (APACHE II) score, systemic inflammatory response syndrome (SIRS) score, bedside index for severity in acute pancreatitis (BISAP) score, and harmless acute pancreatitis score (HAPS).

The Ranson criteria are one of the earlier scoring systems that was used in evaluating AP severity. However, this system requires 48 hours of data collection before full evaluation and consists of 11 different parameters.[67] Although still currently used, the Ranson score was reported to be a poor predictor of severity compared with clinical judgment following a meta-analysis of 110 studies.[69] However, it still carries a significant correlation with mortality.[70]

The APACHE II score uses 12 physiologic measurements in addition to age and health status to yield a generic score for severity of disease.[71] It is calculated on admission and daily thereafter for the first 72 hours, with a score of 8 or higher representing severe AP. During the first 48 hours, an increasing score is highly suggestive of development of severe AP, whereas a decreasing score is highly suggestive of mild AP.[72] Various attempts to improve the score have led to the addition of measurement variables and the development of the APACHE-O and APACHE-III scores. Despite its utility in predicting the need for intensive care treatment and superiority to the Ranson score, APACHE II maintains its limitations in that it can distinguish neither interstitial from necrotizing pancreatitis nor sterile from infected necrosis.[72,73] It was recently reported that, although a score generated in the first 24 hours has a strong negative predictive value for severe AP of 86%, it has a modestly positive predictive value of only

43%.[72] Nevertheless, the APACHE II score is still currently used given its high accuracy in assessing the severity and outcome of AP.[68,70]

The SIRS score determines the severity of AP by assessing the degree of widespread systemic inflammation, which may result in multiple organ dysfunction syndrome.[74,75] Unlike other scores, it can be easily measured at the bedside daily and uses 4 parameters (heart rate, respiratory rate, temperature, and white blood cell count). The score scale ranges from 0 to 4, and a score of 2 or more yields a positive.[75] In a study of 759 patients with AP, those who developed persistent SIRS for longer than 48 hours had a significantly higher incidence of multiorgan dysfunction and mortality than those with transient SIRS lasting less than 48 hours (25% and 8% respectively).[72,74] Persistent SIRS at day 3 resulted in 1 or more adverse outcomes in 80% of the patients with AP.[75] A study by Singh and colleagues[76] showed that patients with 3 or 4 SIRS criteria had more severe pancreatitis compared with those with 2 SIRS criteria and that almost all patients without SIRS on the first day of hospitalization had mild AP. At present, the SIRS score remains an inexpensive and easily measurable bedside tool that can favorably assess the severity of AP compared with other cumbersome scoring systems.

CTSI (formerly the Balthazar score) is a score that has been developed and modified to evaluate the severity of AP based on degree of necrosis, inflammation, and the presence of fluid collections on CT scan without intravenous contrast.[60,77] CTSI assigns 0 to 4 points for grade A to E pancreatitis in addition to 0 to 6 points for necrosis (0 for no necrosis, 2 for up to 30%, 4 for 30%–50%, and 6 for >50%). CTSI showed a significant correlation between incidence of morbidity and mortality and severity index assigned to stratified patients.[73] The CTSI can also be used as an early prognostic tool for AP local complications and mortality.[78,79] A study by Leung and colleagues[79] showed that a CTSI score of 5 or more correlated with an extended hospitalization as well as a higher incidence of morbidity and mortality. Although CTSI score has been shown to be a better predictor for severity of AP than Ranson or APACHE II scores, it does not significantly correlate with the development of organ failure.[80] A modified version, the Mortele CTSI, proved to be an easier calculation and was more strongly correlated with patient outcome parameters such as hospital length of stay, need for intervention, incidents of infection, organ failure, and mortality.[81] However, most recently, Raghuwanshi and colleagues[80] found that the revised Atlanta classification provide a more accurate assessment for patient mortality and organ failure than both the Balthazar and the Mortele indices.

The revised Atlanta classification system was introduced in 2012 to better define and classify the clinical diagnosis, CT findings, and severity of disease of AP in 2 subtypes: interstitial edematous pancreatitis and necrotizing pancreatitis.[82] Although the revised Atlanta classification system cannot distinguish between moderately severe and severe AP within 48 hours after onset, it provides a more accurate assessment for patient mortality and organ failure than both the Balthazar and the Mortele indices.[67,80]

Other scoring systems that were developed, but are not as commonly used, to evaluate the severity of AP include the HAPS score, BISAP score, and other organ failure–based scores (ie, the Marshall organ dysfunction score, the Bernard score, the sequential organ failure assessment [SOFA], and the logistic organ dysfunction system score).[67]

Treatment

Acute pancreatitis

Nonoperative management

1. Aggressive fluids replacement: aggressive fluids resuscitation with 250 to 500 mL/h crystalloid solution should be administered to all patients presenting with AP in the

first 12 to 24 hours. Caution should be exercised in patients with known cardiovascular or renal conditions or other comorbid factors that may preclude them from receiving aggressive fluids replacement.[12] Lactated ringer is usually the preferred crystalloid replacement therapy, although it is relatively contraindicated in patients presenting with AP secondary to hypercalcemia. Fluids requirements should be reassessed frequently in the first 6 hours following presentation and for the next 24 to 48 hours, and the rate should be readjusted based on the BUN and hematocrit level. Improvement in vital signs and urine output can serve as an indicator of adequate fluids resuscitation. Previous studies have shown that aggressive fluid resuscitation in the first 12 to 24 hours is associated with marked reduction in mortality and morbidity.[12,83,84] Patients with AP require close monitoring, especially in the first 24 to 72 hours. This monitoring includes the patients' vital signs, urine output, and electrolytes and serum glucose levels. Patients developing progressive hypoxia and or tachycardia might require closer monitoring in an intensive care unit setting.[12]

2. Nutrition: patients with AP can stay nil by mouth and be managed with intravenous fluids. In patients with mild AP, oral feeding can be started immediately if there is no nausea and vomiting, and abdominal pain has resolved.[12] Initiation of feeding with a low-fat solid diet seems to be as safe as a clear liquid diet.[84] Early feeding was found to be associated with reduced length of hospital stay and decreased gastrointestinal symptoms.[85] In moderate to severe AP, oral feeding might not be tolerated early in the course of the disease because of nausea, vomiting, or postprandial pain. Feeding should be started once the local complications start improving and can be advanced as tolerated.[12] Nasogastric and nasojejunal delivery of enteral feeding seem to be safe and well tolerated.[86]
3. Antibiotics: routine use of prophylactic antibiotics in AP is not recommended. Antibiotics should be given for suspected extrapancreatic infections, such as cholangitis, urinary tract infections, bacteremia, pneumonia, or catheter-acquired infections. However, once cultures from the blood, urine, and other sources are found to be negative, antibiotics should be discontinued. In patients with infected necrosis, studies showed that administering antibiotics known to penetrate pancreatic necrosis, such as carbapenems, quinolones, and metronidazole, are beneficial in delaying and even avoiding interventions with a subsequent improvement in morbidity and mortality.[12] However, studies failed to confirm the advantage of prophylactic antibiotics in preventing infection in sterile necrosis and hence they are not recommended.[12,87] Moreover, administration of prophylactic antifungal therapy is not recommended.[12,88]
4. Hypercalcemia and hypertriglyceridemia: although hypercalcemia is a less common cause of AP, treatment should be directed at normalizing serum calcium and determining the underlying cause. For patients with hypertriglyceridemia, controlling triglyceride level should be achieved. Diet with restricted triglycerides and sugar, exercise, fibrates, niacin, and n-3 fatty acids can be offered. Apheresis has also been offered with some success.[89]

Operative management

1. ERCP: in patients presenting with acute gallstone pancreatitis and concurrent acute cholangitis, ERCP is highly recommended within 24 hours of admission. Further indications include CBD obstruction, dilatation of the CBD, or increased liver enzyme levels without cholangitis. However, ERCP is not needed early in most patients with gallstone pancreatitis, who lack laboratory or clinical evidence of ongoing biliary obstruction.[12,90] In patients with high probability of a retained

stone in the CBD based on persistently increased bilirubin level or evidence of stone on imaging, ERCP should be offered.[91] In those with intermediate probability, preoperative evaluation with EUS or MRCP can be used or, alternatively, laparoscopic cholecystectomy with intraoperative cholangiogram (LC-IOC) should be performed based on the availability of resources and expertise.[91,92] Positive preoperative evaluation, or in cases of visualization of a CBD stone during LC-IOC, postoperative ERCP is indicated.[91,93,94] If ERCP fails, surgical exploration of the CBD should be considered.

In gastric bypass patients, conventional ERCP becomes challenging given the length of the roux limb.[95,96] Choi and colleagues[95] found that percutaneous gastrostomy ERCP is more effective than double-balloon enteroscopy-assisted ERCP for bariatric patients, although it is associated with higher morbidity. A study by Schreiner and colleagues[97] showed that deep enteroscopy-assisted ERCP should be offered if the ligament of Treitz to jejunojejunal anastomosis limb length is less than 150 cm versus a laparoscopy-assisted ERCP for longer roux limbs. At present, it is suggested that laparoscopic ERCP seems to be the most reasonable approach if laparoscopic cholecystectomy is planned.[98] In contrast, balloon enteroscopy or gastrostomy ERCP can represent suitable alternatives.[98]

2. Surgical intervention: patients presenting with mild AP with gallbladder stones require a cholecystectomy during the same admission to prevent another recurrence of AP.[12,99,100] Interval cholecystectomy after mild biliary pancreatitis was shown to be associated with an increased risk of readmission with recurrent attacks of biliary pancreatitis.[100] In contrast, early laparoscopic cholecystectomy was associated with short hospital stay in patients with mild AP.[100,101] Same-admission cholecystectomy was further emphasized by the Pancreatitis of biliary origin: Optimal timiNg of CHOlecystectomy (PONCHO) (same-admission versus interval cholecystectomy for mild gallstone pancreatitis) trial, which showed that, compared with interval cholecystectomy, same-admission cholecystectomy reduced the rate of recurrent gallstone-related complications in patients with mild gallstone pancreatitis, with a very low risk of cholecystectomy-related complications.[102] The 2016 guidelines from the European Association for the Study of the Liver (EASL) clinical practice guidelines on the prevention, diagnosis, and treatment of gallstones currently recommends waiting 72 hours to allow for the confirmation of the diagnosis of mild AP and to perform any additional investigations and treatments, such as MRCP, EUS, or ERCP as indicated.[103] If not possible because of patient-related comorbidities, surgical management should be offered no later than 2 to 4 weeks after discharge to prevent another attack of biliary pancreatitis.[104] In contrast, in patients with severe AP or AP that is associated with cholangitis, cholecystectomy can be deferred until active inflammation subsides (4–6 weeks after AP attack).[99,103,105] Further randomized controlled trials are still warranted to establish the optimal timing for cholecystectomy in this subset of patients.

   Other patients who might benefit from cholecystectomy following an acute attack of pancreatitis are those with evidence of biliary sludge. Although patients with biliary sludge are typically asymptomatic, Lee and colleagues[106] reported that biliary sludge could be an under-recognized cause of acute idiopathic pancreatitis, and further reports showed that those patients can benefit from cholecystectomy.[107]

   Intraoperative cholangiogram can be performed during laparoscopic cholecystectomy if there are concerns of retained stones in the bile duct.

   In patients presenting with infected necrosis and/or symptomatic sterile necrosis, open necrosectomy/debridement used to be the treatment of choice. This treatment was associated with high mortality and the consensus was to delay surgical debridement. However, recent studies suggest that antibiotics alone can successfully treat most patients with infected necrosis.[108] Unstable patients with infected necrosis should undergo urgent surgical debridement, which can be achieved by minimally invasive necrosectomy through the means of endoscopic, radiologic, or laparoscopic approaches or even open surgery once the necrosis is walled off.[108–111]

Chronic pancreatitis

Nonoperative management

1. General recommendations: initial management includes cessation of alcohol intake, cessation of smoking, pancreatic enzyme supplements, octreotide, antioxidants, and analgesia.[30] Previous studies have shown that patients with CP who continue to drink have increased mortalities; up to 50% in 5 years according to one study.[29,112] Smoking has been shown to accelerate the progress of CP and may increase the risk of pancreatic cancer, independent of alcohol consumption.[113] Pancreatic enzyme supplements have been used to suppress the pancreatic exocrine secretion to relieve pain, although their success remains marginal at most.[114–117] In contrast, octreotide has been shown to have antiinflammatory properties and may also protect pancreatic cells, decrease intraductal pressure, and decrease proteolysis. However, because of potential side effects, such as hypoglycemia and biliary stasis, octreotide has not been widely accepted and its effectiveness has not been demonstrated consistently.[118]
2. Pain control: as previously discussed, pain tends to be the presenting symptom in most cases. The first step in easing pain is to address the underlying CP to reduce further damage to the pancreas.

   A trial of nonnarcotic analgesia can be initiated in patients with an early stage of the disease. If the pain does not respond to nonnarcotics, becomes more intense, or becomes progressively debilitating, judicious use of narcotic analgesia is then recommended.[119] Patients with previous addictive behaviors are at risk for dependence, abuse, or addiction. Hence, less-potent narcotics, such as tramadol, are commonly prescribed. Because dependence is an important consideration in CP, a single provider should be identified as the patient's designated prescriber.[29]

   Other agents that can aid the management of the chronic pain syndrome include tricyclic antidepressants, selective serotonin reuptake inhibitors, serotonin-norepinephrine reuptake inhibitors, and gabaoentoids.[29,51] Of those, pregabalin is established as an effective adjuvant therapy for pain in patients with CP.[120]

   Celiac nerve blocks with alcohol or steroids have been reported with limited success.[121] EUS-guided celiac blocks use local anesthesia with bupivacaine with or without steroids. Those blocks are temporary and last a few weeks and are, therefore, not recommended.[30,122] Further endoscopic interventions are discussed later.
3. Radiotherapy: most recently, a pilot study evaluated the role of radiotherapy in CP and suggested that it can play a role in pain control.[123]
4. Other new modalities: other modalities of pain relief include a cholecystokinin (CCK) receptor antagonist-A. A study in Japan showed that oral administration of the CCK antagonist may be useful in the treatment of patients with acute, painful attacks of chronic pancteatitis.[124]

Operative management

1. Increased pressure in the pancreatic duct secondary to a sphincteric dysfunction or strictures has been postulated as one of the mechanisms that can precipitate

pain in patients with CP. Hence, pancreatic sphincterotomy, stent placement, pancreatic duct drainage, stone extraction, and pseudocyst drainage have all been reported with varying degrees of success.[125,126] In a large series of 1018 patients followed for 5 years, endoscopic intervention resulted in pain relief in 86% of the group but only in 65% in an intention-to-treat analysis. One-quarter of the patients required surgery secondary to failure of endoscopic therapy.[127] No significant difference between the patient groups with strictures, stones, or both were reported. Another study reported that pain secondary to tropical pancreatitis responded better to endoscopic therapy than pain secondary to alcohol pancreatitis.[128] A few studies have compared endoscopic drainage procedures with surgical interventions. A randomized trial by Varadarajulu and colleagues[129] showed similar efficacy and less cost for endoscopic drainage compared with surgical cystogastrostomy. However, another small randomized controlled trial found that surgical drainage was more effective in relieving obstruction and achieving pain, and another study found surgery to be more cost-effective compared with endoscopic intervention.[130,131] Nonetheless, endoscopic interventions are typically attempted first, especially at larger centers before surgery.

2. Extracorporeal shockwave lithotripsy (ESWL): used for rapid fragmentation of pancreatic duct stone to facilitate endoscopic extraction. A previous meta-analysis examining 17 studies showed that ESWL is effective in clearance of stones from the pancreatic duct and in pain relief.[132] A subsequent study showed similar findings and reported that ESWL without endoscopic drainage is both effective and more cost-effecient.[133] Patients with small pancreatic duct stones or diffuse punctate stones are not eligible for ESWL. The role of ESWL needs to be further investigated in larger studies to further establish its role in the management of CP.
3. Surgical intervention: for patients who fail medical and/or endoscopic management, surgical therapy is considered. Surgical decompression procedures have been generally recommended for patients with pain refractory to medical management who have a dilated main pancreatic duct. Longitudinal pancreaticojejunostomy is currently recommended for patients with pain and dilated pancreatic duct. Studies have shown that short-term pain relief is achieved in approximately 80% of the patients with very low associated morbidity and mortality.[134] Surgical drainage was reported to be more effective than endoscopic treatment in patients with obstruction of the pancreatic duct caused by CP.[130,135] In a randomized trial by Cahen and colleagues,[130] 36% of the patients who underwent a surgical drainage procedure were pain free compared with only 14% of patients treated with endoscopy. Similar complication rates, length of hospital stay, and changes in pancreatic function were found in both groups.

   Pancreatic resection via pancreaticoduodenectomy, distal pancreatectomy with hemi gastrectomy, total pancreatectomy, and duodenal-preserving resection of the pancreatic head have all been described. Whipple procedure has been considered in patients with duodenal obstruction of inflammatory mass where cancer cannot be excluded preoperatively.[118] However, Whipple procedure was more frequently associated with postoperative diabetes and lower quality of life.[136] The Berger procedure, which aims to preserve the duodenum, and the Frey procedure, which aims to preserve the duodenum and the pylorus, are both associated with lower morbidity and mortality and show a high rate of sustained pain relief and return of productivity compared with pancreaticoduodenectomy procedures.[137] Those procedures have been reported to provide similar relief to patients receiving the modified Puestow procedure, although they provided long-term relief at the expense of more perioperative and postoperative complications.[118,138] Distal pancreatectomy is rarely performed and has a very limited role in management of pain, unless the disease is limited to the pancreatic tail, and is associated with decreased mortality compared with proximal pancreatectomies according to a recent analysis.[139] Total pancreatectomy has been performed, coupled with autotransplant of islet cells. Islet cells are separated from the pancreas and then infused into the portal vein, where they implant in the liver and can reduce the severity of diabetes after pancreatectomy. This procedure is considered a last resort in a select group of patients who have failed medical management. Studies have shown that there was a significant reduction in pain severity and frequency.[140,141] A previous study reported that 45% of patients who underwent this procedure were initially insulin dependent, although insulin dependence decreased over time.[140] This procedure is also considered in younger patients presenting with hereditary CP, whereas older patients with long-standing disease can be managed with surgical resection to decrease the risk of developing adenocarcinoma.[39]

Denervation procedures can be achieved through an open surgical approach or a percutaneous approach to interrupt the afferent nerves returning from the pancreas to the celiac ganglion and splanchnic nerves.[134,142] Although pain relief with denervation procedures has been reported, it is mostly of short duration and the studies evaluating this intervention are limited. A controlled trial comparing denervation procedures with other surgical options is warranted.[134]

To summarize, patients with debilitating pain who failed medical management may be candidates for surgical resection. Medical management can include a drainage procedure or a duodenum-preserving surgical resection. Total pancreatectomy with islet autotransplant is reserved as a last resort in a select group of patients. The role of surgical denervation is still ill-defined and needs further studies to examine its role in the surgical management of CP.

REFERENCES

1. Sankaran SJ, Xiao AY, Wu LM, et al. Frequency of progression from acute to chronic pancreatitis and risk factors: a meta-analysis. Gastroenterology 2015;149(6):1490–500.e1.
2. Yadav D, O'Connell M, Papachristou GI. Natural history following the first attack of acute pancreatitis. Am J Gastroenterol 2012;107(7):1096–103.
3. Schneider A, Löhr JM, Singer MV. The M-ANNHEIM classification of chronic pancreatitis: introduction of a unifying classification system based on a review of previous classifications of the disease. J Gastroenterol 2007;42(2):101–19.
4. Kloppel G. Morphology of acute pancreatitis in relation to etiology and pathogenesis. In: Malfertheiner P, Domínguez-Muñoz JE, Schulz HU, et al, editors. Diagnostic procedures in pancreatic disease. Berlin: Springer; 1997.
5. Vege SS, Yadav D, Chari ST. Pancreatitis. Oxford (United Kingdom): Blackwell Publishing; 2007.
6. Yadav D, Lowenfels AB. The epidemiology of pancreatitis and pancreatic cancer. Gastroenterology 2013;144(6):1252–61.
7. Conwell DL, Lee LS, Yadav D, et al. American Pancreatic Association practice guidelines in chronic pancreatitis: evidence-based report on diagnostic guidelines. Pancreas 2014;43(8):1143–62.
8. Peery AF, Dellon ES, Lund J, et al. Burden of gastrointestinal disease in the United States: 2012 update. Gastroenterology 2012;143(5):1179–87.e1-3.

9. Petrov MS, Shanbhag S, Chakraborty M, et al. Organ failure and infection of pancreatic necrosis as determinants of mortality in patients with acute pancreatitis. Gastroenterology 2010;139(3):813–20.
10. Lankisch PG, Löhr-Happe A, Otto J, et al. Natural course in chronic pancreatitis. Pain, exocrine and endocrine pancreatic insufficiency and prognosis of the disease. Digestion 1993;54(3):148–55.
11. Ammann RW, Akovbiantz A, Largiader F, et al. Course and outcome of chronic pancreatitis. Longitudinal study of a mixed medical-surgical series of 245 patients. Gastroenterology 1984;86(5 Pt 1):820–8.
12. Tenner S, Baillie J, DeWitt J, et al, American College of Gastroenterology. American College of Gastroenterology guideline: management of acute pancreatitis. Am J Gastroenterol 2013;108(9):1400–15, 1416.
13. Gullo L, Migliori M, Oláh A, et al. Acute pancreatitis in five European countries: etiology and mortality. Pancreas 2002;24(3):223–7.
14. Wang GJ, Gao CF, Wei D, et al. Acute pancreatitis: etiology and common pathogenesis. World J Gastroenterol 2009;15(12):1427–30.
15. Moreau JA, Zinsmeister AR, Melton LJ, et al. Gallstone pancreatitis and the effect of cholecystectomy: a population-based cohort study. Mayo Clin Proc 1988; 63(5):466–73.
16. Lowenfels AB, Maisonneuve P, Sullivan T. The changing character of acute pancreatitis: epidemiology, etiology, and prognosis. Curr Gastroenterol Rep 2009;11(2):97–103.
17. Khoo TK, Vege SS, Abu-Lebdeh HS, et al. Acute pancreatitis in primary hyperparathyroidism: a population-based study. J Clin Endocrinol Metab 2009;94(6): 2115–8.
18. Fortson MR, Freedman SN, Webster PD. Clinical assessment of hyperlipidemic pancreatitis. Am J Gastroenterol 1995;90(12):2134–9.
19. Slack S, Abbey I, Smith D. Abdominal pain and hyperamylasaemia–not always pancreatitis. BMJ Case Rep 2010;2010. https://doi.org/10.1136/bcr.02.2010. 2747.
20. Christoforidis E, Goulimaris I, Kanellos I, et al. Post-ERCP pancreatitis and hyperamylasemia: patient-related and operative risk factors. Endoscopy 2002; 34(4):286–92.
21. El Nakeeb A, El Hanafy E, Salah T, et al. Post-endoscopic retrograde cholangiopancreatography pancreatitis: risk factors and predictors of severity. World J Gastrointest Endosc 2016;8(19):709–15.
22. Wilcox CM, Phadnis M, Varadarajulu S. Biliary stent placement is associated with post-ERCP pancreatitis. Gastrointest Endosc 2010;72(3):546–50.
23. Elmunzer BJ, Waljee AK, Elta GH, et al. A meta-analysis of rectal NSAIDs in the prevention of post-ERCP pancreatitis. Gut 2008;57(9):1262–7.
24. Sadr-Azodi O, Mattsson F, Bexlius TS, et al. Association of oral glucocorticoid use with an increased risk of acute pancreatitis: a population-based nested case-control study. JAMA Intern Med 2013;173(6):444–9.
25. Singh S, Chang HY, Richards TM, et al. Glucagonlike peptide 1-based therapies and risk of hospitalization for acute pancreatitis in type 2 diabetes mellitus: a population-based matched case-control study. JAMA Intern Med 2013;173(7): 534–9.
26. Lankisch PG, Dröge M, Gottesleben F. Drug induced acute pancreatitis: incidence and severity. Gut 1995;37(4):565–7.
27. Dassopoulos T, Ehrenpreis ED. Acute pancreatitis in human immunodeficiency virus-infected patients: a review. Am J Med 1999;107(1):78–84.

28. Dragovic G. Acute pancreatitis in HIV/AIDS patients: an issue of concern. Asian Pac J Trop Biomed 2013;3(6):422–5.
29. Mergener K, Baillie J. Chronic pancreatitis. Lancet 1997;350(9088):1379–85.
30. Forsmark CE. Management of chronic pancreatitis. Gastroenterology 2013; 144(6):1282–91.e3.
31. Yadav D, Hawes RH, Brand RE, et al. Alcohol consumption, cigarette smoking, and the risk of recurrent acute and chronic pancreatitis. Arch Intern Med 2009; 169(11):1035–45.
32. Samokhvalov AV, Rehm J, Roerecke M. Alcohol consumption as a risk factor for acute and chronic pancreatitis: a systematic review and a series of meta-analyses. EBioMedicine 2015;2(12):1996–2002.
33. Tarnasky PR, Hoffman B, Aabakken L, et al. Sphincter of Oddi dysfunction is associated with chronic pancreatitis. Am J Gastroenterol 1997;92(7):1125–9.
34. Ewald N, Marzeion AM, Bretzel RG, et al. Endoscopic sphincterotomy in patients with stenosis of ampulla of Vater: three-year follow-up of exocrine pancreatic function and clinical symptoms. World J Gastroenterol 2007;13(6):901–5.
35. Schlosser W, Rau BM, Poch B, et al. Surgical treatment of pancreas divisum causing chronic pancreatitis: the outcome benefits of duodenum-preserving pancreatic head resection. J Gastrointest Surg 2005;9(5):710–5.
36. Pitchumoni CS. Special problems of tropical pancreatitis. Clin Gastroenterol 1984;13(3):941–59.
37. Schneider A, Suman A, Rossi L, et al. SPINK1/PSTI mutations are associated with tropical pancreatitis and type II diabetes mellitus in Bangladesh. Gastroenterology 2002;123(4):1026–30.
38. Bhatia E, Choudhuri G, Sikora SS, et al. Tropical calcific pancreatitis: strong association with SPINK1 trypsin inhibitor mutations. Gastroenterology 2002;123(4): 1020–5.
39. Rebours V, Lévy P, Mosnier JF, et al. Pathology analysis reveals that dysplastic pancreatic ductal lesions are frequent in patients with hereditary pancreatitis. Clin Gastroenterol Hepatol 2010;8(2):206–12.
40. Sharer N, Schwarz M, Malone G, et al. Mutations of the cystic fibrosis gene in patients with chronic pancreatitis. N Engl J Med 1998;339(10):645–52.
41. Witt H, Luck W, Hennies HC, et al. Mutations in the gene encoding the serine protease inhibitor, Kazal type 1 are associated with chronic pancreatitis. Nat Genet 2000;25(2):213–6.
42. Witt H, Kage A, Luck W, et al. Alpha1-antitrypsin genotypes in patients with chronic pancreatitis. Scand J Gastroenterol 2002;37(3):356–9.
43. Novis BH, Young GO, Bank S, et al. Chronic pancreatitis and alpha-1-antitrypsin. Lancet 1975;2(7938):748–9.
44. Witt H. Chronic pancreatitis and cystic fibrosis. Gut 2003;52(Suppl 2):ii31–41.
45. Masaryk TJ, Achkar E. Pancreatitis as initial presentation of cystic fibrosis in young adults. A report of two cases. Dig Dis Sci 1983;28(10):874–8.
46. Borum M, Steinberg W, Steer M, et al. Chronic pancreatitis: a complication of systemic lupus erythematosus. Gastroenterology 1993;104(2):613–5.
47. Bess MA, Edis AJ, van Heerden JA. Hyperparathyroidism and pancreatitis. Chance or a causal association? JAMA 1980;243(3):246–7.
48. Cox DW, Breckenridge WC, Little JA. Inheritance of apolipoprotein C-II deficiency with hypertriglyceridemia and pancreatitis. N Engl J Med 1978; 299(26):1421–4.
49. Banks PA. Acute pancreatitis: diagnosis. In: Lankisch PG, Banks PA, editors. Pancreatitis. New York: Springer-Verlag; 1998.

50. Frøkjær JB, Olesen SS, Drewes AM. Fibrosis, atrophy, and ductal pathology in chronic pancreatitis are associated with pancreatic function but independent of symptoms. Pancreas 2013;42(7):1182–7.
51. Gupte AR, Forsmark CE. Chronic pancreatitis. Curr Opin Gastroenterol 2014; 30(5):500–5.
52. Ammann RW, Muellhaupt B. The natural history of pain in alcoholic chronic pancreatitis. Gastroenterology 1999;116(5):1132–40.
53. Yadav D, Agarwal N, Pitchumoni CS. A critical evaluation of laboratory tests in acute pancreatitis. Am J Gastroenterol 2002;97(6):1309–18.
54. Toouli J, Brooke-Smith M, Bassi C, et al. Guidelines for the management of acute pancreatitis. J Gastroenterol Hepatol 2002;17(Suppl):S15–39.
55. Dervenis C, Johnson CD, Bassi C, et al. Diagnosis, objective assessment of severity, and management of acute pancreatitis. Santorini consensus conference. Int J Pancreatol 1999;25(3):195–210.
56. Domínguez-Muñoz JE, D Hardt P, Lerch MM, et al. Potential for screening for pancreatic exocrine insufficiency using the fecal elastase-1 test. Dig Dis Sci 2017;62(5):1119–30.
57. Ammori BJ, Boreham B, Lewis P, et al. The biochemical detection of biliary etiology of acute pancreatitis on admission: a revisit in the modern era of biliary imaging. Pancreas 2003;26(2):e32–5.
58. Venneman NG, Buskens E, Besselink MG, et al. Small gallstones are associated with increased risk of acute pancreatitis: potential benefits of prophylactic cholecystectomy? Am J Gastroenterol 2005;100(11):2540–50.
59. Finstad TA, Tchelepi H, Ralls PW. Sonography of acute pancreatitis: prevalence of findings and pictorial essay. Ultrasound Q 2005;21(2):95–104 [quiz: 150, 153–4].
60. Balthazar EJ, Robinson DL, Megibow AJ, et al. Acute pancreatitis: value of CT in establishing prognosis. Radiology 1990;174(2):331–6.
61. Arvanitakis M, Delhaye M, De Maertelaere V, et al. Computed tomography and magnetic resonance imaging in the assessment of acute pancreatitis. Gastroenterology 2004;126(3):715–23.
62. Stimac D, Miletić D, Radić M, et al. The role of nonenhanced magnetic resonance imaging in the early assessment of acute pancreatitis. Am J Gastroenterol 2007;102(5):997–1004.
63. Koo BC, Chinogureyi A, Shaw AS. Imaging acute pancreatitis. Br J Radiol 2010; 83(986):104–12.
64. Grendell JH, Cello JP. Chronic pancreatitis. In: Sleisenger MH, Fordtran JS, editors. Gastrointestinal disease. 5th edition. Philadelphia: WB Saunders; 1993. p. 1654–81.
65. Busireddy KK, AlObaidy M, Ramalho M, et al. Pancreatitis-imaging approach. World J Gastrointest Pathophysiol 2014;5(3):252–70.
66. Catalano MF, Sahai A, Levy M, et al. EUS-based criteria for the diagnosis of chronic pancreatitis: the Rosemont classification. Gastrointest Endosc 2009; 69(7):1251–61.
67. Otsuki M, Takeda K, Matsuno S, et al. Criteria for the diagnosis and severity stratification of acute pancreatitis. World J Gastroenterol 2013;19(35):5798–805.
68. Cho JH, Kim TN, Chung HH, et al. Comparison of scoring systems in predicting the severity of acute pancreatitis. World J Gastroenterol 2015;21(8):2387–94.
69. De Bernardinis M, Violi V, Roncoroni L, et al. Discriminant power and information content of Ranson's prognostic signs in acute pancreatitis: a meta-analytic study. Crit Care Med 1999;27(10):2272–83.

70. Simoes M, Alves P, Esperto H, et al. Predicting acute pancreatitis severity: comparison of prognostic scores. Gastroenterology Res 2011;4(5):216–22.
71. Knaus WA, Draper EA, Wagner DP, et al. APACHE II: a severity of disease classification system. Crit Care Med 1985;13(10):818–29.
72. Greenberg JA, Hsu J, Bawazeer M, et al. Clinical practice guideline: management of acute pancreatitis. Can J Surg 2016;59(2):128–40.
73. Balthazar EJ. Acute pancreatitis: assessment of severity with clinical and CT evaluation. Radiology 2002;223(3):603–13.
74. Mofidi R, Duff MD, Wigmore SJ, et al. Association between early systemic inflammatory response, severity of multiorgan dysfunction and death in acute pancreatitis. Br J Surg 2006;93(6):738–44.
75. Kumar A, Chari ST, Vege SS. Can the time course of systemic inflammatory response syndrome score predict future organ failure in acute pancreatitis? Pancreas 2014;43(7):1101–5.
76. Singh VK, Wu BU, Bollen TL, et al. Early systemic inflammatory response syndrome is associated with severe acute pancreatitis. Clin Gastroenterol Hepatol 2009;7(11):1247–51.
77. Balthazar EJ, Freeny PC, vanSonnenberg E. Imaging and intervention in acute pancreatitis. Radiology 1994;193(2):297–306.
78. Vriens PW, van de Linde P, Slotema ET, et al. Computed tomography severity index is an early prognostic tool for acute pancreatitis. J Am Coll Surg 2005;201(4):497–502.
79. Leung TK, Lee CM, Lin SY, et al. Balthazar computed tomography severity index is superior to Ranson criteria and apache II scoring system in predicting acute pancreatitis outcome. World J Gastroenterol 2005;11(38):6049–52.
80. Raghuwanshi S, Gupta R, Vyas MM, et al. CT evaluation of acute pancreatitis and its prognostic correlation with CT severity index. J Clin Diagn Res 2016;10(6):TC06–11.
81. Mortele KJ, Wiesner W, Intriere L, et al. A modified CT severity index for evaluating acute pancreatitis: improved correlation with patient outcome. AJR Am J Roentgenol 2004;183(5):1261–5.
82. Banks PA, Bollen TL, Dervenis C, et al. Classification of acute pancreatitis–2012: revision of the Atlanta classification and definitions by international consensus. Gut 2013;62(1):102–11.
83. Gardner TB, Vege SS, Chari ST, et al. Faster rate of initial fluid resuscitation in severe acute pancreatitis diminishes in-hospital mortality. Pancreatology 2009;9(6):770–6.
84. Working Group IAP/APA Acute Pancreatitis Guidelines. IAP/APA evidence-based guidelines for the management of acute pancreatitis. Pancreatology 2013;13(4 Suppl 2):e1–15.
85. Vaughn VM, Shuster D, Rogers MAM, et al. Early versus delayed feeding in patients with acute pancreatitis: a systematic review. Ann Intern Med 2017;166(12):883–92.
86. Petrov MS, Kukosh MV, Emelyanov NV. A randomized controlled trial of enteral versus parenteral feeding in patients with predicted severe acute pancreatitis shows a significant reduction in mortality and in infected pancreatic complications with total enteral nutrition. Dig Surg 2006;23(5–6):336–44 [discussion: 344–5].
87. Jiang K, Huang W, Yang XN, et al. Present and future of prophylactic antibiotics for severe acute pancreatitis. World J Gastroenterol 2012;18(3):279–84.

88. Trikudanathan G, Navaneethan U, Vege SS. Intra-abdominal fungal infections complicating acute pancreatitis: a review. Am J Gastroenterol 2011;106(7): 1188–92.
89. Piolot A, Nadler F, Cavallero E, et al. Prevention of recurrent acute pancreatitis in patients with severe hypertriglyceridemia: value of regular plasmapheresis. Pancreas 1996;13(1):96–9.
90. Moretti A, Papi C, Aratari A, et al. Is early endoscopic retrograde cholangiopancreatography useful in the management of acute biliary pancreatitis? A meta-analysis of randomized controlled trials. Dig Liver Dis 2008;40(5):379–85.
91. Almadi MA, Barkun JS, Barkun AN. Management of suspected stones in the common bile duct. CMAJ 2012;184(8):884–92.
92. Maple JT, Ben-Menachem T, Anderson MA, et al. The role of endoscopy in the evaluation of suspected choledocholithiasis. Gastrointest Endosc 2010;71(1): 1–9.
93. Varadarajulu S, Eloubeidi MA, Wilcox CM, et al. Do all patients with abnormal intraoperative cholangiogram merit endoscopic retrograde cholangiopancreatography? Surg Endosc 2006;20(5):801–5.
94. Vadlamudi R, Conway J, Mishra G, et al. Identifying patients most likely to have a common bile duct stone after a positive intraoperative cholangiogram. Gastroenterol Hepatol (N Y) 2014;10(4):240–4.
95. Choi EK, Chiorean MV, Coté GA, et al. ERCP via gastrostomy vs. double balloon enteroscopy in patients with prior bariatric Roux-en-Y gastric bypass surgery. Surg Endosc 2013;27(8):2894–9.
96. Nagem RG, Lázaro-da-Silva A, de Oliveira RM, et al. Gallstone-related complications after Roux-en-Y gastric bypass: a prospective study. Hepatobiliary Pancreat Dis Int 2012;11(6):630–5.
97. Schreiner MA, Chang L, Gluck M, et al. Laparoscopy-assisted versus balloon enteroscopy-assisted ERCP in bariatric post-Roux-en-Y gastric bypass patients. Gastrointest Endosc 2012;75(4):748–56.
98. Souto-Rodríguez R, Alvarez-Sánchez MV. Endoluminal solutions to bariatric surgery complications: a review with a focus on technical aspects and results. World J Gastrointest Endosc 2017;9(3):105–26.
99. Larson SD, Nealon WH, Evers BM. Management of gallstone pancreatitis. Adv Surg 2006;40:265–84.
100. van Baal MC, Besselink MG, Bakker OJ, et al. Timing of cholecystectomy after mild biliary pancreatitis: a systematic review. Ann Surg 2012;255(5):860–6.
101. Gurusamy KS, Nagendran M, Davidson BR. Early versus delayed laparoscopic cholecystectomy for acute gallstone pancreatitis. Cochrane Database Syst Rev 2013;(9):CD010326.
102. da Costa DW, Bouwense SA, Schepers NJ, et al. Same-admission versus interval cholecystectomy for mild gallstone pancreatitis (PONCHO): a multicentre randomised controlled trial. Lancet 2015;386(10000):1261–8.
103. European Association for the Study of the Liver (EASL). Electronic address: easloffice@easloffice.eu. EASL clinical practice guidelines on the prevention, diagnosis and treatment of gallstones. J Hepatol 2016;65(1):146–81.
104. Forsmark CE, Baillie J, AGA Institute Clinical Practice and Economics Committee, AGA Institute Governing Board. AGA institute technical review on acute pancreatitis. Gastroenterology 2007;132(5):2022–44.
105. Uhl W, Müller CA, Krähenbühl L, et al. Acute gallstone pancreatitis: timing of laparoscopic cholecystectomy in mild and severe disease. Surg Endosc 1999;13(11):1070–6.

106. Lee SP, Nicholls JF, Park HZ. Biliary sludge as a cause of acute pancreatitis. N Engl J Med 1992;326(9):589–93.
107. Räty S, Pulkkinen J, Nordback I, et al. Can laparoscopic cholecystectomy prevent recurrent idiopathic acute pancreatitis?: A prospective randomized multicenter trial. Ann Surg 2015;262(5):736–41.
108. Freeman ML, Werner J, van Santvoort HC, et al. Interventions for necrotizing pancreatitis: summary of a multidisciplinary consensus conference. Pancreas 2012;41(8):1176–94.
109. van Baal MC, van Santvoort HC, Bollen TL, et al. Systematic review of percutaneous catheter drainage as primary treatment for necrotizing pancreatitis. Br J Surg 2011;98(1):18–27.
110. Bakker OJ, van Santvoort HC, van Brunschot S, et al. Endoscopic transgastric vs surgical necrosectomy for infected necrotizing pancreatitis: a randomized trial. JAMA 2012;307(10):1053–61.
111. Vege SS, Baron TH, Mayo Clinic College of Medicine, Rochester, MN 55905, USA. vege.santhi@mayo.edu. Management of pancreatic necrosis in severe acute pancreatitis. Clin Gastroenterol Hepatol 2005;3(2):192–6.
112. Steer ML, Waxman I, Freedman S. Chronic pancreatitis. N Engl J Med 1995; 332(22):1482–90.
113. Maisonneuve P, Lowenfels AB, Müllhaupt B, et al. Cigarette smoking accelerates progression of alcoholic chronic pancreatitis. Gut 2005;54(4):510–4.
114. Brown A, Hughes M, Tenner S, et al. Does pancreatic enzyme supplementation reduce pain in patients with chronic pancreatitis: a meta-analysis. Am J Gastroenterol 1997;92(11):2032–5.
115. Mössner J, Secknus R, Meyer J, et al. Treatment of pain with pancreatic extracts in chronic pancreatitis: results of a prospective placebo-controlled multicenter trial. Digestion 1992;53(1–2):54–66.
116. Halgreen H, Pedersen NT, Worning H. Symptomatic effect of pancreatic enzyme therapy in patients with chronic pancreatitis. Scand J Gastroenterol 1986;21(1): 104–8.
117. Winstead NS, Wilcox CM. Clinical trials of pancreatic enzyme replacement for painful chronic pancreatitis–a review. Pancreatology 2009;9(4):344–50.
118. Trikudanathan G, Navaneethan U, Vege SS. Modern treatment of patients with chronic pancreatitis. Gastroenterol Clin North Am 2012;41(1):63–76.
119. Enweluzo C, Tlhabano L. Pain management in chronic pancreatitis: taming the beast. Clin Exp Gastroenterol 2013;6:167–71.
120. Olesen SS, Bouwense SA, Wilder-Smith OH, et al. Pregabalin reduces pain in patients with chronic pancreatitis in a randomized, controlled trial. Gastroenterology 2011;141(2):536–43.
121. Busch EH, Atchison SR. Steroid celiac plexus block for chronic pancreatitis: results in 16 cases. J Clin Anesth 1989;1(6):431–3.
122. Gress F, Schmitt C, Sherman S, et al. Endoscopic ultrasound-guided celiac plexus block for managing abdominal pain associated with chronic pancreatitis: a prospective single center experience. Am J Gastroenterol 2001;96(2):409–16.
123. Guarner L, Navalpotro B, Molero X, et al. Management of painful chronic pancreatitis with single-dose radiotherapy. Am J Gastroenterol 2009;104(2): 349–55.
124. Shiratori K, Takeuchi T, Satake K, et al, Study Group of Loxiglumide in Japan. Clinical evaluation of oral administration of a cholecystokinin-A receptor antagonist (loxiglumide) to patients with acute, painful attacks of chronic pancreatitis: a multicenter dose-response study in Japan. Pancreas 2002;25(1):e1–5.

125. Binmoeller KF, Jue P, Seifert H, et al. Endoscopic pancreatic stent drainage in chronic pancreatitis and a dominant stricture: long-term results. Endoscopy 1995;27(9):638–44.
126. Ashby K, Lo SK. The role of pancreatic stenting in obstructive ductal disorders other than pancreas divisum. Gastrointest Endosc 1995;42(4):306–11.
127. Rösch T, Daniel S, Scholz M, et al. Endoscopic treatment of chronic pancreatitis: a multicenter study of 1000 patients with long-term follow-up. Endoscopy 2002; 34(10):765–71.
128. Pai CG, Alvares JF. Endoscopic pancreatic-stent placement and sphincterotomy for relief of pain in tropical pancreatitis: results of a 1-year follow-up. Gastrointest Endosc 2007;66(1):70–5.
129. Varadarajulu S, Bang JY, Sutton BS, et al. Equal efficacy of endoscopic and surgical cystogastrostomy for pancreatic pseudocyst drainage in a randomized trial. Gastroenterology 2013;145(3):583–90.e1.
130. Cahen DL, Gouma DJ, Nio Y, et al. Endoscopic versus surgical drainage of the pancreatic duct in chronic pancreatitis. N Engl J Med 2007;356(7):676–84.
131. Laramée P, Wonderling D, Cahen DL, et al. Trial-based cost-effectiveness analysis comparing surgical and endoscopic drainage in patients with obstructive chronic pancreatitis. BMJ Open 2013;3(9):e003676.
132. Guda NM, Partington S, Freeman ML. Extracorporeal shock wave lithotripsy in the management of chronic calcific pancreatitis: a meta-analysis. JOP 2005; 6(1):6–12.
133. Dumonceau JM, Costamagna G, Tringali A, et al. Treatment for painful calcified chronic pancreatitis: extracorporeal shock wave lithotripsy versus endoscopic treatment: a randomised controlled trial. Gut 2007;56(4):545–52.
134. Gachago C, Draganov PV. Pain management in chronic pancreatitis. World J Gastroenterol 2008;14(20):3137–48.
135. Díte P, Ruzicka M, Zboril V, et al. A prospective, randomized trial comparing endoscopic and surgical therapy for chronic pancreatitis. Endoscopy 2003; 35(7):553–8.
136. Diener MK, Rahbari NN, Fischer L, et al. Duodenum-preserving pancreatic head resection versus pancreatoduodenectomy for surgical treatment of chronic pancreatitis: a systematic review and meta-analysis. Ann Surg 2008;247(6): 950–61.
137. McClaine RJ, Lowy AM, Matthews JB, et al. A comparison of pancreaticoduodenectomy and duodenum-preserving head resection for the treatment of chronic pancreatitis. HPB (Oxford) 2009;11(8):677–83.
138. Lieb JG, Forsmark CE. Review article: pain and chronic pancreatitis. Aliment Pharmacol Ther 2009;29(7):706–19.
139. Hill JS, McPhee JT, Whalen GF, et al. In-hospital mortality after pancreatic resection for chronic pancreatitis: population-based estimates from the nationwide inpatient sample. J Am Coll Surg 2009;209(4):468–76.
140. Bramis K, Gordon-Weeks AN, Friend PJ, et al. Systematic review of total pancreatectomy and islet autotransplantation for chronic pancreatitis. Br J Surg 2012; 99(6):761–6.
141. Garcea G, Pollard CA, Illouz S, et al. Patient satisfaction and cost-effectiveness following total pancreatectomy with islet cell transplantation for chronic pancreatitis. Pancreas 2013;42(2):322–8.
142. Stone HH, Chauvin EJ. Pancreatic denervation for pain relief in chronic alcohol associated pancreatitis. Br J Surg 1990;77(3):303–5.

Pneumoperitoneum

Tiffany Nicole Tanner, MD*, Bradley Rounsborg Hall, MD,
Jacob Oran, MD

KEYWORDS

• Pneumoperitoneum • Peritonitis • Management

KEY POINTS

- Develop a differential diagnosis for patients with pneumoperitoneum.
- Understand the basic management strategies for patients with pneumoperitoneum.
- Know when patients with pneumoperitoneum need operative exploration.

INTRODUCTION

Pneumoperitoneum has a wide differential diagnosis and presents with varying degrees of severity; however, not all etiologies require operative intervention. It is imperative that all patients with this diagnosis are evaluated by a surgeon. A thorough history, physical examination, and workup, aimed at localization of the source of pneumoperitoneum will ultimately determine the necessary treatments, including the need for operative intervention. We aim to provide the reader with a working knowledge regarding the evaluation and treatment of patients with pneumoperitoneum.

OVERVIEW

Pneumoperitoneum is ultimately the result of tissue ischemia, erosion, infection, or mechanical and/or thermal injury and has a wide differential diagnosis that includes cancer, iatrogenic injury, infection, and ulcerative disease, to name a few. Patients may present with a wide range of symptoms with varying severities of illness and physical examination findings. Perforated viscus is the most common etiology (85%–95% of cases) and operative intervention is required for many patients.[1,2] When evaluating a patient with pneumoperitoneum, the etiology is not always known before surgery, but an appropriate history and workup may identify the organ most likely responsible. For patients who undergo operative exploration with an unknown etiology, the definitive cause may not be known until biopsy and pathology results return. We intend to

Disclosures: The authors have nothing to disclose.
Department of Surgery- Section of General Surgery, 983280 Nebraska Medical Center Omaha, NE 68198-3280, USA
* Corresponding author.
E-mail address: ttanner@unmc.edu

Surg Clin N Am 98 (2018) 915–932
https://doi.org/10.1016/j.suc.2018.06.004
surgical.theclinics.com

cover the salient points regarding pneumoperitoneum; however, the broadness of this topic is prohibitive in covering all possible scenarios related to pneumoperitoneum. This section focuses on pneumoperitoneum as it relates to the following organs or situations:

- Abdominal esophagus
- Stomach
- Small intestine
- Colon and rectum
- Pneumatosis intestinalis
- Postoperative pneumoperitoneum

It is important to note that pneumoperitoneum may be the result of etiologies that do not require operative treatment. These causes are listed in **Table 1**.[1–9] Further discussion of these maladies is outside the scope of this article, but they remain of importance for the surgeon to be aware.

CLINICAL PRESENTATION

Patients with pneumoperitoneum may present with a varied symptoms, but infrequently are asymptomatic. Symptoms vary based on the location of perforation but may include abdominal pain, chest pain, nausea, or vomiting. Patients with pneumoperitoneum frequently develop symptoms acutely and may progress to fulminant sepsis if not treated promptly within hours to days.[1]

WORKUP

An upright chest radiograph frequently establishes the diagnosis of pneumoperitoneum, but is less likely to determine the exact etiology (**Fig. 1**).[1] A thorough history eliciting the temporal relationship of symptoms and disease progression is critical to determine the appropriate treatment strategy for all patients with pneumoperitoneum. Patients should be questioned about pertinent risk factors and medical history. The physical examination should focus on the abdomen and the identification of findings that narrow the differential diagnosis and guide management. Laboratory tests should be obtained to determine if hematologic or electrolyte abnormalities, or coagulopathy

Table 1
Nonsurgical causes of pneumoperitoneum

Thoracic	Chronic obstructive pulmonary disease/Severe coughing[3] Mechanical ventilation[3] Cardiopulmonary resuscitation[4] Pneumothorax, tracheal rupture[2]
Abdominal	Spontaneous bacterial peritonitis[5] Scleroderma/Collagen vascular disease[2,6] Pneumatosis cystoides intestinalis[2] Percutaneous endoscopic gastrostomy[2] Chronic peritoneal dialysis[2,7]
Gynecologic	Vaginal instrumentation[8] Coitus[2]
Miscellaneous	Amyloidosis[9] Diving with decompression[2] Cocaine use[2]

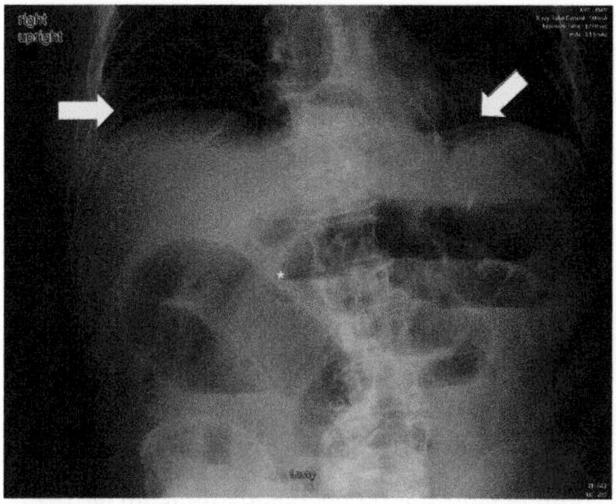

Fig. 1. Upright chest radiograph demonstrating pneumoperitoneum beneath the diaphragm (*arrows*) along with Rigler sign (*star*).

are present that may complicate surgical intervention, and allow the provider to estimate severity of illness.

In addition to an upright chest radiograph, a left lateral decubitus film may demonstrate free air between the abdominal wall and the lateral edge of the liver; however, the sensitivity of an upright chest radiograph is superior.[1,10] For patients with pneumoperitoneum who receive a supine radiograph, visualization of both the inner and outer walls of bowel, known as the "Rigler sign," is indicative of free air and can be easily overlooked (**Fig. 2**).[1] The most sensitive imaging modality for pneumoperitoneum is a computed tomography (CT) scan (**Fig. 3**), which may identify a specific organ or area of concern.[1]

Pneumoperitoneum Due to Esophageal Perforation

Overview

Pneumoperitoneum as a result of esophageal perforation (EP) is rare but carries a mortality rate near 20%.[11–14] Several factors play a role in determining patient outcomes including time of diagnosis (early vs late), etiology, location, presence of

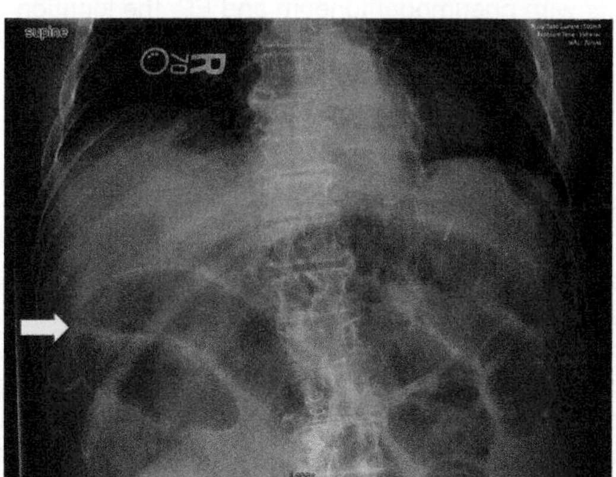

Fig. 2. A supine abdominal radiograph demonstrating Rigler sign (*arrow*).

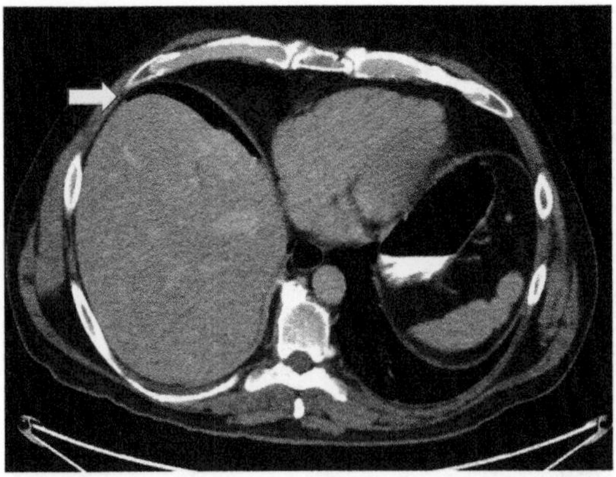

Fig. 3. Abdominal CT scan demonstrating pneumoperitoneum (*arrow*).

comorbidities, and type of treating hospital.[11,12,15,16] Considering that pneumoperitoneum due to cervical and thoracic EP is relatively rare, we will focus only on distal EP.

Relevant anatomy

The abdominal esophagus is 3 to 4 cm in length and courses to the left of the vertebral column. The blood supply originates from the left gastric artery. The esophagus narrows just superior to the gastroesophageal junction (GEJ) and is the site of 12% to 37% of EPs. At this site, EP has the highest mortality, ranging from 0% to 43%.[12,13] The abdominal esophagus is difficult to access given its posterior and superior location. Mobilization of the stomach is necessary to visualize the esophagus, placing other structures at risk, such as the anterior and posterior branches of the vagus nerve. For patients with EP, contamination will make this exposure more difficult.

Clinical presentation

The clinical presentation of EP mimics other causes of pneumoperitoneum and is dependent on the time to presentation and the level of injury.[12] There needs to be a high index of suspicion for perforation if a patient has a combination of chest pain, dysphagia, dyspnea, subcutaneous emphysema, epigastric pain, fever, tachycardia, or tachypnea after any esophageal instrumentation, or history of vomiting or retching.[12,15] For patients with pneumoperitoneum and EP, the location of the perforation is likely in either the distal third of the thoracic esophagus or the abdominal esophagus.

Workup

The gold standard for diagnosing and localizing an EP has historically been a water-soluble contrast esophagram with a sensitivity of 75% to 80%.[17] Some advocate for follow-up barium contrast esophagram within hours if the first esophagram was negative and there remains a high clinical suspicion for EP.[12,18] The use of CT with contrast has largely surpassed contrast esophagram. The sensitivity is upward of 92% to 100%, and it provides additional information to estimate the degree of contamination and identify other pathology.[19] In prior years, esophagoduodenoscopy (EGD) was used sparingly with the concern that insufflation will worsen a small perforation or make localization of the perforation more difficult.[12] However, in more recent studies, the use of EGD has become more acceptable, and those advocating for its use have not noted any worsening of these injuries.[14]

Treatment

Spontaneous and iatrogenic perforations Treatment options for EP include endoluminal stenting, operative management, and in select cases, nonoperative management. Esophageal stenting is reserved for patients who are diagnosed early with a contained perforation and minimal contamination in the absence of distal obstruction. Abdominal EPs are relative contraindications to stenting because stents near the GEJ may migrate; however, stenting can be considered for patients who are unsuitable for immediate operative management, such as coagulopathic patients or patients with poorly controlled portal hypertension.[20] Drainage procedures should also accompany placement of a stent to eliminate extraluminal fluid collections, and it is useful to perform a contrast study to ensure the leak is sealed.[13,14,16,20–23] For patients who undergo operative intervention, several technical principles apply[12,15,20,24,25]:

- Debridement of devitalized and necrotic tissue
- Adequate drainage
- Generous myotomy to fully identify the proximal and distal extent of the mucosal tear
- Two-layer closure, including the mucosa (with absorbable suture) and outer muscle layer
- Buttressing of the repair[11,12,15,20]

Patients with spontaneous perforations should be closed primarily regardless of time interval due to the significant increase in mortality with stenting.[13,23] Nonoperative management can be used for select patients with well-contained iatrogenic injuries in the absence of sepsis. However, patients who have abdominal perforations, or pneumoperitoneum, in general, are not contained perforations, and are not candidates for nonoperative management.[12,20,26,27]

Achalasia There is a reported 1% to 5% rate of perforation with pneumatic dilation performed for achalasia.[12,15] Treatment of a perforation in the setting of achalasia requires the surgeon to perform a myotomy on the opposite side of the esophagus extending 6 to 8 cm proximal to the GEJ and 3 cm distal onto the stomach.[28] This is typically followed by a partial fundoplication covering both the myotomy and the perforation.[12,20]

Esophageal cancer EP in the setting of cancer carries significant morbidity and mortality.[13] Therapy should be tailored to the patient's stage. If the patient has resectable disease, esophagectomy should be considered.[11,12,15] Other options include palliation, drainage and diversion with cervical esophagostomy, and possible stenting with drainage.[11,13,15,29]

Clinical outcomes

In general, recent studies still show a wide range of reported overall mortality from EP, ranging from 1% to 26%.[11–16,20,23,29,30] More recent studies show a continued increase in mortality when EP is left untreated for longer than 24 hours.[12,15,16,29] Stenting EPs show promise, but are not an option with abdominal perforations and in those who present with pneumoperitoneum.[13]

Pneumoperitoneum Due to Gastric and Duodenal Perforations

Overview

Etiologies of pneumoperitoneum from gastric and duodenal sources overlap in many ways. Primary causes include iatrogenic, postoperative, malignant, and benign causes. The advent of H2 blockers and proton pump inhibitors has greatly decreased the role of surgery in the management of peptic ulcer disease (PUD).[31]

Relevant anatomy

The lesser curve of the stomach is attached to the liver via the gastrohepatic ligament. Care should be taken to identify a potential replaced or aberrant left hepatic artery traversing the gastrohepatic ligament. At the superior and lateral aspect of the greater curve is the spleen, which is attached to the stomach via the short gastrics. Dissecting through the gastrocolic ligament exposes the lesser sac, providing access to the posterior stomach and the pancreas.

Aside from its first portion, the duodenum is only partially invested by peritoneum. It has arterial vascular supply from both the celiac and superior mesenteric arteries (SMA). The common bile duct and pancreatic duct converge to form the ampulla of Vater in the second portion of the duodenum. The duodenum ends at the ligament at Treitz where it becomes intraperitoneal, giving rise to the jejunum.

Clinical presentation

The presentation of foregut perforations is similar to other hollow viscus perforations. Patients typically present with acute upper abdominal pain that progresses to peritonitis. Patients who have peritonitis may have reflex emesis (60%–72%) or hiccoughs (29%).[32]

Workup

The workup as outlined previously should be used.

Treatment

Peptic ulcer The most common cause of pneumoperitoneum is a perforated peptic ulcer (75% of cases).[33] Although proton pump inhibitors have dramatically reduced the incidence of PUD, bleeding and perforation complications have not decreased significantly.[34] Perforated PUD occurs in 2% to 14% of patients with complicated PUD, and has a 24% mortality rate.[34,35] Nonoperative management, including resuscitation, nasogastric tube (NGT) decompression, intravenous antibiotics, and acid suppression, has been attempted with similar mortality compared with operative repair; however, 28% of patients ultimately required surgical intervention, and 35% experience a longer hospital stay.[36] Patients older than 70 are also less likely to respond to nonoperative management.[36] Nonoperative management with drainage of intra-abdominal fluid collections is currently elected for patients who cannot tolerate general anesthesia or have a sealed retroperitoneal perforation.[37]

Laparoscopic surgery can be considered when expertise is available. Compared with open surgery, laparoscopic approaches are as effective, with similar operative times and complication rates; however, laparoscopic repairs have reduced length of stay and less postoperative pain.[34,38–40] All surgeries should include drainage of the extraluminal space of enteric contents, securing the perforation, and restoring alimentary flow. Temporary diversion of gastric contents with an NGT may be necessary. The NGT should be used until normal bowel function has returned. Feeding tube placement may be considered at the time of the initial operation.[32]

Gastric ulcer The treatment of gastric ulcer depends on the size and location of the perforation along with patient factors. Gastric ulcers can be broken down into 4 types: types I and IV, which are less likely to be acid mediated, and more likely to be associated with malignancy, and types II and III, which are more likely to be acid mediated. Surgery is the treatment of choice for PUD perforations and options include:

- Primary closure with or without omental patch
- Ulcer excision with vagotomy
- Highly selective vagotomy or vagotomy with pyloroplasty

- Partial distal gastrectomy
- Partial distal gastrectomy with vagotomy

Patients with sepsis, peritonitis, age older than 65, multiple comorbidities, small defect, or late presentation may be appropriate candidates for primary closure with omental patch[35]; however, although many patients are treated this way, patients who present with either a type I or type IV ulcer, stenosis, or bleeding should be considered for gastric resection or acid-reducing surgery.[32] Turner and colleagues[41] previously recommended gastric resection for prepyloric ulcers due to concern for postoperative pyloric stenosis; however, small ulcers have been treated with primary repair with omental patch.

Giant gastric ulcers (larger than 3 cm) account for 1% of all gastric ulcers and have an increased risk of malignancy (10%–20%).[42] The preferred options for repair include partial gastrectomy and omental patching.[42] Partial gastrectomy allows for exclusion of the malignancy and has a lower recurrence rate; however, the perioperative mortality rate may be higher.[42,43] Patients should be tested for *Helicobacter pylori*, and treated if present, to reduce recurrence rates.[32,37] It is imperative to perform a follow-up EGD with biopsy of gastric ulcers that were treated but never biopsied to rule out gastric cancer.[37]

Duodenal ulcer For small and D1 duodenal perforations, appropriate operations include patch repair or primary closure with or without vagotomy.[32] For perforations near the ampulla of Vater, an enterectomy is inappropriate because the vasculature supplying this area also supplies the pancreas. Instead, options include the following:

- Omental patching
- Drainage of enteric secretions and bypassing the area of injury by placing a large percutaneous drain into the duodenum through the perforation
- Excision of ulcer with restoration of gastrointestinal continuity with a Billroth or Roux-en-Y

A pyloric exclusion procedure in addition to a gastrojejunostomy may be performed.[44] Pyloric exclusion can be included with drainage of the stomach through an NGT or gastrostomy tube in addition to large-bore drains being placed next to the defect and feeding jejunostomy.[45] This is frequently the case for ulcers in which the tissue is too friable for repair or for large ulcers in which the defect is larger than 2 cm.[44] Large ulcers can be difficult to manage and are associated with a high leak rate and mortality.[46]

Gastric cancer Perforation in the setting of a malignant peptic ulcer is rare but can be managed either in a 1-stage (gastrectomy at index operation) or 2-stage (conservative treatment initially, followed by definitive gastrectomy) approach. Although the stability of the patient largely dictates the approach, there may be potential operative and oncologic mortality benefits for patients able to undergo a 2-staged resection.[47] Improved mortality is likely secondary to completion of appropriate staging, and performance of the gastrectomy by a surgeon with experience in esophagogastric cancer surgery when the patient's condition has improved.[48]

Endoscopic perforation Perforation after EGD or endoscopic retrograde cholangiopancreatography (ERCP) is rare (0.3%–1.3% occurrence rate), but carries a high mortality rate.[49,50] The perforations can be classified by their location, and typically require surgery due to the large size of the injury.[50] Periampullary perforations that are the result of sphincterotomies are often amenable to nonoperative management.[50] This is reserved for patients who are clinically improving and have contained extraluminal gas on imaging.[50] Placement of percutaneous endoscopic gastrostomy tube can be a common cause of pneumoperitoneum, with estimates of up to 25% of these procedures resulting in pneumoperitoneum.[2] Most air resolves within a week, and nonoperative management is appropriate for patients who are clinically stable without peritoneal signs.[2]

Pneumoperitoneum Due to Small Intestine Perforation

Pneumoperitoneum due to small intestine perforation (SIP) can occur along the length of the entire small bowel, and may be the result of several causes, including trauma, vascular ischemia, obstruction, malignancy, or iatrogenic injury during surgery. Pneumoperitoneum is found in only 50% of cases of small bowel perforations.[51]

Relevant anatomy

The small intestine begins at the duodenum and ends at the ileocecal valve. The jejunum and ileum account for approximately 3 to 5 m of intestine, with the jejunum responsible for most of the small bowel absorptive capacity.[52] The jejunum and ileum receive blood from only the SMA, which crosses anterior to the third portion of the duodenum before entering the intestinal mesentery. The SMA also gives rise to the ileocolic artery that provides blood to the distal ileum and proximal colon.

Clinical presentation

Patients with pneumoperitoneum due to SIP will typically present with nonfocal abdominal pain that progresses to peritonitis if left untreated.[53] Nausea and/or vomiting may be present due to intra-abdominal irritation, ileus, or obstruction. Fevers, tachycardia, and hypotension are more concerning features, and indicate a more severely ill patient. A thorough physical examination may help determine the etiology (ie, an irregular pulse may increase the suspicion of embolic phenomenon); however, there are no specific symptoms or signs that indicate the patient has an SIP.

Workup

The standard workup as described previously should be used.

Medical management

In select situations, this may be pursued in patients not able or willing to undergo operative intervention. Percutaneous drains are useful to drain contaminated intra-abdominal fluid; however, these do not address the perforation.

Surgical management

Surgical treatment is sought in many patients with intestinal perforation. The appropriate procedure varies based on the location of perforation. For perforations in the small bowel with defects encompassing less than half the bowel circumference, debridement of the wound edges followed by a 1-layer or 2-layer closure is reasonable; however, if a larger defect is present, an enterectomy may be required.

Meckel diverticulum Meckel diverticulum is one of the most common malformations of the small intestine, and has an incidence of 2% to 4%.[54] Meckel diverticulum is frequently located 100 cm from the ileocecal valve and may contain ectopic gastric, pancreatic, or colonic mucosa.[53,54] These patients present at a median age of 5 years, but may present from 7 days to 43 years old.[54] Patients may present with appendicitis-like inflammation or ectopic tissue may ulcerate the adjacent small bowel and lead to perforation.[53,54] Surgical management may be laparoscopic or open and can include simple diverticulectomy or wedge excision of the adjacent ileum or a segmental small bowel resection.[54]

Acute mesenteric ischemia Acute mesenteric ischemia (AMI) is defined as a group of diseases that are characterized by an interruption of the blood supply to the bowel leading to ischemia and inflammatory changes that can lead to necrosis and perforation of the intestines. This disease process is broken into occlusive or nonocclusive mesenteric ischemia (NOMI). The primary etiology for occlusive disease is an arterial embolism (50%), mesenteric arterial thrombosis (15%–25%), or venous thrombosis (5%–15%).[55] This is a rare disease; however, it can cause pneumoperitoneum from a perforation within an ischemic segment of bowel. Patients classically present with pain out of proportion to examination findings, and should be assumed to be AMI until disproven.[56] A careful history can help determine the cause. Patients who present with chronic postprandial abdominal pain and weight loss or thrombus should be considered.[55] Patients who have poor cardiac performance NOMI should be suspected, and patients who have a presentation of a mixture of nausea, vomiting, diarrhea, and cramping.[55] Patients with atrial fibrillation are at risk for an embolic AMI.[55] Once suspected, patients should undergo a CT angiography immediately, as a delay in diagnosis can increase mortality.[55] Regardless of the cause, the presence of pneumoperitoneum is indicative of intestinal perforation and indicates advanced disease necessitating rehydration, systemic antibiotics with operative intervention, and, if possible, reestablishing vascular flow to the intestines. Planned reassessment of the bowel with further resection or anastomosis and stoma may be appropriate.[55]

Pneumoperitoneum Due to Colorectal Perforation

Pneumoperitoneum due to perforation of the colon and rectum can develop in the setting of other illnesses, such as cancer or colitis, or may be due to many vascular, infectious, or inflammatory etiologies. Iatrogenic causes include delayed thermal injury, endoscopic procedures and biopsies, and laparoscopy, to name a few. Perforations of the colon and rectum are distinguished from other causes of pneumoperitoneum in that diversion of the fecal stream can be used to minimize the associated morbidity and mortality.[56]

Relevant anatomy

The ascending and descending colon are in the retroperitoneal space. An important landmark is the white line Toldt, which represents the joining of the mesocolon and retroperitoneum. Mobilization of the colon by dissecting along this line may be necessary to visualize or resect the colon. The tenia coli converge to form a single connective band in 2 locations: one at the base of the cecum, serving as a landmark to identify the appendix, and at the transition from distal sigmoid colon to proximal rectum. The junction of the transverse colon and descending colon is a watershed region that is prone to ischemia and poor anastomotic healing. The rectum is located in the pelvis, with the anterior upper two-thirds intraperitoneal with the remainder being extraperitoneal.

Clinical presentation

Patients with colonic or rectal perforation typically develop progressive abdominal pain, which is usually focal initially, but leads to peritonitis if untreated. Signs and symptoms are also dependent on the time of presentation. Patients who present late (days) after perforation are more likely to become systemically ill, whereas patients who present early may have only mild symptoms.

Surgical management

Treatment of perforation of the colon or rectum is dependent on the causative etiology in many cases. Many patients require operative intervention. In the setting of contamination, bowel necrosis, or significant inflammation, primary anastomosis is at higher risk of leak, and one should consider creation of colostomies at the index procedure. In the absence of inflammation, necrosis, or contamination, stable patients with a small perforation may be candidates for primary repair; however, consideration for diverting loop ileostomy should be sought.[57,58] In patients found to have rectal perforation, fecal diversion is typically undertaken.[59]

Toxic megacolon Toxic megacolon (TM) if differentiated from other forms of colonic distention in that patients with toxic megacolon develop a severe systemic response and are severely ill. Etiologies may be either inflammatory or infectious, but *Clostridium difficile* infection (CDI) is becoming a more common cause of TM, with up to 3% of patients diagnosed with CDI developing TM.[60–62] For patients with TM due to CDI, mortality is at least 30%.[61] Pneumoperitoneum in the setting of CDI is a sign of advanced disease, and perforation increases the operative mortality rate fivefold compared with patients who have not yet perforated.[63] During surgery, the colon may grossly appear normal on the outside of the bowel, but this should not sway the surgeon from performing a total abdominal colectomy, as partial colectomy for CDI is associated with higher recurrence, morbidity, and mortality rates.[64] Loop ileostomy and intraoperative colonic lavage has been proposed as an alternative to total abdominal colectomy in this patient population; however, there is not enough evidence to support its use over total abdominal colectomy and it should thus be pursued only in select situations by experienced surgical personnel.[65]

Endoscopic perforation Pneumoperitoneum after colonoscopy occurs in up to 0.3% of diagnostic and 3% of interventional endoscopic procedures, and the incidence of perforation has remained stable over many years.[2,66] Not all cases of pneumoperitoneum following colonoscopy warrant immediate surgical intervention; however, they do warrant inpatient admission for intravenous antibiotics, serial abdominal examinations, and observation until symptoms either resolve or progress. Patients with pneumoperitoneum associated with endoscopy often experience some level of abdominal discomfort shortly after their endoscopic procedure, and a number of these patients may be classified as having postpolypectomy syndrome, especially in cases in which electrocautery was used, so long as they are stable and without peritonitis.[67] Patients who develop fevers, peritonitis, or otherwise clinically worsen, warrant operative intervention. At the time of surgery, careful examination of the bowel is required to ensure that all injuries are adequately treated.

Large bowel obstruction Large bowel obstruction is often attributed to a malignant etiology; however, it also may be the result of other etiologies, such as diverticulitis. Although self-expanding metal stents have gained favor in bridging patients to surgery in the setting of uncomplicated large bowel obstructions, the presence of pneumoperitoneum may contraindicate their use in this setting.[68,69] Perforations that occur in the setting of a large bowel obstruction may occur either at the site of the obstruction or upstream in the proximal colon, most commonly in the cecum. Operative intervention is warranted in patients able and willing to undergo surgery. Intraoperatively, special consideration should be given to a potential malignant etiology. For patients who have an identifiable perforation at the site of obstruction, an oncologic resection, including the associated lymphatics and mesentery, should be considered if there is high suspicion for malignant etiology. For patients who have an obstructive lesion and perforation at different locations, an extended colonic resection, and potentially a total abdominal colectomy, should be considered. Historically, a multistaged approach was used to restore continuity in patients with malignant bowel obstructions; however, the perceived benefits of this approach are negated by the risks inherent to subsequent operations, thus, a single-staged surgery is acceptable. Currently, the decision to perform primary anastomosis relies more heavily on presence of comorbidities, malnutrition, and intra-abdominal contamination or peritonitis.[70]

Ischemic colitis Ischemic colitis is the most common form of gastrointestinal ischemia, and primarily effects the colon.[71] There are multiple causes; however, all causes are secondary impaired perfusion of the colon that can lead to mucosal injury or full-thickness necrosis and perforation.[71] Most cases of ischemia are transient and do not lead to full-thickness necrosis, and therefore do not require operative intervention.[71] Seventy-five percent of ischemic colitis occurs in the left colon and splenic flexure.[71] This area is considered a "watershed" region because it is where the superior and inferior mesenteric artery meet, and is most sensitive to decreased blood flow. Treatment is aimed at the underlying cause and requires volume resuscitation, bowel rest, and broad-spectrum antibiotics. Pneumoperitoneum is rare, but is indicative of perforation and is an indication for operative intervention.[71] The extent of bowel resection must rely on preoperative imaging or endoscopy, because the ischemia is usually limited to mucosa or submucosa, and the serosa will often appear normal, so mucosal evaluation is recommended.[71] The decision to return for a second look, diversion, or to perform an anastomosis should be guided by the patient's clinical picture.[71]

Diverticulitis Diverticulitis is complicated in roughly 10% to 25% of all cases.[72] Neither the presence nor the quantity of pneumoperitoneum in the setting of diverticulitis mandates an operation. However, the patient's clinical condition, physical examination, and the characteristics of intra-abdominal abscesses in conjunction with pneumoperitoneum will dictate the need for operative intervention versus medical management. Medical management includes bowel rest, parental antibiotics, and percutaneous drainage of an abscess if appropriate. Options for surgical management include the following:

- Primary resection and anastomosis
- Two-staged procedure (emergency Hartman pouch followed by elective reversal if suitable)
- Laparoscopic lavage

Primary resection and anastomosis with or without a defunctioning ileostomy has been performed in the setting of Hinchey class III (purulent peritonitis) and IV (feculent peritonitis), with studies showing similar morbidity and mortality; however, there is concern for bias in these studies.[72] Laparoscopic lavage has recently been proposed as an alternative to colectomy in patients with Hinchey class III or IV. These patients had similar mortality but an increased risk of intra-abdominal abscess.[72] A significant number of patients required subsequent colectomy, and 4% of patients had a missed sigmoid carcinoma.[72,73] In their guidelines for sigmoid diverticulitis from 2014 patients, Hinchey class III or IV, the American Society of Colon and Rectal Surgeons indicate that operative therapy without resection is generally not considered an appropriate alternative to colectomy. When choosing colectomy with primary anastomosis with or without diversion versus end ostomy, patient, intraoperative factors, and surgeon preference is used to determine the best operative therapy.[74–76]

Appendicitis Appendicitis is one of the most common surgical emergencies. Lifetime risk is 7% to 9% and nearly 20% of patients present with perforated appendicitis, and the rate of concurrent pneumoperitoneum is 0% to 7%.[77,78] For patients who present early, operative intervention is indicated; however, for patients with complicated appendicitis (perforation, abscess, phlegmon), it is unclear if early operative intervention is truly superior to nonoperative management, as some studies suggest early appendectomy may be superior to nonoperative management due to a 25% failure rate of nonoperative management.[79,80] For patients who worsen with no-operative management, surgery is indicated.

Pneumatosis intestinalis Pneumatosis intestinalis (PI) is the presence of gas within the wall of the intestines (**Figs. 4** and **5**). It is rare with an incidence of 0.03% worldwide.[81] The disease presents anywhere from an incidental finding to a life-threatening condition. A retrospective review of all PI seen on CT scans found that PI was primarily found in the colon (47%), followed by small bowel (27%), both the colon and small bowel (7%), stomach (5%), and the entire intestinal tract with portal venous gas (14%).[82] Most patients were managed nonoperatively with a 6% mortality rate.[82] Most patients taken to surgery had bowel ischemia.[82] In general, the nonsurvivors had the following[82]:

- Higher APACHE II scores
- Portal venous gas
- Acidosis
- Elevated serum creatinine, bilirubin, and lactate

Concerning CT findings included the following[83]:

- Small bowel PI
- Dilation of the affected bowel
- Bowel obstruction
- Fat stranding/inflammatory changes
- Decreased bowel enhancement
- Portal venous gas
- Mesenteric edema

Pneumoperitoneum in addition to PI, or the pattern of the PI, was not found to be statistically different between benign and clinically worrisome PI. The most concerning clinical findings were as follows[82–84]:

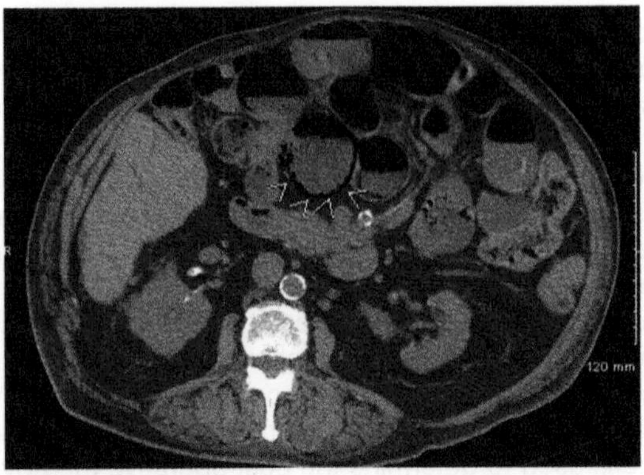

Fig. 4. PI as demonstrated on axial CT scan.

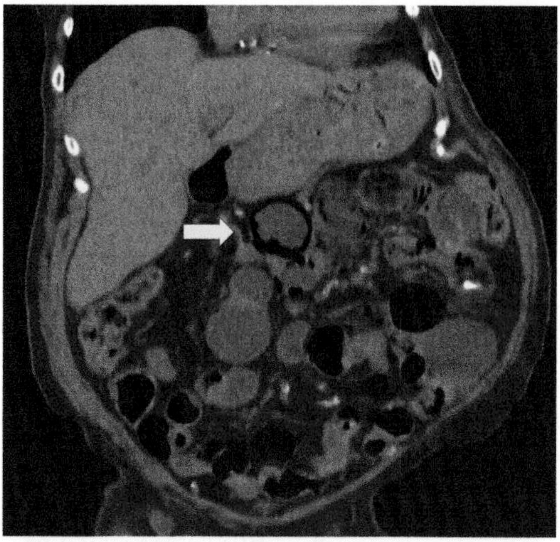

Fig. 5. PI (*arrow*) as demonstrated on coronal CT scan.

- Elevated serum lactate and international normalized ratio
- Sepsis
- Peritonitis

Overall, PI is a rare condition that can be managed expectantly with operative intervention reserved for patients with signs of perforation, peritonitis, or abdominal sepsis.[81]

Postoperative Pneumoperitoneum

Postoperative pneumoperitoneum (POP) creates a dilemma, as it is difficult to distinguish between benign and complicated POP, with concern being for ongoing leak or contamination. Previous studies have reported on the expected duration of POP; however, the duration of benign POP varied, lasting days to weeks.[2,85–93] Laparoscopic surgery uses carbon dioxide, and has limited entry of atmospheric air into the abdomen. Since the absorption of carbon dioxide is rapid compared with free air, one should expect smaller volumes of POP after laparoscopic procedures and faster resolution, compared with open surgery.[86,87,89,92] In 1997, Schauer and colleagues[89] reported that air from laparoscopic cholecystectomy dissipated after 24 hours. CT imaging confirms that patients who undergo laparoscopy should have minimal free air several days after surgery.[89] Milone and colleagues[93] obtained upright radiographs on all open and laparoscopic patients on postoperative days (PODs) 2 and 3, and suggested free air on upright plain film on PODs 2 and 3 is concerning for possible gastrointestinal perforation or leak.

Patients who have undergone laparotomy and then CT scans have shown pneumoperitoneum until POD 5, although the volume is small and widely distributed with air commonly near the umbilical and epigastric regions or around surgical drains.[85–87,91] In general, pneumoperitoneum is not an unexpected finding on postoperative imaging; however, large amounts of free air may be concerning, especially if free fluid also is present.[85–87,91]

SUMMARY

Pneumoperitoneum is typically the result of a perforated hollow viscus. It has a wide differential diagnosis and clinical presentation. Treatment is guided by the patient's presentation and clinical course. Although nonoperative management may be used, many of these patients will require surgery to make a definitive diagnosis and obtain source control.

REFERENCES

1. Pinto A, Miele V, Schilliro ML, et al. Spectrum of signs of pneumoperitoneum. Semin Ultrasound CT MR 2016;37(1):3–9.
2. Mularski RA, Sippel JM, Osborne ML. Pneumoperitoneum: a review of nonsurgical causes. Crit Care Med 2000;28(7):2638–44.
3. Beilin B, Shulman DL, Weiss AT, et al. Pneumoperitoneum as the presenting sign of pulmonary barotrauma during artificial ventilation. Intensive Care Med 1986; 12(1):49–51.
4. Hartoko TJ, Demey HE, Rogiers PE, et al. Pneumoperitoneum—a rare complication of cardiopulmonary resuscitation. Acta Anaesthesiol Scand 1991;35(3): 235–7.
5. Wakeen MJ, Zimmerman SW, Bidwell D. Viscus perforation in peritoneal dialysis patients: diagnosis and outcome. Perit Dial Int 1994;14(4):371–7.
6. Ritchie M, Caravelli J, Shike M. Benign persistent pneumoperitoneum in scleroderma. Dig Dis Sci 1986;31(5):552–5.
7. Chang JJ, Yeun JY, Hasbargen JA. Pneumoperitoneum in peritoneal dialysis patients. Am J Kidney Dis 1995;25(2):297–301.
8. Jacobs VR, Mundhenke C, Maass N, et al. Sexual activity as cause for nonsurgical pneumoperitoneum. JSLS 2000;4(4):297.
9. Matsuda M, Nishikawa N, Okano T, et al. Spontaneous pneumoperitoneum: an unusual complication of systemic reactive AA amyloidosis secondary to rheumatoid arthritis: case report. Amyloid 2003;10(1):42–6.
10. Stapakis JC, Thickman D. Diagnosis of pneumoperitoneum: abdominal CT vs. upright chest film. J Comput Assist Tomogr 1992;16(5):713–6.
11. Bayram AS, Erol MM, Melek H, et al. The success of surgery in the first 24 hours in patients with esophageal perforation. Eurasian J Med 2015;47(1):41.
12. Brinster CJ, Singhal S, Lee L, et al. Evolving options in the management of esophageal perforation. Ann Thorac Surg 2004;77(4):1475–83.
13. Schweigert M, Sousa HS, Solymosi N, et al. Spotlight on esophageal perforation: a multinational study using the Pittsburgh esophageal perforation severity scoring system. J Thorac Cardiovasc Sur 2016;151(4):1002–11.
14. Ben-David K, Behrns K, Hochwald S, et al. Esophageal perforation management using a multidisciplinary minimally invasive treatment algorithm. J Am Coll Surg 2014;218(4):768–74.
15. Chirica M, Champault A, Dray X, et al. Esophageal perforations. J Visc Surg 2010;147(3):e117–28.
16. Kuppusamy MK, Hubka M, Felisky CD, et al. Evolving management strategies in esophageal perforation: surgeons using nonoperative techniques to improve outcomes. J Am Coll Surg 2011;213(1):164–71.
17. Foley MJ, Ghahremani GG, Rogers LF. Reappraisal of contrast media used to detect upper gastrointestinal perforations: comparison of ionic water-soluble media with barium sulfate. Radiology 1982;144(2):231–7.
18. Hogan BA, Winter D, Broe D, et al. Prospective trial comparing contrast swallow, computed tomography and endoscopy to identify anastomotic leak following oesophagogastric surgery. Surg Endosc 2008;22(3):767–71.

19. di Castelguidone ED, Merola S, Pinto A, et al. Esophageal injuries: spectrum of multidetector row CT findings. Eur J Radiol 2006;59(3):344–8.
20. Carrott PW, Low DE. Advances in the management of esophageal perforation. Thorac Surg Clin 2011;21(4):541–55.
21. El Hajj II, Imperiale TF, Rex DK, et al. Treatment of esophageal leaks, fistulae, and perforations with temporary stents: evaluation of efficacy, adverse events, and factors associated with successful outcomes. Gastrointest Endosc 2014;79(4):589–98.
22. Dasari BV, Neely D, Kennedy A, et al. The role of esophageal stents in the management of esophageal anastomotic leaks and benign esophageal perforations. Ann Surg 2014;259(5):852–60.
23. Persson S, Elbe P, Rouvelas I, et al. Predictors for failure of stent treatment for benign esophageal perforations-a single center 10-year experience. World J Gastroenterol 2014;20(30):10613.
24. Fischer A, Thomusch O, Benz S, et al. Nonoperative treatment of 15 benign esophageal perforations with self-expandable covered metal stents. Ann Thorac Surg 2006;81(2):467–72.
25. Gupta NM, Kaman L. Personal management of 57 consecutive patients with esophageal perforation. Am J Surg 2004;187(1):58–63.
26. Cameron JL, Kieffer RF, Hendrix TR, et al. Selective nonoperative management of contained intrathoracic esophageal disruptions. Ann Thorac Surg 1979;27(5):404–8.
27. Altorjay A, Kiss J, Vörös A, et al. Nonoperative management of esophageal perforations. Is it justified? Ann Surg 1997;225(4):415.
28. Urbani M, Mathisen DJ. Repair of esophageal perforation after treatment for achalasia. Ann Thorac Surg 2000;69(5):1609–11.
29. Sudarshan M, Elharram M, Spicer J, et al. Management of esophageal perforation in the endoscopic era: is operative repair still relevant? Surgery 2016;160(4):1104–10.
30. Keeling WB, Miller DL, Lam GT, et al. Low mortality after treatment for esophageal perforation: a single-center experience. Ann Thorac Surg 2010;90(5):1669–73.
31. Chung KT, Shelat VG. Perforated peptic ulcer-an update. World J Gastroenterol 2017;9(1):1.
32. Rigopoulos A, Ramboiu S, Georgescu I. A critical evaluation of surgical treatment of perforated ulcer. Curr Health Sci J 2011;37(2):75.
33. Le YT. Acute peritonitis. Physiopathology, etiology, diagnosis, development, treatment. Rev Prat 1993;43(2):259–62.
34. Ge B, Wu M, Chen Q, et al. A prospective randomized controlled trial of laparoscopic repair versus open repair for perforated peptic ulcers. Surgery 2016;159(2):451–8.
35. Gachabayov M, Babyshin V, Durymanov O, et al. Surgical scales: primary closure versus gastric resection for perforated gastric ulcer—a surgical debate. Niger J Surg 2017;23(1):1–4.
36. Crofts TJ, Park KG, Steele RJ, et al. A randomized trial of nonoperative treatment for perforated peptic ulcer. N Engl J Med 1989;320(15):970–3.
37. Søreide K, Thorsen K, Søreide JA. Strategies to improve the outcome of emergency surgery for perforated peptic ulcer. Br J Surg 2014;101(1):e51–64.
38. Siu WT, Leong HT, Law BK, et al. Laparoscopic repair for perforated peptic ulcer: a randomized controlled trial. Ann Surg 2002;235(3):313.

39. Tan S, Wu G, Zhuang Q, et al. Laparoscopic versus open repair for perforated peptic ulcer: a meta-analysis of randomized controlled trials. Int J Surg 2016; 33:124–32.
40. Sanabria A, Villegas MI, Morales Uribe CH. Laparoscopic repair for perforated peptic ulcer disease. Cochrane Database Syst Rev 2013;(2):CD004778.
41. Turner WW, Thompson WM, Thal ER. Perforated gastric ulcers: a plea for management by simple closures. Arch Surg 1988;123(8):960–4.
42. Vashistha N, Singhal D, Makkar G, et al. Management of giant gastric ulcer perforation: report of a case and review of the literature. Case Rep Surg 2016;2016: 4681989.
43. Tsugawa K, Koyanagi N, Hashizume M, et al. The therapeutic strategies in performing emergency surgery for gastroduodenal ulcer perforation in 130 patients over 70 years of age. Hepatogastroenterology 2001;48(37):156–62.
44. Søreide K, Thorsen K, Harrison EM, et al. Perforated peptic ulcer. Lancet 2015; 386(10000):1288–98.
45. Kutlu OC, Garcia S, Dissanaike S. The successful use of simple tube duodenostomy in large duodenal perforations from varied etiologies. Int J Surg Case Rep 2013;4(3):279–82.
46. Gupta S, Kaushik R, Sharma R, et al. The management of large perforations of duodenal ulcers. BMC Surg 2005;5(1):15.
47. Hata T, Sakata N, Kudoh K, et al. The best surgical approach for perforated gastric cancer: one-stage vs. two-stage gastrectomy. Gastric Cancer 2014; 17(3):578–87.
48. Mouly C, Chati R, Scotté M, et al. Therapeutic management of perforated gastroduodenal ulcer: literature review. J Visc Surg 2013;150(5):333–40.
49. Chertoff J, Khullar V, Burke L. Duodenal perforation following esophagogastroduodenoscopy (EGD) with cautery and epinephrine injection for peptic ulcer disease: an interesting case of nonoperative management in the medical intensive care unit (MICU). Int J Surg Case Rep 2015;10:121–5.
50. Motomura Y, Akahoshi K, Gibo J, et al. Immediate detection of endoscopic retrograde cholangiopancreatography-related periampullary perforation: fluoroscopy or endoscopy? World J Gastroentero 2014;20(42):15797.
51. Hines J, Rosenblat J, Duncan DR, et al. Perforation of the mesenteric small bowel: etiologies and CT findings. Emerg Radiol 2013;20(2):155–61.
52. Crane RK. Intestinal absorption of sugars. Physiol Rev 1960;40(4):789–825.
53. Harden RM, Alexander WD, Kennedy I. Isotope uptake and scanning of stomach in man with 99mTc-pertechnetate. Lancet 1967;289(7503):1305–7.
54. Papparella A, Nino F, Noviello C, et al. Laparoscopic approach to Meckel's diverticulum. World J Gastroenterol 2014;20(25):8173.
55. Bala M, Kashuk J, Moore EE, et al. Acute mesenteric ischemia: guidelines of the World Society of Emergency Surgery. World J Emerg Surg 2017;12(1):38.
56. Cameron JL, Cameron AM. Current surgical therapy E-book. Philadelphia: Elsevier Health Sciences; 2013.
57. Curran TJ, Borzotta AP. Complications of primary repair of colon injury: literature review of 2,964 cases. Am J Surg 1999;177(1):42–7.
58. Rotholtz NA, Laporte M, Lencinas S, et al. Laparoscopic approach to colonic perforation due to colonoscopy. World J Surg 2010;34(8):1949–53.
59. Iqbal CW, Chun YS, Farley DR. Colonoscopic perforations: a retrospective review. J Gastrointest Surg 2005;9(9):1229–36.
60. Autenrieth DM, Baumgart DC. Toxic megacolon. Inflamm Bowel Dis 2012;18(3): 584–91.

61. Earhart MM. The identification and treatment of toxic megacolon secondary to pseudomembranous colitis. Dimens Crit Care Nurs 2008;27(6):249–54.
62. Ausch C, Madoff RD, Gnant M, et al. Aetiology and surgical management of toxic megacolon. Colorectal Dis 2006;8(3):195–201.
63. Sheth SG, LaMont JT. Toxic megacolon. Lancet 1998;351(9101):509–13.
64. Bhangu A, Nepogodiev D, Gupta A, et al. Systematic review and meta-analysis of outcomes following emergency surgery for *Clostridium difficile* colitis. Br J Surg 2012;99(11):1501–13.
65. Neal MD, Alverdy JC, Hall DE, et al. Diverting loop ileostomy and colonic lavage: an alternative to total abdominal colectomy for the treatment of severe, complicated *Clostridium difficile* associated disease. Ann Surg 2011;254(3):423–9.
66. Reumkens A, Rondagh EJ, Bakker CM, et al. Post-colonoscopy complications: a systematic review, time trends, and meta-analysis of population-based studies. Am J Gastroenterol 2016;111(8):1092–101.
67. Damore LJ, Rantis PC, Vernava AM, et al. Colonoscopic perforations. Dis Colon Rectum 1996;39(11):1308–14.
68. Finan PJ, Campbell S, Verma R, et al. The management of malignant large bowel obstruction: ACPGBI position statement. Colorectal Dis 2007;9(s4):1–7.
69. Yeo HL, Lee SW. Colorectal emergencies: review and controversies in the management of large bowel obstruction. J Gastrointest Surg 2013;17(11):2007–12.
70. Frago R, Ramirez E, Millan M, et al. Current management of acute malignant large bowel obstruction: a systematic review. Am J Surg 2014;207(1):127–38.
71. Washington C, Carmichael JC. Management of ischemic colitis. Clin Colon Rectal Surg 2012;25(4):228–35.
72. Cirocchi R, Afshar S, Di Saverio S, et al. A historical review of surgery for peritonitis secondary to acute colonic diverticulitis: from Lockhart-Mummery to evidence-based medicine. World J Emerg Surg 2017;12:14.
73. Schultz JK, Yaqub S, Wallon C, et al. Laparoscopic lavage vs primary resection for acute perforated diverticulitis: the SCANDIV randomized clinical trial. JAMA 2015;314(13):1364–75.
74. Feingold D, Steele S, Lee S, et al. Practice parameters for the treatment of sigmoid diverticulitis. Dis Colon Rectum 2014;57(3):284–94.
75. Penna M, Markar SR, Mackenzie H, et al. Laparoscopic lavage versus primary resection for acute perforated diverticulitis: review and meta-analysis. Ann Surg 2018;267(2):252–8.
76. Langenfeld SJ. Mandatory exploration is not necessary for patients with acute diverticulitis and free intraperitoneal air. J Trauma Acute Care Surg 2013;74(5):1376.
77. Körner H, Söndenaa K, Söreide JA, et al. Incidence of acute nonperforated and perforated appendicitis: age-specific and sex-specific analysis. World J Surg 1997;21(3):313–7.
78. Şahin S, Cavusoglu T, Kubat M, et al. A rare cause of pneumoperitoneum: perforated appendicitis. J Ayub Med Coll Abbottabad 2016;28(2):415–6.
79. Simillis C, Symeonides P, Shorthouse AJ, et al. A meta-analysis comparing conservative treatment versus acute appendectomy for complicated appendicitis (abscess or phlegmon). Surgery 2010;147(6):818–29.
80. Young KA, Neuhaus NM, Fluck M, et al. Outcomes of complicated appendicitis: is conservative management as smooth as it seems? Am J Surg 2018;215(4):586–92.
81. Jenkins M, Courtney H, Pope E, et al. A case report and approach to management in pneumatosis intestinalis. Ann Med Surg (Lond) 2017;23:25–7.

82. Morris MS, Gee AC, Cho SD, et al. Management and outcome of pneumatosis intestinalis. Am J Surg 2008;195(5):679–83.
83. Goyal R, Lee HK, Akerman M, et al. Clinical and imaging features indicative of clinically worrisome pneumatosis: key components to identifying proper medical intervention. Emerg Radiol 2017;24(4):341–6.
84. Hawn MT, Canon CL, Lockhart ME, et al. Serum lactic acid determines the outcomes of CT diagnosis of pneumatosis of the gastrointestinal tract. Am Surg 2004;70(1):19.
85. Earls JP, Dachman AH, Colon E, et al. Prevalence and duration of postoperative pneumoperitoneum: sensitivity of CT vs left lateral decubitus radiography. Am J Roentgenol 1993;161(4):781–5.
86. Gayer G, Jonas T, Apter S, et al. Postoperative pneumoperitoneum as detected by CT: prevalence, duration, and relevant factors affecting its possible significance. Abdom Imaging 2000;25(3):301–5.
87. Gayer G, Hertz M, Zissin R. Postoperative pneumoperitoneum: prevalence, duration, and possible significance. Semin Ultrasound CT MR 2004;25(3):286–9.
88. Gottfried EB, Plumser AB, Clair MR. Pneumoperitoneum following percutaneous endoscopic gastrostomy: a prospective study. Gastrointest Endosc 1986;32(6):397–9.
89. Schauer PR, Page CP, Ghiatas AA, et al. Incidence and significance of subdiaphragmatic air following laparoscopic cholecystectomy. Am Surg 1997;63(2):132–6.
90. Harrison I, Litwer H, Gerwig WH Jr. Studies on the incidence and duration of postoperative pneumoperitoneum. Ann Surg 1957;145(4):591.
91. Malgras B, Placé V, Dohan A, et al. Natural history of pneumoperitoneum after laparotomy: findings on multidetector-row computed tomography. World J Surg 2017;41(1):56–63.
92. Millitz K, Moote DJ, Sparrow RK, et al. Pneumoperitoneum after laparoscopic cholecystectomy: frequency and duration as seen on upright chest radiographs. AJR Am J Roentgenol 1994;163(4):837–9.
93. Milone M, Di Minno MN, Bifulco G, et al. Diagnostic value of abdominal free air detection on a plain chest radiograph in the early postoperative period: a prospective study in 648 consecutive patients who have undergone abdominal surgery. J Gastrointest Surg 2013;17(9):1673–82.

Acid Peptic Disease

Jason W. Kempenich, MD*, Kenneth R. Sirinek, MD, PhD

KEYWORDS

• Peptic ulcer disease • Bleeding ulcer • Perforated ulcer • Obstructing ulcer
• *Helicobacter pylori*

KEY POINTS

- The surgical management of peptic ulcer disease has changed drastically due to advances in acid suppression therapy and the discovery and treatment of *Helicobacter pylori*.
- Complications of peptic ulcer disease include bleeding, perforation, and obstruction and are still a significant cause of morbidity and mortality.
- Surgical management is rarely necessary in patients bleeding from peptic ulcer disease.
- Because of advances in medical, endoscopic, and angiographic therapy, surgery is most often used in the emergent setting of a patient with a perforated ulcer.

INTRODUCTION: NATURE OF THE PROBLEM

As the understanding of the pathophysiology of peptic ulcer disease (PUD) developed through the 1970s and 1980s, surgical treatment has become less frequent. The major decline has been in elective surgery for intractable disease, but the number of emergent operations has also decreased.[1] The annual incidence of PUD requiring medical or surgical treatment ranges between 0.10% and 0.19% and is declining.[2,3] Despite this decline, the complications of PUD (which include bleeding, perforation, and obstruction) still account for approximately 150,000 hospital admissions per year in the United States.[4] Although bleeding is the most common complication (ratio of 6:1), perforation carries the highest mortality risk of up to 30%.[4]

PATHOPHYSIOLOGY

Mucosal disruption in patients with acid peptic disease can be due to either infection, barrier disruption, or gastric acid hypersecretion. Risk factors for developing PUD include *Helicobacter pylori* infection, alcohol consumption, tobacco use, cocaine and amphetamine use, nonsteroidal anti-inflammatory drugs (NSAIDs), fasting,

Disclosure: The authors have nothing to disclose.
Department of Surgery, University of Texas Health Science Center at San Antonio, 7703 Floyd Curl Drive, San Antonio, TX 78229, USA
* Corresponding author.
E-mail address: kempenich@uthscsa.edu

Surg Clin N Am 98 (2018) 933–944
https://doi.org/10.1016/j.suc.2018.06.003 surgical.theclinics.com

Zollinger-Ellison syndrome, cancer treatment with angiogenesis inhibitors, and bariatric surgery (**Fig. 1**).[4]

PUD in most patients is a result of *H pylori* infection or chronic NSAID or aspirin use. *H pylori* infection causes both a direct bacterial effect and a secondary host inflammatory response inflicting damage to the mucosa of the stomach and duodenum. Of the patients infected with *H pylori*, 10% to 15% will have hypersecretion of gastric acid leading to antral or duodenal ulcers secondary to inhibition of somatostatin secretion, thereby stimulating gastrin release. The remaining majority of patients infected with *H pylori* will have gastric ulcers associated with hypochlorhydria and mucosal atrophy. NSAIDs damage the gastric mucosa by inhibiting Cyclooxygenase-1 prostaglandins, which provide a protective effect on the gastric mucosa.[2]

Most peptic ulcers heal with gastric acid suppression, most commonly by administration of a proton pump inhibitor (PPI) alone or with *H pylori* treatment for 6 to 8 weeks. More than 85% of NSAID-induced ulcers will heal within 6 to 8 weeks after cessation of the offending drug along with gastric acid suppression.[2] The effectiveness of this

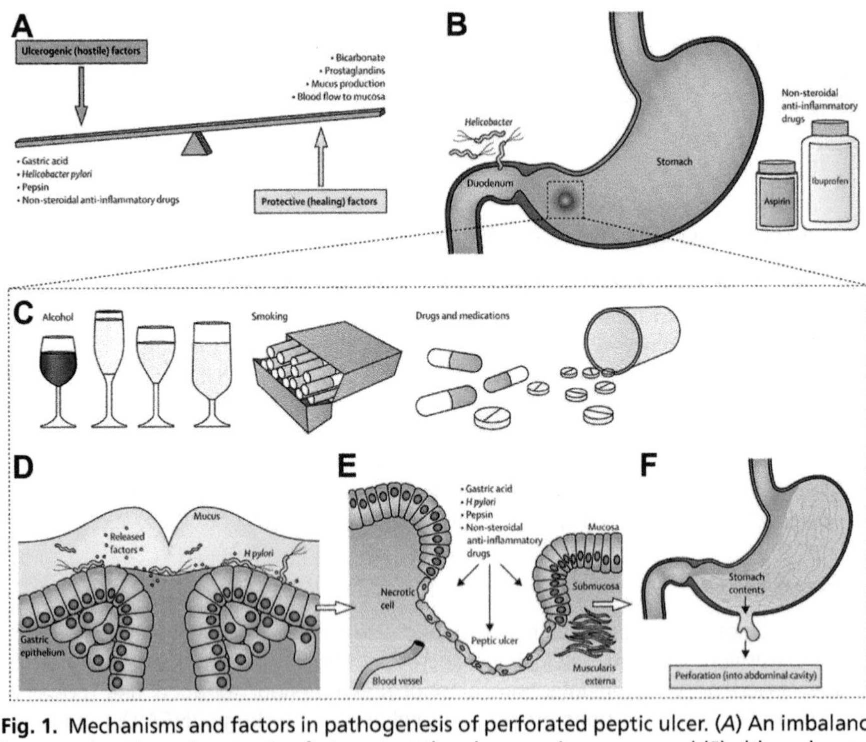

Fig. 1. Mechanisms and factors in pathogenesis of perforated peptic ulcer. (*A*) An imbalance between hostile and protective factors start the ulcerogenic process, and (*B*) although many cotributors are known, *Helicobacter* infection and use of NSAIDs appear of importance in disturbing the protective mucosal layer and (*C*) expose the gastric epithelium to acid. Several additional factors (*D*) may augment the ulcerogenic process (such as smoking, alcohol use, and use of several drugs) that leads to erosion (*E*). Eventually, the serosal lining is breached (*F*), and when perforated, the stomach content, including acidic fluid, will enter the abdominal cavity, giving rise to intense pain, local peritonitis that may become generalized, and eventually lead to a systemic inflammatory response syndrome and sepsis with the risk of multiorgan failure and mortality. (*Adapted from* Søreide K, Thorsen K, Harrision EM, et al. Perforated peptic ulcer. Lancet 2015;386(10000):1291; with permission.)

medical therapy has markedly changed the overall treatment algorithm resulting in less surgical intervention compared with the past.[1]

Those patients who are shown to be *H pylori* negative and also have no evidence of NSAID use are classified as having idiopathic ulcers. The pathogenesis of idiopathic ulcers is unknown.[4] In North America, this is a growing problem with estimates of 11% to 44% of patients with PUD that cannot be explained by either *H pylori* infection or NSAID use.[5] Some reports suggest that patients with idiopathic ulcers may have a more fulminant clinical course compared with those with either *H pylori* or NSAID-induced ulcers.[5]

ANATOMY

Clinical Presentation/Examination

Patients with a duodenal or gastric ulcer will have symptoms similar to those seen with gastroesophageal reflux disease, which include heartburn, epigastric pain, and referred pain to the back or left shoulder (**Fig. 2**). Patients with a duodenal ulcer may feel hungry or have nocturnal abdominal pain associated with the circadian secretion of gastric acid. Patients with a gastric ulcer tend to present with postprandial abdominal pain, nausea, vomiting, and weight loss.

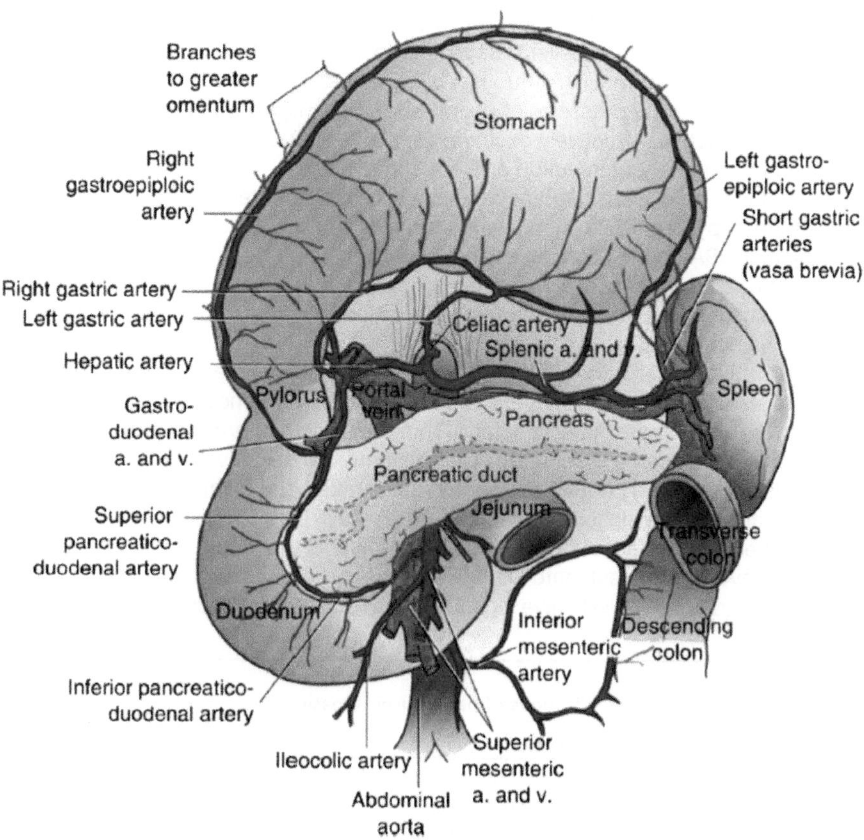

Fig. 2. Arterial supply of the foregut. (*From* Zuidema G. Shackelford's surgery of the alimentary tract. 4th edition. Philadelphia: WB Saunders; 1995; with permission.)

Patients presenting with an ulcer perforation will often describe a sudden onset of epigastric pain. On physical examination of the abdomen, they have acute abdominal tenderness, which then progresses to guarding and rigidity. Patients may have tachycardia with or without hypotension secondary to peritonitis. Patients with a bleeding ulcer may present with abdominal pain, hematemesis, and/or melena along with tachycardia and hypotension due to acute blood loss. Gastric outlet obstruction is a rare complication of PUD. These patients may present with severe dehydration and a metabolic alkalosis secondary to prolonged vomiting. The diagnosis of PUD and its associated complications may be missed clinically in the elderly, obese, or immunocompromised patient due to the presence of only minimal symptoms.

SIGNS AND SYMPTOMS

Diagnostic Procedures

After performing a history and physical examination in a patient suspected of having PUD, a diagnostic workup should exclude other causes of the abdominal pain (**Table 1**). Initial diagnostic workup should include an acute abdominal series, a complete blood count, blood chemistry evaluation as well as liver function tests and pancreatic enzyme levels.

Esophagogastroduodenoscopy (EGD) is the diagnostic procedure of choice. Given the pivotal role it plays, all patients with PUD should be tested for *H pylori*. Direct biopsy of the antrum during EGD with rapid urease test (CLO test) and the measurement of stool antigen are both excellent diagnostic tests. Prior PPI use does increase the risk of a false negative result. A mucosal biopsy specimen sent for histologic examination to determine the presence of *H pylori* is another option. A serum *H pylori* antibody test, if negative, effectively excludes an active *H pylori* infection, but if positive, only confirms a history of infection and not active disease.

A patient with a nonperforated peptic ulcer should be treated with gastric acid suppression therapy (eg, PPI) along with cessation of the offending medication or behavior (eg, NSAID use, tobacco use, alcohol intake) and treatment of *H pylori* infection if confirmed. Ulcers of the duodenum do not need to be biopsied during an EGD; however, ulcers of the stomach should be biopsied routinely to exclude an ulcerated gastric malignancy.

For patients exhibiting signs of sepsis, an arterial blood gas measurement and blood lactate level may be helpful. An acute abdominal series may show free air, but it is not as sensitive as computed tomography (CT) of the abdomen and pelvis for identification and localization of the source of perforation (98% sensitive).[4] Patients who are in extremis should have intravenous access established and be appropriately resuscitated. Urinary catheter insertion to monitor urine output and placement of invasive monitoring equipment should be considered additional measures to guide resuscitation. Some investigators estimate that 30% to 35% of patients who go to the operating room for perforated PUD will have signs of shock and sepsis resulting in death in half

Table 1
Signs and symptoms of complications of peptic ulcer disease

Bleeding	Perforation	Obstruction
Hematemesis	Epigastric pain	Preceding ulcer symptoms
Melena	Sudden onset	Nausea
± Abdominal pain	Abdominal guarding & rigidity	Vomiting
Tachycardia	Tachycardia	Metabolic alkalosis
Hypotension	Hypotension	

of these patients.[4] If the diagnosis is clear, surgical intervention should not be delayed for a confirmatory test such as a CT scan. One Danish cohort study of 2688 patients with a perforated ulcer found that every hour of delay from admission to surgical intervention resulted in a 2.4% increase in postoperative mortality.[6]

Ulcers that are recurrent or refractory to treatment or those occurring in the jejunum not associated with a gastrojejunostomy (marginal ulcer) should raise suspicion that the patient may have Zollinger-Ellison (gastrinoma) syndrome. These gastrinoma patients have hypersecretion of gastrin due to neuroendocrine tumors of the duodenum or pancreas. Other symptoms include abdominal pain, diarrhea, and weight loss. If the diagnosis is suspected, a fasting serum gastrin level should be obtained with the patient off of PPIs for at least 72 hours (PPIs cause elevation of serum gastrin). If elevated, a secretin provocation test can then be performed. A paradoxic increase in the serum gastrin of 200 pg/dL or greater is considered diagnostic for the presence of a gastrinoma.

TREATMENT

Eradication of Helicobacter pylori

Treatment of *H pylori* is paramount in infected patients with PUD to avoid future ulcer recurrence. Unfortunately, this task has become more difficult because of bacterial drug resistance.[2] A recent consensus statement on *H pylori* eradication recommends use of the traditional treatment strategy with triple therapy using a PPI, amoxicillin, and clarithromycin only in regions with favorable bacterial sensitivities to clarithromycin. In regions with resistance to clarithromycin or if sensitivities are unknown, a recent consensus statement recommends first-line therapy to include a PPI and metronidazole combined with either bismuth and tetracycline or amoxicillin and clarithromycin (**Table 2**). In addition, all treatment regimens should be given for 14 days to improve *H pylori* eradication rates.[7] The complete updated treatment guidelines are contained in **Table 2**.

Table 2
Recommendations for *Helicobacter pylori* eradication (all patients should be treated for 14 d)

First Line	
Bismuth quadruple (PBMT)	PPI + bismuth + metronidazole + tetracycline
Concomitant nonbismuth (PAMC)	PPI + amoxicillin + metronidazole + clarithromycin
Prior Treatment Failure	
Bismuth quadruple (PBMT)	PPI + bismuth + metronidazole + tetracycline
Levofloxacin-containing therapy	PPI + amoxicillin + levofloxacin
Dosages	
PPI	Double-dose bid (ie, esomeprazole 40 mg bid)
Bismuth subsalicylate	262 mg, 2 tablets qid
Colloidal bismuth subcitrate	120 mg, 2 tablets bid
Bismuth biskalcitrate	140 mg, 3 tablets qid
Metronidazole	500mg qid (bismuth regimens) 500mg bid (non-bismuth regimens)
Tetracycline	500 mg qid
Amoxicillin	1000 mg bid
Clarithromycin	500 mg bid
Levofloxacin	500 mg/day

Adapted from Fallone CA, Chiba N, van Zanten SV, et al. The Toronto consensus for the treatment of Helicobacter pylori infection in adults. Gastroenterology 2016;151(1):52–3; with permission.

Perforation

The effectiveness of gastric acid suppression therapy by H2 receptor antagonists and PPIs as well as the discovery and treatment of *H* pylori has been well documented.[1] PPIs act irreversibly on the final common pathway to gastric acid secretion, the proton pump, with excellent results.[3] The successful medical treatment of PUD has caused surgeons to reassess what is the best operation to treat patients with a perforated ulcer.

Following its introduction in the early twentieth century, most surgeons treated a patient with a perforated ulcer with the patch technique because of its reduced morbidity and mortality compared with gastric resection. The downside of this more conservative surgical approach has been a significant incidence of ulcer recurrence. With the goal of reducing the risk of ulcer recurrence, other procedures to reduce both gastric acid secretion and ulcer recurrence were used, which include pyloroplasty with truncal vagotomy, antrectomy with truncal vagotomy, and a parietal cell vagotomy combined with an omental patch.[8] The clinical success of gastric acid suppression with medication and treatment of *H* pylori infection for patients with PUD has greatly impacted the modern general surgeon's experience with these classic surgical procedures for PUD.[1]

As previously stated, ulcer perforation is the leading cause of death in patients with PUD. The most expedient surgical technique should be used to effectively deal with the perforation and at the same time obtain control of the intra-abdominal sepsis. Most perforations occur in the duodenum or prepyloric antrum and should undergo an omental patch repair (**Fig. 3**). A tongue of healthy omentum is selected and secured as a plug with several (usually 3) sutures that incorporate bites of healthy tissue on either side of the ulcer. These sutures are used to fix the tongue of omentum to the area of perforation, taking care not to strangulate the omentum while adequately plugging the perforation. The patch can be performed laparoscopically or by the open technique. A recent review of the Cochrane database by Sanabria and colleagues[9] found no difference in outcomes between laparoscopic versus open management

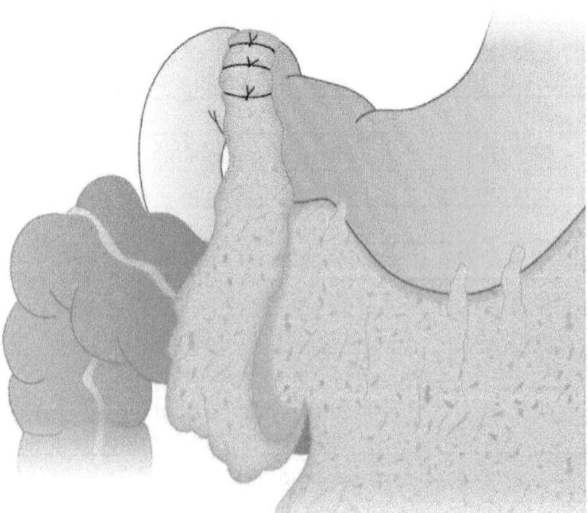

Fig. 3. Graham patch repair of perforated duodenal ulcer. A tongue of omentum is fixed with sutures over a perforation of the duodenum. (*From* Baker RJ. Perforated duodenal ulcer. In: Fischer JE, Bland KI, editors. Mastery of surgery. 5th edition. Philadelphia: Lippincott Williams & Wilkins; 2007. p. 898; with permission.)

of patients with a perforated ulcer. Biopsy is unnecessary because these ulcers are rarely associated with malignancy. In the past, if the patient was stable, some surgeons performed an acid-suppressing operation (ie, parietal cell vagotomy) along with an omental patch.[8] However, the effectiveness of gastric acid suppression therapy has made this procedure physiologically unnecessary. The patient should be treated with an intravenous PPI and tested for *H pylori* and treated if positive. Endoscopy should be performed 6 to 8 weeks after surgery and completion of *H pylori* therapy. Gastric ulcers that do not heal with appropriate therapy should raise suspicion for malignancy.

Giant peptic ulcers of the duodenum (>3 cm in diameter) that perforate present a unique technical challenge given their location proximal to the ampulla of Vater. Partial gastrectomy with either a Roux-en-Y or Billroth II reconstruction can be daunting and ill advisable secondary to a scarred and fibrotic duodenum. Multiple solutions have been advocated, including an omental patch, a loop of jejunum as a serosal patch, or placement of a drainage tube through the perforation. The authors advocate an omental patch repair combined with a "triple tube" technique, with or without pyloric exclusion. A "triple tube" technique is performed by placing a tube in the stomach for drainage as well as a retrograde jejunostomy tube that is fed back into the duodenum for decompression. Finally, a feeding catheter jejunostomy is placed for enteral feeding. Pylorus exclusion can be accomplished by either suturing the pylorus with an absorbable suture in a purse-string manner or by stapling across the distal stomach with a noncutting stapler just proximal to the pylorus. As the duodenum heals, the gastric staple line or pyloric sutures will open, and continuity will be restored to the gastrointestinal (GI) tract. Peritoneal drains are usually placed around the perforation site to control leakage of duodenal contents.

Gastric ulcer types I, IV, and V are not associated with gastric acid hypersecretion (**Table 3**). The preferred treatment of these perforated gastric ulcers is excision or wedge resection; however, a partial gastrectomy may be required depending on both the ulcer location and the extent of the disease. Because these ulcers are not associated with gastric acid hypersecretion, there is no need for a vagotomy. In the absence of *H pylori* infection or NSAID use, a gastric malignancy should be suspected (type I and IV ulcers). In patients diagnosed with these ulcers who have not had an excision or resection, follow-up EGD is essential to both document ulcer healing and exclude gastric cancer because 13% of gastric perforations may be secondary to a malignancy.[4]

Marginal ulceration has become a more common clinical problem secondary to the obesity epidemic in the United States and the subsequent large number of patients who have undergone a Roux-en-Y gastric bypass. The cause of a marginal ulcer perforation in these patients may be secondary to chronic ischemia of the

Table 3
Modified Johnson classification of gastric ulcer types

Type	Location	Acid Hypersecretion
I	Lesser curve at incisura	No
II	Gastric ulcer with duodenal ulcer	Yes
III	Prepyloric	Yes
IV	High on lesser curve	No
V	Any location	No, cause = NSAID

anastomosis due to surgical technique, tobacco use, inappropriate NSAID use, *H pylori* infection, or a large gastric pouch. Treatment consists of an omental patch or primary closure and an omental patch with placement of a gastrostomy tube in the gastric remnant (the portion of stomach still connected to the duodenum) for feeding access. Resection of the gastrojejunal anastomosis should be avoided in the acute setting because this would leave very little gastric pouch (the small portion of stomach in continuity with the esophagus) to anastomose to the jejunum. A better approach would be an omental patch, intraperitoneal drains, enteral feeding access, and reassess the need for further surgical intervention following resolution of the acute process.

In response to the potential comorbidities and severe sepsis seen in patients with a perforated ulcer, Moller and colleagues[10] developed a perioperative protocol based on the Surviving Sepsis Campaign. The Surviving Sepsis Campaign includes screening for sepsis, initial cardiovascular and pulmonary stabilization, early administration of broad-spectrum antibiotics, admission to an intensive care unit, early goal-directed intravenous fluid therapy, and thorough monitoring of vital parameters, including utilization of invasive means when appropriate. They showed a significant decrease in mortality from 27% to 17% ($P = .005$) with this protocol.

Nonoperative management of the patient with a perforated ulcer was described as early as the 1930s but it fell out of favor as a treatment option until more recently. Donovan and colleagues[8] reasoned that if most PUD is infectious and curable with antibiotics, those patients who do not exhibit generalized peritonitis could be treated nonoperatively. Their reasoning was based on several observational reports and their own experience where, at operation, the omentum had already sealed the perforation in half of their patients. They recommend nonoperative treatment in appropriately selected patients wherein the cause of the peptic ulcer perforation is most likely secondary to *H* pylori infection or NSAID use.

The patient must be hemodynamically stable, with no generalized peritonitis, and have a gastrografin study showing either a small-contained perforation or a sealed ulcer. If the patient is suitable for nonoperative treatment, the protocol includes gastric decompression with a nasogastric tube, intravenous broad-spectrum antibiotics, intravenous PPI therapy (see bleeding section for dose), and serial abdominal examinations to ensure that the patient does not develop peritoneal signs suggesting free perforation. If the patient develops generalized peritonitis or worsening sepsis, they most likely have had a leak of gastric contents into the abdominal cavity and should be taken expeditiously to the operating room for a definitive surgical procedure (**Table 4**).

Caution is advised when using a nonoperative approach in patients who are either immunocompromised, who are on steroids, or who have debilitating comorbidities. As

Table 4
Nonoperative management of perforated peptic ulcer disease

Eligibility	Protocol	Indications to Abort
• Hemodynamically stable • Localized tenderness • Sealed perforation on gastrografin study • No severe comorbidities • Immunocompetent • Cause likely *H pylori* or NSAID use	• Nasogastric decompression • Broad-spectrum antibiotics • Intravenous PPI • Serial abdominal examinations • Assess *H pylori* status	• Generalized peritonitis • Worsening sepsis

previously mentioned, any delay in operative treatment in a patient with free perforation increases the risk of postoperative death. The difficult task for the surgeon is deciding which patient is a candidate for the nonoperative approach. In general, these patients should be clinically stable and less symptomatic than would be expected of a patient who has free air on abdominal imaging. In appropriately selected patients, the morbidity and mortality rates for nonoperative treatment of a perforated peptic ulcer are comparable to those for surgery.[11] Patients should be treated with a PPI and for *H pylori* infection with follow-up EGD in 6 weeks.

Finally, some may have concerns that lifelong PPI use may have deleterious side effects compared with definitive surgical management of gastric acid secretion. Although there have been some studies correlating long-term PPI use with chronic kidney disease, dementia, bone fracture, and small intestinal bacterial overgrowth, the data are often confounding and far from definitive. In patients who have had complications from acid peptic disease, long-term PPI use is both effective and recommended, particularly in those patients who do not have a reversible cause.[12]

Bleeding

Hospital admissions for upper GI bleeding due to PUD are on the decline; however, mortality has remained constant at 5% to 10%.[2] Endoscopic treatment of a patient with a bleeding peptic ulcer has become the cornerstone in the algorithm for both diagnosis and treatment. The downside of endoscopic treatment has been recurrent or continued bleeding from the ulcer. Five percent to 10% of patients treated endoscopically will rebleed.[13,14] When compared with urgent surgery, Lau and colleagues[13] showed that endoscopic treatment of recurrent ulcer bleeding was as effective with less morbidity and had a comparable mortality. Factors predicting failure of endoscopic treatment were hypotension during the rebleeding event and patients with large ulcers measuring greater than 2 cm.

Although massive upper GI bleeding in the past was an indication for emergent surgical management, angiographic embolization has largely supplanted surgery's role in this setting. In a retrospective review of patients with rebleeding ulcers treated with surgery versus transcatheter arterial embolization (TAE), Erikson and colleagues[15] found that although the TAE group was older with more comorbidities, the 30-day mortality was lower in the TAE group. Similar results have been found by other investigators.[14] In their review of the literature, Loffroy and colleagues[14] found endovascular treatment to be successful in 93% of patients. Therefore, embolization has become the procedure of choice when endoscopic management is not feasible, for the patient with a rebleeding ulcer or for initial massive GI hemorrhage.

Besides hemorrhage control, treatment of the patient with a bleeding ulcer requires aggressive intravenous volume resuscitation, evaluation and treatment of *H pylori* infection, and an intravenous PPI. Administration of a high-dose PPI intravenously works within hours versus days when given orally. Theoretically, the PPI has a major impact on decreasing the rebleeding rate through gastric acid suppression to prevent lysis of blood clots. High dose for either omeprazole or pantoprazole is an initial 80 mg intravenous bolus followed by a continuous infusion at 8 mg/h for 72 hours.[2]

Idiopathic ulcers may also be a predictor for recurrent ulcer bleeding over time. Wong and colleagues[5] showed in a small prospective cohort study that those patients who were *H pylori* negative with idiopathic ulcers had a 42.3% incidence of recurrent ulcer bleeding compared with 11.2% (*P*<.0001) in the *H pylori* ulcer group. They also found an increase in mortality in the idiopathic ulcer group of 87.6% versus 37.3% over the 7-year period.

If a patient presents with upper GI bleeding from a peptic ulcer that is not amenable to endoscopic therapy and TAE is not clinically available, surgery is then the only option. Following a midline laparotomy, bleeding ulcers in the stomach can be excised or wedge resected. If the ulcer is in a location that is not amenable to excision, an anterior gastrotomy with oversewing of the bleeding can be performed.

Bleeding from a posterior ulcer in the second portion of the duodenum is a result of erosion into the gastroduodenal artery (GDA). A Kocher maneuver is performed, and a linear incision is made on the anterior duodenum extending through the pylorus and onto the anterior stomach to expose the posterior duodenum. The GDA is then ligated at 3 points: superior, inferior, and medially along the body of the pancreas. One must be careful to avoid accidentally ligating the common bile duct (CBD). A probe can be prophylactically placed into the CBD through the ampulla of Vater to prevent this technical error. A cholangiogram can be performed if there is any doubt concerning injury to the CBD. After hemostasis has been achieved, the pylorus can be closed transversely in the same manner as a pyloroplasty to avoid narrowing. The GDA can also be ligated distal to its origin from the common hepatic artery and at its bifurcation into the superior pancreaticoduodenal and right gastroepiploic arteries.

The need for surgical management as described above has become exceedingly rare because TAE has become the mainstay of treatment to control bleeding from the GDA. Most centers have adopted this technique because of its effectiveness, lower morbidity compared with surgery, and successful treatment in patients with large-volume hemorrhage where EGD is virtually impossible.

Obstruction

Gastric outlet obstruction due to a recurrent ulcer and scarring is rare after eradication of *H pylori* and modern gastric acid suppression.[4] Although rare, these patients present a clinical challenge for the surgeon because they are routinely malnourished given the chronic nature of their disease. CT imaging with oral contrast is often the initial diagnostic test performed in these patients to identify obstruction or stricture as well as evaluate for evidence of malignancy. If there is any uncertainty, a gastrografin study may be helpful to further characterize the presence and degree of stricture. An EGD is indicated to assess appearance and, the degree of gastric outlet obstruction and to obtain biopsies to exclude malignancy. After initial evaluation, nutritional deficiencies and serum electrolyte deficits must be corrected. In the event of a benign peptic stricture, endoscopic balloon dilatation has become the mainstay of treatment, especially in those patients with a reversible and treatable cause such as *H pylori* infection or chronic NSAID use.[16] The use of balloon dilatation in idiopathic PUD is controversial. If repeated dilatation fails in these patients, surgical intervention should be considered.[16,17]

Before surgical intervention, it is appropriate to correct nutritional deficiencies with either a nasoenteral feeding tube or total parenteral nutrition. Surgical options include truncal vagotomy with either a pyloroplasty, an antrectomy, or a gastrojejunostomy. A pyloroplasty or gastrectomy may be technically difficult in these patients because of significant scarring, fibrosis, and inflammation from a chronic, refractory disease process. Gastrojejunostomy with a truncal vagotomy avoids the difficult duodenum and is a good technical option in this setting but has a higher incidence of recurrent ulcer disease. In addition, although rare, a malignancy could be missed. If the surgeon is not experienced with performing a truncal vagotomy or the patient has other complicating factors, maintenance on lifetime acid suppression therapy with a PPI is an acceptable treatment option in lieu of truncal vagotomy.

SUMMARY

The management of PUD has evolved significantly over the last 40 years. Although acid suppression therapy and the discovery and treatment of *H pylori* have made chronic ulcer disease less common, acute ulcer perforation, bleeding, and obstruction require the surgeon to have significant knowledge of the multiple treatment algorithms appropriate for the elective and acute care of these patients.

REFERENCES

1. Schwesinger WH, Page CP, Sirinek KR, et al. Operations for peptic ulcer disease: paradigm lost. J Gastrointest Surg 2001;5(4):438–43.
2. Lanas A, Chan FKL. Peptic ulcer disease. Lancet 2017;390(10094):613–24.
3. Teitelbaum EN, Hungness ES, Mahvi DM. Stomach. In: Courtney M, Townsend J, Beauchamp DR, et al, editors. Sabiston textbook of surgery. 20th edition. Philadelphia: Elsevier; 2017. p. 1188–236.
4. Søreide K, Thorsen K, Harrision EM, et al. Perforated peptic ulcer. Lancet 2015; 386(10000):1288–98.
5. Wong GL-H, Wong VW-S, Chan Y, et al. High incidence of mortality and recurrent bleeding in patients with *Helicobacter pylori*-Negative Idiopathic Bleeding Ulcers. Gastroenterology 2009;137(2):525–31.
6. Buck DL, Vester-Andersen M, Møller MH. Surgcial delay is a critical determinant of survival in perforated peptic ulcer. Br J Surg 2013;100(8):1045–9.
7. Fallone CA, Chiba N, van Zanten SV, et al. The Toronto consensus for the treatemtn of helicobacter pylori infection in adults. Gastroenterology 2016;151(1): 51–69.
8. Donovan AJ, Berne TV, Donovan JA. Perforated. Arch Surg 1998;133(11): 1166–71.
9. Sanabria A, Villegas MI, Urive CHM. Laparoscopic repair for perforated peptic ulcer disease. Cochrane Database Syst Rev 2013;(2):CD004778.
10. Moller MH, Adamsen S, Thomsen RW, et al. Multicentre trial of a perioperative protocol to reduce mortality in patients with peptic ulcer perforation. Br J Surg 2011;98(6):802–10.
11. Marshall C, Ramaswamy P, Bergin FG, et al. Evaluation of a protocol for the non-operative management of perforated peptic ulcer. The Br J Surg 1999;86(1): 131–4.
12. Freedberg DE, Kim LS, Yang Y-X. The risks and beneftis of long-term use of proton pump inhibitors: expert review and best practice advice from the American Gastroneterological Association. Gastroenterology 2017;152(4): 706–15.
13. Lau JYW, Sung JJY, Y-h Lam, et al. Endoscopic retreatment compared with surgery in patient swith recurrent bleeding after initial endoscopic control of bleeding ulcers. N Engl J Med 1999;340(10):751–6.
14. Loffroy R, Rao P, Ota S, et al. Embolization of acute nonvariceal upper gastrointestinal hemorrhage resistant to endoscopic treatment: results and predictors of recurrent bleeding. Cardiovasc Intervent Radiol 2010;33(6): 1088–100.
15. Eriksson L, Ljungdahl M, Sundborn M, et al. Transcatheter arterial embolization versus surgery in the treatment of upper gastrointestinal bleeding after therapeutic endoscopy failure. J Vasc Interv Radiol 2008;19(10):1423–8.

16. Cherian PT, Cherian S, Singh P. Long-term follow-up of patients with gastric outlet obstruction related to peptic ulcer disease treated with endoscopic balloon dilatation and drug therapy. Gastrointest Endosc 2007;66(3):491–7.
17. Gibson JB, Behrman SW, Fabian TC, et al. Gastric outlet obstruction resulting from peptic ulcer disease requiring surgical intervention is infrequently associated with *Helicobacter pylori* infection. J Am Coll Surg 2000;191(1):32–7.

Small Bowel Obstruction

Katie Love Bower, MD, MSc*, Daniel I. Lollar, MD,
Sharon L. Williams, MD, Farrell C. Adkins, MD, David T. Luyimbazi, MD,
Curtis E. Bower, MD

KEYWORDS

- Small bowel obstruction • Intestinal obstruction • Enterolysis • Adhesiolysis
- Water soluble contrast challenge

KEY POINTS

- Identify patients early who need urgent surgery and who will fail nonoperative management to avoid undue morbidity and mortality. If no indication for urgent operation, computed tomography scan with/without intravenous contrast is recommended.
- Nonoperative management includes bowel rest, nasogastric tube decompression, serial examinations/laboratory tests, and water- soluble contrast challenge.
- Conditions such as age greater than 65, post Roux-en-Y gastric bypass, inflammatory bowel disease, malignancy, virgin abdomen, diabetes, pregnancy, hernia, early postoperative state, and malnutrition deserve special consideration.
- Open and laparoscopic exploration are safe and effective, depending on the surgeon's experience and the etiology for obstruction.
- Regardless of operative approach, timing is paramount. Examine the abdominal cavity, identify/alleviate obstruction source(s), run the bowel to assess for viability, confirm resolution of obstruction(s), and identify/repair injuries.

INTRODUCTION: NATURE OF THE PROBLEM

The concept management of patients with small bowel obstruction (SBO) became more complicated in 1981 when Bizer and colleagues[1] reported that nonoperative management was successful in a significant percentage of patients. Our approach has changed considerably since then owing to advancements in imaging technology, the prevalence of adhesion disease, the prominence of laparoscopy, and the development of protocols to help ensure timely intervention. What has not changed is the need to avoid nontherapeutic surgery, as well as unnecessary delay when surgery is required. Morbidity and mortality owing to SBO increase when there is an undue delay in operation and decrease with the institution of appropriately timed surgery.[2]

Disclosure: The authors have nothing to disclose.

Carilion Clinic and Virginia Tech Carilion School of Medicine, Carilion Clinic Department of Surgery, 1906 Belleview Avenue, Med. Ed., 3rd Floor, Suite 332, Roanoke, VA 24014, USA
* Corresponding author.
E-mail address: klbower1@carilionclinic.org

Surg Clin N Am 98 (2018) 945–971
https://doi.org/10.1016/j.suc.2018.05.007 surgical.theclinics.com

The most common reason for litigation in SBO malpractice claims is failure to diagnose and treat in a timely manner.[3] The challenge for the emergency general surgeon is identifying as quickly as possible the 24% of patients presenting with SBO who will not resolve without surgery.[4]

RELEVANT ANATOMY AND PATHOPHYSIOLOGY

When considering SBO, it is important to understand the difference between functional disorders that lead to nonpropulsion through the gut and mechanical disorders that impede otherwise normal propulsive effort. Gastrointestinal paralysis (ileus) secondary to enteritis that may be attributable to surgery, medication, infection, or inflammation is the most common imitator of a SBO in terms of presenting symptoms, physical examination findings, and static imaging findings. It is often brought to the attention of a surgeon when a radiologist states that SBO cannot be ruled out based on radiographic patterns. Ileus results in dysfunctional peristalsis, which is not correctable with surgery, and it often falls on the surgeon to differentiate between the two. Relevant history including identification of risk factors for ileus, trends in the abdominal examination and laboratory results, and dynamic contrast imaging findings help to make the call.

SBO is due to intraluminal or extraluminal mechanical compression (**Table 1**). Adhesion disease is the most common cause of mechanical SBO in developed countries.[5] Less common causes include hernia, malignancy, and various infectious and inflammatory disorders.

CLINICAL PRESENTATION AND PHYSICAL EXAMINATION

SBO is included in the differential diagnosis when a patient presents with nausea, vomiting, abdominal pain, abdominal distension, and constipation. Rarely are all of these symptoms present. Pain attributed to mechanical SBO is intermittent, described

Table 1
Intraluminal or extraluminal mechanical compression causes for SBO

>70% Mechanical SBOs	Adhesion Disease[5]
Less common causes:	Abdominal wall or internal hernia Anastomotic stricture Volvulus Neoplasm Sclerosis Abscess Perforation Malrotation Fecalith Gallstone[6] Bezoar[7] Foreign bodies
Less common causes: Inflammatory disorders	Crohn's disease Immunologic disorders Pelvic inflammatory disease Endometriosis
Less common causes: Infectious disorders	Tuberculosis Parasites

Abbreviation: SBO, small bowel obstruction.

as crampy or colicky owing to increased peristalsis against the physical obstruction. Patients can present with diarrhea even in the presence of a complete SBO owing to this increased intestinal activity.[5]

Primary Evaluation

- Exclude the presence of bowel ischemia, sepsis, and perforation, and ensure adequate resuscitation.

Patients with SBO are often hypovolemic from vomiting and/or dehydration. Basic resuscitation should be implemented:

- Evaluate vital signs;
- Obtain adequate intravenous (IV) access;
- Assess volume status;
- Start IV fluid as warranted;
- Determine whether invasive monitoring or urinary catheterization are indicated;
- Obtain blood specimens for complete blood count, comprehensive metabolic panel, and lactic acid level;
- Timely initiation of antibiotics if sepsis suspected[8];
- Insert a nasogastric (NGT) if the patient is vomiting and/or the abdomen is distended; and
- Hold narcotics and other central nervous system depressants to maintain reliability of the abdominal examination.

Initial laboratory assays should include a complete blood count with differential and a metabolic panel, to aid in evaluation of electrolyte and acid–base disturbances, liver and kidney function, as well as systemic signs of malperfusion and infection. Hypokalemia and contraction alkalosis are common, as well as metabolic acidosis owing to bicarbonate loss and tissue hypoperfusion. A metabolic acidosis with a wide anion gap should prompt an evaluation for lactic acidosis, which could indicate mesenteric ischemia or global hypoperfusion owing to hypovolemia. Mesenteric ischemia is more likely if the lactate level does not return to normal quickly after fluid resuscitation. Beware, though: a normal or decreasing lactate level does not rule out mesenteric ischemia. Cells that succumb to ischemic necrosis are unable to perform anaerobic metabolism and, thus, will no longer produce lactate. Further, when outflow for a diseased segment of small bowel is congested or obstructed, there could be ischemic necrosis without a leukocytosis or acidosis, because these inflammatory markers are prevented from entering the systemic circulation.

History and Physical Examination

History and physical examination will have a prominent role in determining the etiology of the SBO and whether there are immediate indications for surgery. The duration and severity of symptoms, such as acute abdominal pain, nausea, and obstipation, are requisite. These nonspecific symptoms need to be considered in context with previous episodes, how often they occur, and whether there has been weight loss, gastrointestinal bleeding, or prior abdominal surgery.

Past surgical history should focus on prior abdominopelvic operations, specifically inquiring about procedures that can predispose to internal hernias such as bowel resection or intestinal bypass. Previous episodes of SBO, timing of these episodes relative to prior operations, how the episodes were managed, and outcomes ought to be documented, because this information can influence operative management strategy for the current episode. The probability that a patient who previously underwent nonoperative management will require readmission for recurrent SBO increases with each episode.[9–11] If there has been more than 1 episode in a year, the episodes are recurring with increasing frequency, or resolution of symptoms between episodes is incomplete, surgical intervention is warranted. Recurrent SBO after multiple laparotomies for lysis of adhesions can present a unique operative challenge.[5] The level of difficulty in lysing adhesions and evaluating gastrointestinal anatomy increases exponentially owing to fibrosis that becomes more diffuse with each subsequent operation, thus, increasing the risk of technical complications.

Determining whether resolution of symptoms has occurred between episodes often requires meticulous investigation regarding the patient's ability to eat as well as more mild symptoms the patient may be experiencing on a regular basis that do not prompt her or him to seek medical attention. Such patients alter their diet to cope with symptoms. Although they report they are tolerating solid food, they may not volunteer that tolerance requires changes in the types, amounts, or textures of food consumed, the frequency with which they are able to eat, or coping mechanisms they must use such as saturating food with fluid during consumption. Determining whether there has been weight loss is pivotal. A patient with recurring episodes of even mild partial SBO who is also suffering weight loss has a serious problem that will lead to eventual death from malnutrition-related complications if not recognized and intervened upon while the patient is physiologically capable of tolerating surgery. Refer to Nutrition Considerations, elsewhere in this article.

Physical examination findings are pertinent to the diagnosis of mechanical SBO as well as decisions regarding diagnostics and management. Abdominal distension suggests an abnormal accumulation of air or fluid. Tympany over a distended area indicates the presence of air, whereas dullness indicates fluid. Peritoneal signs and focal abdominal tenderness suggest inflammation owing to compromised or perforated bowel. Abdominal wall or inguinal hernias may represent transition points for SBO, especially if incarcerated or tender to palpation. Abdominal pain out of proportion to the examination suggests mesenteric ischemia. A digital rectal examination should be performed, because occult or gross blood may represent mucosal ischemia and a distal obstruction could be identified and alleviated without further workup or intervention.

Signs of sepsis, such as tachycardia, hypotension, leukocytosis, or acidosis with evidence of focal tenderness or peritonitis, should compel a greater sense of urgency toward operative management.[12,13] "Compromised bowel in the setting of SBO is *unlikely* if the patient has a WBC [white blood cell count of] less than 16,000/mL, and no fever, and no pain or tenderness, and no tachycardia, and no ominous radiologic findings."[5]

DIAGNOSIS

Secondary Evaluation

- Obtain a computed tomography (CT) scan of the abdomen and pelvis with and without IV contrast; consider enteric contrast.
- Identify the potential etiology for SBO and its likelihood of resolution with nonoperative management.
- Pursue urgent operative management if static imaging findings suggest perforation or ischemia.
- Assess and manage comorbid conditions present on admission that could impact outcomes of both operative management and nonoperative management, such as cardiopulmonary disease and malnutrition.

- Findings on radiographic imaging should be interpreted by the surgeon within the context of the patient's presentation and examination.
- CT scans cannot reliably predict who will fail nonoperative management.

Imaging

Clinical features cannot be relied on to exclude SBO[14] or to determine whether complications are present.[15,16] Thus, imaging has assumed a prominent role in guiding management.[12,13,17,18]

Computed tomography

Unless there are unquestionable clinical indications for operative exploration, a CT of the abdomen with and without IV contrast is recommended when SBO is suspected, because it can provide information regarding location, grade, severity, and etiology,[12,13,17,19–22] and help to avoid "inadvertent nonoperative management" in the presence of strangulation.[13] CT scans can sometimes guide the choice of laparoscopic versus open surgical intervention, in the event features associated with matted or single-band adhesions are present.[23] In combination with clinical assessment parameters, CT scans can affirm that an operation will be beneficial and it can provide reassurance in a stable patient that a complication is less likely to be present at the time of the study.[16] Unfortunately, its impotent ability to predict failure of nonoperative management has been repeatedly demonstrated.[12–14,16,24–37]

- Enteral contrast for CT imaging: Enteral contrast can optimize the study for SBO, but it is not required for diagnosis. It is not routinely given to patients unable to tolerate oral intake. In cases where intestinal ischemia is present, bowel wall enhancement is more readily identified without enteral contrast.[19,38] The American College of Radiology (ACR) recommends that oral contrast not be used if high-grade SBO is known or suspected because it wastes resources, does not add to diagnostic accuracy, and can lead to vomiting and aspiration. However, it is not contraindicated and may add functional information for suspected intermittent or low-grade SBO.[39,40]
- CT findings that suggest SBO (**Box 1**) include transition point with proximal dilatation and distal decompression of bowel, decompressed colon, and failure of proximal enteral contrast to pass the transition point.
- CT findings that suggest bowel ischemia: Intestinal ischemia is more commonly associated with certain causes of SBO, including an obstructing mass, intussusception, hernia, volvulus, and closed loop obstruction.[16] The sensitivity and specificity of CT for high-grade SBO and for identifying bowel ischemia is greater than 90%.[16,19,41–43] There are many radiographic signs that suggest bowel ischemia (**Box 2**), all attributed to congestion of lymphatic fluid, blood, and/or stool with resultant malperfusion.[17,22,24,26,30,44–46]

Box 1
Computed tomography findings that suggest small bowel obstruction

Transition point

Decompressed colon

Failure of proximal enteral contrast to pass

Box 2 Computed tomography findings that suggest bowel ischemia
Altered or absent bowel wall enhancement
Abnormal course of mesenteric vessels, such as a swirl sign with volvulus
Presence of free fluid
Mural thickening
Ascites
Mesenteric edema
Mesenteric venous congestion
Pneumatosis intestinalis
Closed loop obstruction
Portal venous gas
Small bowel feces sign, or fecalization of small bowel

Magnet Resonance Imaging

The sensitivity and specificity of MRI to diagnose and characterize SBO is similar to that of CT scanning; however, it is more expensive and less available. MRI is most appropriate for children, younger patients with multiple prior CT examinations, and pregnant women[39,40]

- Radiographs: Abdominal radiographs can indicate the presence of dilated bowel (>3 cm outer wall to outer wall) with nondilated distal loops and air–fluid levels, all findings indicative of SBO. Pneumoperitoneum may be visualized in SBO complicated by perforation or pneumotosis intestinalis in SBO complicated by mesenteric ischemia. However, the absence of these findings does not rule out SBO or related complications, and it is not always possible to distinguish an adynamic ileus from mechanical obstruction with a radiograph.[22,38] It is not necessary to obtain a radiograph before a CT scan when SBO is suspected [2013 Update https://acsearch.acr.org/docs/69476/Narrative/].[39,47,48]
- Ultrasound examination: Because of the presence of bowel gas and the inability of sonography to detect adhesions,[20] ultrasound examination does not aid clinical management decisions in most cases of SBO. A technique for the ultrasound diagnosis of SBO is described.[49]

Evidence on static imaging of complications such as ischemia, strangulation, perforation, and closed loop should prompt urgent surgical intervention.

- Dynamic contrast study
  - Fluoroscopic small bowel follow through: For low-grade or chronic intermittent SBO, this procedure may establish the diagnosis and can add functional information as an adjunct to CT scans. Findings consistent with SBO are dilated loops proximal to a transition point and delayed transit time of contrast. Enteral contrast studies can determine the level and cause of obstruction, detect minimal adhesions and small intraluminal mass lesions, depict and grade the severity of partial obstruction, and demonstrate sites of multifocal complete obstructions. It should be performed with a water-soluble contrast to avoid complications associated with concretion of barium. Use isoosmolar or low osmolar contrast material if there is a risk of aspiration.[20,39,40]

- Radiographic fluoroscopic small bowel follow through: Also known as the water-soluble contrast challenge (WSCc), this procedure has become a requisite modality when attempting nonoperative management. It decreases the need for surgery in patients who do not meet the criteria for urgent operation and enhances the ability to pursue early intervention for those who fail nonoperative management. Decreases in time to resolution after nonoperative management and hospital duration of stay have been demonstrated after administration of water-soluble enteric contrast as well.[18,50–57] The 2 most common types of water-soluble contrast agents are Gastrografin (Bracco Diagnostics, Inc., Monroe Township, NJ) and Gastroview (Mallinckrodt, Inc., St. Louis, MO). The WSCc is for patients undergoing nonoperative management for SBO, after need for urgent surgery is ruled out.
- The patient ingests 80 to 100 mL diluted in 40 to 50 mL water via NGT after 2 to 6 hours of nasogastric decompression. The patient is reexamined every 4 hours. Unless the patient develops nausea or increasing abdominal pain, the NGT should remain clamped after administration of contrast and have an abdominal radiograph obtained 8 hours later to evaluate for contrast passage beyond the transition point and into the colon. The radiograph can be repeated every 8 to 12 hours as long as the patient's examination, symptoms, laboratory tests, and vital signs improve or remain stable. Lack of passage of contrast to the colon and/or failure to resolve should prompt operative exploration.[18,50,53,54] Patients who are frail, over age 65 years, suffer from chronic obstructive pulmonary disease or other pulmonary insufficiency requiring home oxygen therapy, or have a paraesophageal or hiatal hernia are considered at increased risk of aspiration. Although there is no evidence against this technique for such patients, clinical judgment should be used in terms of implementing the WSCc.[18] Use iso-osmolar or low osmolar contrast material if there is a risk of aspiration[20,39,40]

CLINICAL PATHWAY

Admission

The majority of SBOs (65% to 80%) will resolve without operation.[33,55,58–62] Timely recognition of patients in need of operative intervention is paramount in terms of minimizing morbidity and mortality. Whether or not a patient with suspected SBO should be admitted to a surgical or medical team is a common dilemma. A high rate of nonoperative management suggests selected patients should be safe on a nonsurgical service. Recent retrospective studies, performed at a single institution[63–66] and on a large statewide database,[60] demonstrate an increased duration of stay, higher in-hospital expense, a higher 30-day readmission rate whether operative management or nonoperative management is used, and higher rates of perioperative complications, including mortality, when SBO patients are admitted primarily to a nonsurgical service. In addition, survey data from a single institution demonstrated lower patient satisfaction scores when the primary provider is not a surgeon.[67] These data are subject to the concerns of retrospective studies, namely, selection bias among heterogeneous patient populations. They allude to but do not address the severity and acuity of concurrent medical comorbidities these patients often suffer with their possible SBO, and whether these had an impact on the examined outcomes. When medical comorbidities are present in acute exacerbation, one could postulate that a multidisciplinary approach would be most beneficial regardless of the admitting service. Further, the presence of an in-house surgeon dedicated to emergency general surgery patients is more likely a mitigating factor regarding outcomes associated with expediency of intervention,[68] and less so the specific service (medical vs surgical) to which the patient is admitted. None of these studies discussed the availability of attending surgeon coverage. Although the data to date support the bias that SBO should be managed on a surgical service, prospective data are needed to confirm these suspicions.

Predicting Outcomes

Other than information gained with WSCc, there has been no reliable clinical method for predicting failure of nonoperative management for adhesive SBO.[33,53,69] One center was able to validate the likelihood of preventing delayed operative management for strangulated obstructions in the presence of:

- Obstipation;
- Lack of small bowel feces sign; and
- Mesenteric edema.

Operative exploration was recommended within 12 hours if all 3 of these signs were present owing to a 90% chance of requiring surgery before discharge.[31] A disease severity score for SBO has been developed and validated by the American Association for the Surgery of Trauma. It has not been widely implemented, but can be helpful in predicting outcomes including mortality,[70] as well as providing a guideline for documentation that aids in risk stratification when evaluating outcomes for institutions and individual surgeons.

Operative Management

If the indicators for urgent surgical intervention are present (sepsis, peritonitis, perforation, ischemia, strangulation, or etiology for SBO that does not resolve without operative intervention), the patient should undergo operative management after a brief period of resuscitation, within 1 to 2 hours from diagnosis. There is no literature to support delaying surgical intervention owing to additional adhesion formation.[35] Patients treated surgically for adhesive SBO have a lower recurrence rate and a longer time to recurrence than those who undergo nonoperative management.[71–73]

The bowel obstruction on which the sun should not set or rise without surgical intervention is the one that presents with a history of obstipation for 8 to 12 hours, significant distension of the bowel, and no recent improvement of either. This is especially true if the patient also has unrelenting severe abdominal pain, fever, leukocytosis, and/or tachycardia, indicating strangulation.

Nonoperative Management

If there are no indications for urgent surgical intervention, nonoperative management can safely and effectively be pursued,[1,5,12,13,18] most notably in the presence of an adhesive SBO.[74] Within 48 hours, 88% of patients with an adhesive SBO can be expected to resolve without surgery.[61] Nonoperative management requires premeditated vigilance, allowing a trend to be observed under serial clinical assessments. Many acute care surgery services institute algorithms or protocols that help to make the observation period more efficient.[12,13,17,18] The various published guidelines for initial nonoperative management of adhesive SBO have the following elements in common:

- Bowel rest, NPO.
- NGT decompression.
- Serial abdominal examinations documented every 4 to 6 hours.
- Serial laboratory tests, including complete blood count, basic metabolic panel, and lactic acid every 6 hours.

- Water-soluble contrast challenge, radiographic fluoroscopic small bowel follow through:
  - Once contrast reaches colon, trial clear liquid diet and advance as tolerated.
- Urgent exploration with worsening examination, development of peritonitis or sepsis, or if there are signs of evolving bowel ischemia.

Morbidity and mortality associated with SBO can be decreased by earlier identification of patients who will fail nonoperative management.[25] Although there is no consensus in the literature about the optimal duration of a nonoperative management trial, studies have suggested an SBO be observed no longer than 3 to 5 days, and the most stringent recommendations are to observe for a maximum of 72 hours. If nonoperative management exceeds 3 days, the patient's hospital duration of stay is extended, bowel resection is more likely, 30-day morbidity increases, and risk of death increases by more than 60%.[17,18,75,76] Early surgical intervention, defined to be within 24 hours of admission, is associated with a 53% relative decrease in mortality.[35] Long-term recurrence of an SBO after WSCc is similar to that of patients who underwent initially successful nonoperative management without WSCc.[77]

- Nonoperative management is appropriate for adhesive SBO unless there is evidence of bowel compromise or failure to resolve.
- The etiology and its likelihood of resolution need to be considered in non-adhesive SBO before deciding to use nonoperative management.
- When in doubt, operate. Abdominal exploration is sometimes required to rule out life-threatening conditions or to establish a definitive diagnosis.

Fig. 1 is a published algorithm for the management of SBO.[13]

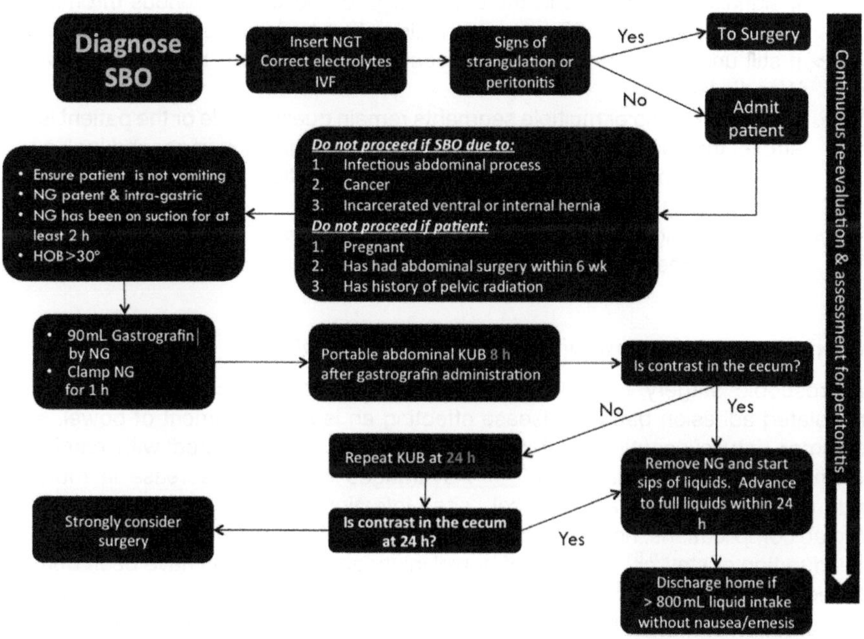

Fig. 1. Decision-making flow diagram. HOB, head of bed; IVF, intravenous fluid; KUB, kidney, ureter, bladder; NG, nasogastric; SBO, small bowel obstruction. (*From* Azagury D, Liu RC, Morgan A, et al. Small bowel obstruction: a practical step-by-step evidence-based approach to evaluation, decision making, and management. J Trauma Acute Care Surg 2015;79(4):663; with permission.)

Technical Considerations

Open exploration and enterolysis through a midline incision is historically the standard approach.

- Use prior incision scar as a guide. With a scalpel, extend the midline skin incision beyond the scarred region. If possible, enter the abdomen through an unoperated area. This technique will help to avoid enterotomy. The use of electrocautery can cause thermal injury to any bowel adherent to the abdominal wall.
- Dissect adherent viscera away from the incision using a scalpel or Metzenbaum scissors to separate the visceral from parietal tissue planes. Blunt dissection can result in tearing of the bowel.
- Identify and alleviate transition point(s).
- Continue to lyse adhesions until the bowel can be examined in its entirety for injury, malperfusion, and resolution of obstruction(s). Start where adhesions are filmy, hypovascular, and the bowel wall is easy to identify, and work toward more difficult areas. Do not spend too much time lysing adhesions in a single location because such tenacity will often result in injury.
- Assess bowel viability. Pink, edematous, and thickened bowel is at low risk for ischemia.[5]
  - Violaceous or cyanotic serosa should be kept warm and observed for improved perfusion over 15 to 20 minutes.
  - Resect short segments of bowel that seem to be unsalvageable. Primary anastomosis is usually feasible and safe.
  - If viability remains questionable along a long segment of bowel, use a sterile Doppler ultrasound probe to evaluate for arterial pulse within the bowel wall. If signals are present and there is no sign of mesenteric venous thrombosis, observation for 15 to 20 minutes should suffice to decide on whether to resect.
  - If still unsure, administer IV fluorescein dye and assess blood supply with a Wood's lamp.
  - If viability of long or multiple segments remain questionable or the patient is unstable, the abdomen can be temporarily closed for planned second look operation. Re-exploration should occur after the patient has been resuscitated, usually within 8 to 24 hours.
  - Before closing, run the bowel from the ileocecal valve to the ligament of Treitz to confirm the absence of, or repair, enterotomies and serosa injuries.

Evidence supports laparoscopic exploration and enterolysis

Laparoscopic surgery for SBO is safe and effective, especially when owing to an isolated adhesion band or disease effecting an isolated segment of bowel, such as tumor, intussusception, or foreign body. It can be attempted with caution in patients with matted adhesions.[78–80] Advantages include a decrease in mortality and morbidity, such as surgical site infections, respiratory complications, cardiac complications, need for bowel resection, venous thromboembolism, and hospital duration of stay.[6,81–83] Rates of bowel injury and reoperation have been demonstrated to be equivalent.[83] Success with a laparoscopic approach requires a specific skill set and may not be appropriate in all patients. It depends on an individual surgeon's experience and comfort level with laparoscopic surgery, as well as an individual patient's anatomy and pathophysiology. Outcomes do not differ between patients treated by surgeons with or without postresidency training in minimally invasive surgery.[6] The only absolute contraindications for laparoscopic surgery are hemodynamic instability or cardiopulmonary impairment.[84] Abdominal distension is not an absolute contraindication, although care must be taken when gaining access to and insufflating the abdominal cavity. Massive bowel distension may not allow for adequate laparoscopic exposure. The timing of operation for laparoscopic surgery is identical to the open approach in all cases. Technical considerations for laparoscopic surgery include the following:

- Position the patient supine with arms spread on a table that allows for Trendelenburg and reverse Trendelenburg positioning, bilateral tilt, and height adjustment. Secure patient to the table with a lap belt.
- Three ports are typically required, and a 30° angled scope will aid exposure.
- Trocar sites should be selected according to surgical history. Initial port placement in the left upper quadrant, or furthest from previous incisions, is recommended. An umbilical port is usually not helpful.
- Ensure sufficient abdominal domain to accommodate insufflation and achieve adequate exposure. If insufflated to a maximum of 12 to 15 mm Hg and visualization is poor or the patient develops hemodynamic instability, convert to an open procedure. Otherwise, perform an initial exploration.
- Choose sites for the second and third ports away from the area of interest to triangulate with the camera.
- Systematically inspect the entire abdominal cavity using atraumatic graspers. Run the bowel from the nondistended segment at the ileocecal valve toward the ligament of Treitz. Avoid grasping serosa if possible, and grasp gently if necessary. Jejunum is more susceptible than ileum to grasper injury, especially if dilated and inflamed.
- Lyse visceroparietal and viscerovisceral adhesions using scissors, forceps, and laparoscopic coagulation shears. Transect adhesive bands.
- If bowel resection and reconstruction is required, this can be performed under direct vision in the extracorporeal space with extension of the port site incision most convenient to the segment of bowel.
- After the obstruction is relieved, run the bowel again to ensure relief of obstruction(s), evaluate viability, and examine for injury.
- Convert to an open procedure at any time that exposure becomes inadequate, laparoscopy seems insufficient, or the patient fails to tolerate the procedure from a hemodynamic standpoint, and preferably before an injury occurs.
- Reasons for conversion to open include the following:
  - Matted adhesions,
  - Inadequate exposure, and
  - Injury to mesentery, bowel, bladder, or other organs.[78]

When bowel injury occurs during laparoscopy for SBO, outcomes are worse than if the patient underwent open surgery without bowel injury.[85]

Nutritional Considerations

Patients with SBO can present in a malnourished state or rapidly progress to malnutrition in the perioperative period. This is especially true in the setting of chronic partial or intermittent SBO. Thus, a history including inadequate oral intake and recent unintended weight loss should be elicited and accounted for during the initial evaluation. Because the most common postoperative complication is ileus,[74] which can be prolonged for a week or more, it is prudent to consider initiating parenteral nutrition early in such patients.

CONFOUNDING CONDITIONS

Geriatric

Geriatric patients will usually tolerate an operation, but not the complication

Because of medical comorbidities, especially in the emergency setting, patients older than 60 and 80 years have twice and thrice the risk of adverse outcomes after surgery, respectively, relative to younger adults.[86] They also have less physiologic reserve. Older patients with SBO who fail nonoperative management may have a higher mortality rate than those who undergo immediate surgery, and, therefore, should be managed aggressively if they do not resolve quickly.[87] Patients greater than 65 years of age who received the same intensity of treatment for SBO as younger adult patients at 1 institution had similar outcomes, including overall complication rates, but were more likely to have postoperative cardiac complications and be discharged to a subacute care facility.[88]

- Age alone should not determine management.
- Preoperative cardiac risk stratification should be considered and optimized when possible, but urgent surgery should not be delayed for this purpose.
- Preadmission functional status assessment should be included in the history and physical examination.
- Goals of care, code status, and discharge disposition should be discussed at the time of admission.

Pregnancy

Maternal demise results in fetal demise 100% of the time

SBO in pregnancy is rare; it is estimated that a practicing surgeon may manage 1 to 2 cases in a career. One-half of reported SBO cases during pregnancy are due to adhesions and the other half are due to internal hernia, volvulus, mesenteric band, and ileal pouch compression. The operative rate of pregnant patients with all cause SBO is greater than 90% and some of these cases have been successfully delayed to allow the fetus to mature. Maternal mortality rate is similar to nonpregnant adults. Fetal mortality averages 21% and is more likely with surgery in the first trimester.[89]

- Indications for urgent operative management are the same as for nonpregnant adults.
- Urgent MRI is advised absent immediate indications for surgery.
- SBO owing to a cause other than adhesions should undergo urgent operative management.
- Adhesive SBO should undergo trial of nonoperative management with a low threshold for operation.
- Surgery for partial or incomplete adhesive SBO can be delayed for fetal maturity if there is no clinical evidence of a complication.
- Pregnancy is not an absolute contraindication to ionizing radiation from radiographs or CT scans; however, the risks and benefits of fetal exposure to radiation need to be carefully weighed. Refer to ACR Practice Parameters for imaging pregnant patients[90] (available: https://www.acr.org/-/media/ACR/Files/Practice-Parameters/pregnant-pts.pdf).
- Safety analyses on use of gastrointestinal contrast in pregnancy have not been done, and those on IV contrast agents have been limited. See the ACR Manual on Contrast Media (pp. 58 to 59 and 98 to 101).[91]

Virgin Abdomen

For SBO in the absence of prior abdominopelvic surgery, traditional dictum mandated operative exploration without a trial of observation. There is a greater chance the etiology will not resolve without surgery. However, 60% of these cases have been found to be due to inflammatory adhesions. Thus, nonoperative management may be acceptable in select patients, such as those without leukocytosis and no free fluid or transition point on CT scanning.[92,93] Other than adhesions, the most common cause of SBO in the virgin abdomen is hernia.[5] Rare causes include metastatic disease, Chron's disease, gallstone ileus, Meckel's diverticulum, and sclerosing encapsulating peritonitis.[93,94]

Early Postoperative Small Bowel Obstruction

Early postoperative SBO occurs within 4 to 6 weeks after abdominopelvic surgery. Most are due to adhesions and resolve with nonoperative management.[95] Although WSCc has been deemed safe in patients with suspected early postoperative SBO, no therapeutic benefit was demonstrated.[57] After 10 to 14 days postoperatively, adhesions are dense and hypervascular making reoperation treacherous. However, causes of early postoperative SBO after laparoscopic surgery are usually more localized; therefore, reexploration with laparoscopic surgery can be accomplished with fewer complications as compared with open reexploration.[96] Patients with early postoperative SBO who fail to resolve after 2 weeks but do not meet criteria for urgent surgery should be managed with NGT decompression and parenteral nutrition until they pass the 6-week mark, when it would be safer to operate.

Abdominopelvic Malignancy and Palliation

Unlike nonmalignant etiologies, these patients tend to have a subacute clinical picture with a slow insidious onset that is typical of partial SBO. Regardless, complete obstruction and intestinal ischemia are inevitable without correction. Although many patients with a malignant cause for SBO will only be able to have their symptoms managed, a portion of them will present with de novo and treatable tumors. A potentially viable oncologic procedure should not be compromised for treatment of the SBO unless there is no other choice from a standpoint of physiologic stability. If no proper cancer operation can be performed, then focus solely on relieving the obstruction and, hopefully, preventing the next.

For patients who present with SBO due to a nonmetastatic or locally advanced primary small bowel tumor, an operative intervention with curative intent remains the principal tenet of management. The differential for these tumors typically include small bowel neuroendocrine tumors, adenocarcinoma, lymphomas, and gastrointestinal stromal tumors. For such patients, a viable oncologic procedure involves a resection of the involved segment of bowel along with a 5- to 10-cm margin along the intestine proximal and distal to the tumor. The resection must also include all associated mesentery. This ensures an adequate lymphadenectomy and proper evaluation for adjuvant systemic treatment based on final staging.

For patients who present with obstruction from incurable advanced disease, the factors affecting the final treatment plan include established goals of care set forth by the patient with the guidance of the surgeon and the medical oncologist. It is beneficial to involve a palliative care specialist at this juncture as well. The patient's primary malignancy type, cancer staging, previous treatment, performance status, and comorbidities all play an important role.[97] Appropriately identifying which patients will benefit from operative management is crucial, because the morbidity and mortality of a surgical procedure in this population remains significant.[98,99] In a fashion similar to

SBO of nonmalignant etiology, the initial approach is to resuscitate the patient. Nonoperative management with NGT decompression is attempted for 48 hours in the absence of peritonitis or a worsening clinical picture. Those who persist with obstructive symptoms after this timeframe are offered definitive surgical intervention if they are deemed to be suitable surgical candidates. In addition, the case for or against surgical intervention can be guided by nomograms that have identified predictors of 30-day mortality in patients who present with malignant SBO.[100]

Operative Management with Malignancy

Once the decision to operate has been made, the choice of surgical procedure needed to address the obstruction is considered. The options include the following:

- Small bowel resection with primary anastomosis,
- Small bowel bypass,
- Lysis of adhesions, and
- Creation of a small bowel or proximal stoma.

The decision of which techniques to use is based in part on the location of the obstruction, patient comorbidities, and overall prognosis.[101] Adhesions remain a common cause of SBO in patients who have cancer and have undergone a prior operation. Enterolysis is, therefore, a surgical technique that can be used in combination with the other three, or in isolation when no other cause of obstruction is found. With the exception of ovarian cancer where tumor debulking has shown a survival benefit, implementing this approach will be of limited benefit to the patient and will likely result in the tumor growing back.[102,103] Small bowel resection is a preferable approach when the site of obstruction is isolated, the tumor causing the obstruction is intrinsic to bowel, negative margins are a possibility, and the postoperative outcome is potentially curative. A small bowel bypass is preferable if the tumor causing the obstruction cannot be completely resected and multiple sites of bowel obstruction exist. The goal with bypass is palliation.

Nonoperative Management with Malignancy

In the event that a nonoperative decision is made, the options for management involve enteric tube decompression and pharmacologic management. Placement of a NGT offers significant symptom relief, albeit temporary. Prolonged use can lead to poor pulmonary toilet, aspiration pneumonia, erosion of the nasal cartilage, and bleeding. A percutaneous endoscopic gastrostomy can be placed to manage nausea and vomiting in the long term.[104] Because the tube is placed along the anterior wall of the stomach, decompression and relief of symptoms are incomplete and typically require additional palliative measures to address symptoms. Pharmacologic management is centered on control of pain, diminishing intraluminal secretions and peristalsis, and lessening of peritumoral edema.[101,105] Somatostatin analogs inhibit gastrointestinal secretions and decrease bowel motility.[99] Various studies have shown its efficacy over anticholinergic agents in the symptomatic management of malignant SBO.[101,106] This medication is typically administered twice daily subcutaneously and titrated up as needed. Patients who respond can transition to a depot injection of long-acting octreotide that is administered monthly. Among the antiemetics, IV haloperidol, a selective dopamine receptor antagonist, is considered a first choice for patients with malignant SBO.[107] IV administration has a lower risk of sedation and lower cholinergic effects. The anticholinergic agents include scopolamine administered as a transdermal patch and glycopyrrolate. This class of medications may be selected in patients predisposed to somnolence and confusion.[108]

Radiation Enteritis

Radiation therapy for cancers of the cervix, endometrium, rectum, ovary, bladder, and prostate can injure exposed small bowel, causing acute and chronic radiation enteritis. Although acute enteritis is self-limiting and resolves after radiation treatment, chronic enteritis becomes evident within 3 months to 10 years after radiation treatment. It is the product of an obliterative arteritis that leads to intestinal ischemia, then strictures followed by luminal SBO. Partial SBO is the most common clinical manifestation of this disease.[109] Treating SBO from chronic enteritis represents a formidable challenge. For patients with intermittent obstructive symptoms, dietary modification is first attempted. Patients should avoid foods that are high in fiber.[110,111] Surgical intervention for radiation-induced obstructive symptoms carries significant morbidity. Distinguishing healthy tissue from irradiated tissue by gross inspection is unreliable. The risk of a leak is, therefore, high when creating anastomoses between irradiated small bowel; thus, surgical intervention is avoided in the absence of high-grade obstruction.[112] If an operation is indeed necessary, an intestinal bypass rather than a resection may be the preferred approach. It has been shown to lead to long-term alleviation of obstruction with successful palliation in this setting.[113]

Intussusception

Intussusception is uncommon in adults and is an uncommon cause of SBO.[114,115] The presentation of intussusception is variable and can be chronic or acute. Timely diagnosis requires CT imaging and a high index of suspicion, because the symptoms of intussusception are often nonspecific.[116] It is caused by a lead point or structural abnormality in up to 90% of cases. If a patient is asymptomatic with enteroenteric intussusception (as opposed to ileocolonic or colocolonic intussusception, which have a higher frequency of associated malignancy[117–119]), it may be transient, especially in the setting of inflammatory conditions of the small bowel.[120] If there is any doubt about the etiology of an intussusception, formal resection is recommended.[116]

Intussusception can be anterograde where the proximal bowel is carried forward into the distal bowel in the direction of peristalsis. Retrograde intussusception occurs when an anastomosis is pushed proximally in the opposite direction of peristalsis, as is seen after Roux-en-Y reconstruction of the intestine. Owing to the increased number of structural abnormalities involved in adult intussusception, resection is recommended. There is some debate regarding reduction of the intussusceptum before resection in the small bowel where malignancy is less likely. At this point, there is no gold standard and clinical judgment is advised. There have been studies that show laparoscopic intervention, including resection, is safe and feasible.[121] In the case of retrograde intussusception at the site of an anastomosis, reduction alone or reduction with enteropexy are additional surgical options.

Hernias

- Evidence supports laparoscopic enterolysis when possible.
- Increasing evidence supports the use of synthetic mesh for strangulated hernia repair, even with bowel resection.

Hernias are a common cause for incarcerated and strangulated SBO.[122] Any patient presenting with evidence of an SBO should be examined for hernias. A typical workup for these includes physical examination of the abdominal wall, including inguinal and flank areas, as well as CT imaging. Any identified hernia that is suspected of causing symptoms should undergo attempted manual reduction. If this procedure fails, urgent operative intervention is appropriate.

Surgical repair of an SBO owing to a hernia may result in a clean contaminated or contaminated case with nonviable bowel, bowel resection, or frank perforation. Historically, there has been a predilection to avoid placing mesh in these cases owing to the concern for surgical site infection or mesh infection. However, more modern meshes and techniques have challenged this management scheme. Certainly, primary repair of a ventral, incisional, or inguinal hernia has a higher incidence of recurrence that approaches unacceptable rates (63%).[123]

To these authors' knowledge, there are no synthetic, biologic, or biosynthetic meshes that are indicated for use in contaminated or clean contaminated procedures. In recent history, biologic mesh was used in such cases. Over the past decade, mesh construct has evolved and there has been a shift to macroporous models of synthetic mesh. This design seems to have improved the ability of synthetic meshes to survive infections.[124] There is very little literature to offer guidance in this area.

There is evidence to support the use of prosthetic material in urgent inguinal repairs whether there is a need for removal of nonviable tissue (including bowel resection).[125] Ventral and incisional hernia repair in the setting of a clean contaminated or contaminated case is challenging given the structural and physiologic variability with which individual patients present. Comparisons of synthetic mesh and primary suture repair in incarcerated and strangulated ventral and incisional hernias that require bowel resection have demonstrated similar surgical site infection rates but lower recurrence rates with mesh.[123,126] Prophylactic placement of mesh was compared with no mesh in patients undergoing ventral or incisional hernia repair with simultaneous stoma closure. Both had similar surgical site infection rates. In these patients, mesh placement in a clean contaminated procedure did not significantly change the infection rates.[127] Another study compared biologic mesh placement to synthetic mesh placement in Ventral Hernia Working Group class II wounds (essentially higher risk patients with diabetes, previous infections, etc). The biologic mesh had a significantly higher hernia recurrence rate (14.8% vs 0%) when compared with synthetic mesh placement.[128] An inference from this finding is that more complex hernias have higher recurrence rates with biologic mesh.

Because there are no studies to directly answer the question of when and in whom to place mesh during an emergent hernia repair for bowel obstruction, we are left with inference based on data from other studies, reliance on expert opinions, and dependence on our own experience. No meshes carry an indication for contaminated or clean contaminated cases. Mesh placement decreases hernia recurrence rates. Biologic meshes are far more expensive than synthetic and have a higher hernia recurrence rate. Newer synthetic meshes may be safely used in clean contaminated or contaminated procedures, but definitive evidence is lacking.[129] Large registries such as that promulgated by the Americas Hernia Society may add additional data, the analysis of which will help to determine the risks of wound and mesh infections as they are balanced against the increased risks of recurrent hernias in nonmesh repairs.

Bariatric Surgery

The American Society for Metabolic and Bariatric Surgery reports an estimated 196,000 bariatric procedures performed in the United States in 2015 with 23% of them being laparoscopic Roux-en-Y gastric bypass. Bariatric patients can present with obstruction from the same causes as all other patients, but also carry a greater risk of internal hernia, intussusception, and closed loop obstructions owing to surgical creation of mesenteric defects. There is a great deal of discussion regarding the usefulness of closure of mesenteric defects at the initial surgery. Some data suggest that closure of mesenteric defects decreases the risk of subsequent internal herniation after gastric bypass.[130,131] Bariatric patients can also have variable presentation and radiologic findings depending on the limbs of intestine involved and whether a hernia or intussusception is intermittent. Of the 3.9% of bariatric patients studied who required an operation for SBO, 30.1% had adhesion disease, 27.6% had internal hernia, 11.8% had adhesions causing kinking of the biliopancreatic limb, and 9.5% had intussusception of the jejunojejunal anastomosis.[132]

Gastric bypass patients with obstruction can present with chronic intermittent, progressive, or acute symptoms of abdominal pain, nausea, vomiting, bloating ,or obstipation. CT scan results for patients with a history of laparoscopic Roux-en-Y gastric bypass may be subtle. Significantly dilated small bowel with transition point is often a late finding. Some studies report mesenteric swirl, hurricane eye, and mushroom sign, as well as more subtle finding such as engorged mesenteric vessels and small bowel edema, which can be present even when frank obstruction is not observed.[133–135] In addition to leukocytosis and lactic acidosis, which are followed in all patients with SBO, elevated amylase and/or lipase may be a significant finding in this patient population, especially with acute obstruction of the biliopancreatic limb. Thus, amylase or lipase ought to be drawn on all Roux-en-Y gastric bypass patients presenting with abdominal pain, and biliopancreatic limb obstruction should be ruled out if enzymes are elevated or other evidence of pancreatitis is present.[136]

Once SBO is suspected, early operative intervention is recommended for bariatric patients. Early postoperative SBO after Roux-en-Y gastric bypass is rare and requires prompt surgical intervention to prevent morbidity or mortality related to anastomotic leak or disruption.[137] Patients who have undergone Roux-en-Y gastric bypass surgery and have an SBO are 3 times as likely as patients without a history of Roux-en-Y gastric bypass surgery who have an SBO to require surgical intervention.[138] Laparoscopic approach is determined by surgeon preference and patient presentation. Type of surgical intervention depends on operative findings and may require enterolysis, reduction of hernia, repair of abdominal wall defect, and/or repair of mesenteric defects. Retrograde intussusception (antiperistaltic telescoping of the common channel limb into the jejunal anastomosis) is an uncommon late cause of SBO in this population. Options for treating intussusception include reduction, reduction with enteropexy, or resection and revision.[139]

In clinical practice, Roux-en-Y gastric bypass patients with SBO will often present with a history of laparoscopic Roux-en-Y gastric bypass many years prior with effective weight loss after the surgery. The patient may report weeks or months of intermittent abdominal pain and nausea, and usually experience retching rather than vomiting. They rarely appear distended but may complain of bloating. Routine physical examination and laboratory tests are appropriate, including a complete blood count, basic metabolic panel, lactic acid, lipase, and amylase. We recommend reviewing the CT scan with the radiologist to discuss any subtle findings. Have a lower threshold to proceed to the operating room for any suspicious finding. Early intervention is necessary to prevent the loss of significant portions of bowel to ischemia with resulting increased morbidity and mortality. Laparoscopic enterolysis is feasible and safe. Intraoperatively, these cases can be confusing because nearly the entire length of bowel can be involved in the hernia defect. Careful bowel handling and clearly identifying all 3 limbs is essential, because mesenteric or internal hernia can occur at multiple sites.

Inflammatory Bowel Disease

Inflammatory bowel disease, usually Crohn's disease, is a relatively uncommon cause of SBO, accounting for approximately 7% of all SBO.[140] A disease-specific history is essential for any patient with inflammatory bowel disease with SBO to elucidate current symptoms, overall chronicity of disease, current and historical medical therapies, and prior surgical interventions.

For some patients, symptoms of abdominal pain and distention, decreased stool output, and inability to tolerate oral intake may represent the first presentation of the disease. Radiographic imaging, usually by CT scanning as an initial screening examination, may confirm the location of actively diseased segments if enteric contrast is used.[141] Nonoperative management, including bowel rest, IV hydration, and selective bowel decompression, is generally successful; however, IV corticosteroids may be required to aid in decreasing bowel wall inflammation.[142]

Patients with chronic Crohn's disease with a stricturing pattern of disease may present with single or multifocal sites of fibrotic stricture formation leading to SBO. In this setting, nonoperative management may be successful; however, recurrence rates are high. Surgical options include resection and anastomosis or stricturoplasty. Resection and anastomosis is typically used in patients with a single segment of small bowel disease or ileocolonic involvement, with some literature suggesting an improvement in time to recurrence over stricturoplasty. Stricturoplasty remains an effective strategy when multiple short segments or long singular segments of stricture are identified where resection would compromise overall bowel length. The length of stricture usually determines the type of stricturoplasty performed. Short segments (<10 cm) may be managed with a Heineke-Mickulicz–type stricturoplasty, whereas medium segments of stricture 10 to 20 cm in length may be managed with a Finney-type stricturoplasty. Even longer segments of stricture may require a side-to-side isoperistaltic strictuorplasty.[143,144] Preoperative factors such as malnutrition (hypoalbuminemia, weight loss, psoas atrophy), steroid use, free or contained perforation of the bowel, and phlegmonous involvement of a diseased segment are typical contraindications to both primary anastomosis and stricturoplasty. If emergent surgical intervention is required in the face of such conditions, stoma creation should be considered to prevent the morbidity of anastomotic complications.

Patients with chronic Crohn's disease with a penetrating pattern of disease may also present with SBO, but are more likely to have associated inflammatory or phlegmonous changes. In the absence of peritonitis or clinical decline, nonoperative management should be used. Bowel rest, nutritional support, and control of local sepsis (commonly via antibiotics and percutaneous abscess drainage, if necessary) can frequently serve as a bridge to a less morbid, planned resection.[145]

Although the lack of small bowel involvement makes encountering SBO in active ulcerative colitis less likely, adhesive SBO may occur in patients with prior colectomy or proctocolectomy for ulcerative colitis.[146] Nonoperative management should be used routinely, absent indications for urgent surgery. If operative intervention is required, patients with prior reconstruction with an ileal pouch-anal anastomosis (commonly a J- or S-type pouch) may have a dilated pouch that extends out of the pelvis and may easily be injured during enterolysis. In similar patients, it is also important to rule out a distal ileoanal anastomotic stricture as a source of obstruction, which may require operative dilation.[147]

SUMMARY

Identifying patients with SBO who require immediate operative intervention and those who will fail nonoperative management is an ongoing challenge. In the absence of indications for urgent operative intervention, a CT scan with and without IV contrast should be obtained in most patients to identify the location, grade, and etiology of the obstruction. Most SBO will resolve with nonoperative management, including NGT decompression, serial examinations, and a water-soluble contrast challenge. Both open and laparoscopic operative management are acceptable approaches. Malnutrition needs to be identified early and immediately intervened upon, especially if the patient is to undergo operative management. Confounding conditions in SBO patients, such as age greater than 65, post Roux-en-Y gastric bypass, inflammatory bowel disease, malignancy, virgin abdomen, pregnancy, hernia, and early postoperative state deserve special consideration.

REFERENCES

1. Bizer LS, Liebling RW, Delany HM, et al. Small bowel obstruction: the role of nonoperative treatment in simple intestinal obstruction and predictive criteria for strangulation obstruction. Surgery 1981;89(4):407–13.
2. Bickell NA, Federman AD, Aufses AH Jr. Influence of time on risk of bowel resection in complete small bowel obstruction. J Am Coll Surg 2005;201(6):847–54.
3. Choudhry AJ, Haddad NN, Rivera M, et al. Medical malpractice in the management of small bowel obstruction: a 33-year review of case law. Surgery 2016;160(4):1017–27.
4. Foster NM, McGory ML, Zingmond DS, et al. Small bowel obstruction: a population-based appraisal. J Am Coll Surg 2006;203(2):170–6.
5. Dayton MT, Dempsey DT, Larson GM, et al. New paradigms in the treatment of small bowel obstruction. Curr Probl Surg 2012;49(11):642–717.
6. Davies SW, Gillen JR, Guidry CA, et al. A comparative analysis between laparoscopic and open adhesiolysis at a tertiary care center. Am surg 2014;80(3):261–9.
7. Wang PY, Wang X, Zhang L, et al. Bezoar-induced small bowel obstruction: clinical characteristics and diagnostic value of multi-slice spiral computed tomography. World J Gastroenterol 2015;21(33):9774–84.
8. Rhodes A, Evans LE, Alhazzani W, et al. Surviving sepsis campaign: international guidelines for management of sepsis and septic shock: 2016. Crit Care Med 2017;45(3):486–552.
9. Ellis H, Moran BJ, Thompson JN, et al. Adhesion-related hospital readmissions after abdominal and pelvic surgery: a retrospective cohort study. Lancet 1999;353(9163):1476–80.
10. Tingstedt B, Isaksson J, Andersson R. Long-term follow-up and cost analysis following surgery for small bowel obstruction caused by intra-abdominal adhesions. Br J Surg 2007;94(6):743–8.
11. Colonna AL, Byrge NR, Nelson SD, et al. Nonoperative management of adhesive small bowel obstruction: what is the break point? Am J Surg 2016;212(6):1214–21.
12. Maung AA, Johnson DC, Piper GL, et al. Evaluation and management of small-bowel obstruction: an Eastern Association for the Surgery of Trauma practice management guideline. J Trauma Acute Care Surg 2012;73(5 Suppl 4):S362–9.
13. Azagury D, Liu RC, Morgan A, et al. Small bowel obstruction: a practical step-by-step evidence-based approach to evaluation, decision making, and management. J Trauma Acute Care Surg 2015;79(4):661–8.
14. Jang TB, Schindler D, Kaji AH. Predictive value of signs and symptoms for small bowel obstruction in patients with prior surgery. Emerg Med J 2012;29(9):769–70.

15. Jancelewicz T, Vu LT, Shawo AE, et al. Predicting strangulated small bowel obstruction: an old problem revisited. J Gastrointest Surg 2009;13(1):93–9.
16. O'Malley RG, Al-Hawary MM, Kaza RK, et al. MDCT findings in small bowel obstruction: implications of the cause and presence of complications on treatment decisions. Abdom Imaging 2015;40(7):2248–62.
17. Di Saverio S, Coccolini F, Galati M, et al. Bologna guidelines for diagnosis and management of adhesive small bowel obstruction (ASBO): 2013 update of the evidence-based guidelines from the world society of emergency surgery ASBO working group. World J Emerg Surg 2013;8(1):42.
18. Loftus T, Moore F, VanZant E, et al. A protocol for the management of adhesive small bowel obstruction. J Trauma Acute Care Surg 2015;78(1):13–9 [discussion: 9–21].
19. Chuong AM, Corno L, Beaussier H, et al. Assessment of bowel wall enhancement for the diagnosis of intestinal ischemia in patients with small bowel obstruction: value of adding unenhanced CT to contrast-enhanced CT. Radiology 2016;280(1):98–107.
20. Jha AK. Radiological techniques in the diagnosis of strangulating small bowel obstruction. JNMA J Nepal Med Assoc 2013;52(190):420–6.
21. Tirumani H, Vassa R, Fasih N, et al. Small bowel obstruction in the emergency department: MDCT features of common and uncommon causes. Clin Imaging 2014;38(5):580–8.
22. Hayakawa K, Tanikake M, Yoshida S, et al. CT findings of small bowel strangulation: the importance of contrast enhancement. Emerg Radiol 2013;20(1):3–9.
23. Osada H, Watanabe W, Ohno H, et al. Multidetector CT appearance of adhesion-induced small bowel obstructions: matted adhesions versus single adhesive bands. Jpn J Radiol 2012;30(9):706–12.
24. Suri RR, Vora P, Kirby JM, et al. Computed tomography features associated with operative management for nonstrangulating small bowel obstruction. Can J Surg 2014;57(4):254–9.
25. Santillan CS. Computed tomography of small bowel obstruction. Radiol Clin North Am 2013;51(1):17–27.
26. Millet I, Taourel P, Ruyer A, et al. Value of CT findings to predict surgical ischemia in small bowel obstruction: a systematic review and meta-analysis. Eur Radiol 2015;25(6):1823–35.
27. Deshmukh SD, Shin DS, Willmann JK, et al. Non-emergency small bowel obstruction: assessment of CT findings that predict need for surgery. Eur Radiol 2011;21(5):982–6.
28. O'Leary MP, Neville AL, Keeley JA, et al. Predictors of ischemic bowel in patients with small bowel obstruction. Am surg 2016;82(10):992–4.
29. O'Leary EA, Desale SY, Yi WS, et al. Letting the sun set on small bowel obstruction: can a simple risk score tell us when nonoperative care is inappropriate? Am surg 2014;80(6):572–9.
30. He B, Gu J, Huang S, et al. Diagnostic performance of multi-slice CT angiography combined with enterography for small bowel obstruction and intestinal ischaemia. J Med Imaging Radiat Oncol 2017;61(1):40–7.
31. Zielinski MD, Eiken PW, Heller SF, et al. Prospective, observational validation of a multivariate small-bowel obstruction model to predict the need for operative intervention. J Am Coll Surg 2011;212(6):1068–76.
32. van Oudheusden TR, Aerts BA, de Hingh IH, et al. Challenges in diagnosing adhesive small bowel obstruction. World J Gastroenterol 2013;19(43):7489–93.

33. Bueno-Lledo J, Barber S, Vaque J, et al. Adhesive small bowel obstruction: predictive factors of lack of response in conservative management with gastrografin. Dig Surg 2016;33(1):26–32.
34. Pricolo VE, Curley F. CT scan findings do not predict outcome of nonoperative management in small bowel obstruction: retrospective analysis of 108 consecutive patients. Int J Surg 2016;27:88–91.
35. Teixeira PG, Karamanos E, Talving P, et al. Early operation is associated with a survival benefit for patients with adhesive bowel obstruction. Ann Surg 2013; 258(3):459–65.
36. Kulvatunyou N, Pandit V, Moutamn S, et al. A multi-institution prospective observational study of small bowel obstruction: clinical and computerized tomography predictors of which patients may require early surgery. J Trauma Acute Care Surg 2015;79(3):393–8.
37. Leung AM, Vu H. Factors predicting need for and delay in surgery in small bowel obstruction. Am surg 2012;78(4):403–7.
38. Mullan CP, Siewert B, Eisenberg RL. Small bowel obstruction. AJR Am J Roentgenol 2012;198(2):W105–17.
39. DiSantis DJ, Ralls PW, Balfe DM, et al. The patient with suspected small bowel obstruction: imaging strategies. American College of Radiology. ACR appropriateness criteria. Radiology 2000;(215 Suppl):121–4.
40. American College of Radiology. American College of Radiology appropriateness criteria clinical condition: suspected small bowel obstruction. 2013. Available at: https://acsearch.acr.org/docs/69476/Narrative/2013. Accessed December 17, 2017.
41. Frager DH, Baer JW, Rothpearl A, et al. Distinction between postoperative ileus and mechanical small-bowel obstruction: value of CT compared with clinical and other radiographic findings. AJR Am J Roentgenol 1995;164(4):891–4.
42. Megibow AJ, Balthazar EJ, Cho KC, et al. Bowel obstruction: evaluation with CT. Radiology 1991;180(2):313–8.
43. Fukuya T, Hawes DR, Lu CC, et al. CT diagnosis of small-bowel obstruction: efficacy in 60 patients. AJR Am J Roentgenol 1992;158(4):765–9 [discussion: 71–2].
44. Nakashima K, Ishimaru H, Fujimoto T, et al. Diagnostic performance of CT findings for bowel ischemia and necrosis in closed-loop small-bowel obstruction. Abdom Imaging 2015;40(5):1097–103.
45. Geffroy Y, Boulay-Coletta I, Julles MC, et al. Increased unenhanced bowel-wall attenuation at multidetector CT is highly specific of ischemia complicating small-bowel obstruction. Radiology 2014;270(1):159–67.
46. Sandhu PS, Joe BN, Coakley FV, et al. Bowel transition points: multiplicity and posterior location at CT are associated with small-bowel volvulus. Radiology 2007;245(1):160–7.
47. Carpenter CR, Pines JM. The end of X-rays for suspected small bowel obstruction? Using evidence-based diagnostics to inform best practices in emergency medicine. Acad Emerg Med 2013;20(6):618–20.
48. Katz DS, Baker ME, Rosen MP, et al. Expert panel on gastrointestinal imaging. 2013. Available at: https://acsearch.acr.org/docs/69476/Narrative/. Accessed December 17, 2017.
49. Hollerweger A, Wustner M, Dirks K. Bowel obstruction: sonographic evaluation. Ultraschall Med 2015;36(3):216–35 [quiz: 36–8].
50. Goussous N, Eiken PW, Bannon MP, et al. Enhancement of a small bowel obstruction model using the gastrografin(R) challenge test. J Gastrointest Surg 2013;17(1):110–6 [discussion p: 6–7].

51. Assalia A, Schein M, Kopelman D, et al. Therapeutic effect of oral Gastrografin in adhesive, partial small-bowel obstruction: a prospective randomized trial. Surgery 1994;115(4):433–7.
52. Choi HK, Chu KW, Law WL. Therapeutic value of gastrografin in adhesive small bowel obstruction after unsuccessful conservative treatment: a prospective randomized trial. Ann Surg 2002;236(1):1–6.
53. Ceresoli M, Coccolini F, Catena F, et al. Water-soluble contrast agent in adhesive small bowel obstruction: a systematic review and meta-analysis of diagnostic and therapeutic value. Am J Surg 2016;211(6):1114–25.
54. Zielinski MD, Haddad NN, Cullinane DC, et al. Multi-institutional, prospective, observational study comparing the Gastrografin challenge versus standard treatment in adhesive small bowel obstruction. J Trauma Acute Care Surg 2017;83(1):47–54.
55. Branco BC, Barmparas G, Schnuriger B, et al. Systematic review and meta-analysis of the diagnostic and therapeutic role of water-soluble contrast agent in adhesive small bowel obstruction. Br J Surg 2010;97(4):470–8.
56. Galardi N, Collins J, Friend K. Use of early gastrografin small bowel follow-through in small bowel obstruction management. Am surg 2013;79(8):794–6.
57. Khasawneh MA, Ugarte ML, Srvantstian B, et al. Role of gastrografin challenge in early postoperative small bowel obstruction. J Gastrointest Surg 2014;18(2):363–8.
58. Sarraf-Yazdi S, Shapiro ML. Small bowel obstruction: the eternal dilemma of when to intervene. Scand J Surg 2010;99(2):78–80.
59. Wilson MS, Hawkswell J, McCloy RF. Natural history of adhesional small bowel obstruction: counting the cost. Br J Surg 1998;85(9):1294–8.
60. Aquina CT, Becerra AZ, Probst CP, et al. Patients with adhesive small bowel obstruction should be primarily managed by a surgical team. Ann Surg 2016;264(3):437–47.
61. Cox MR, Gunn IF, Eastman MC, et al. The safety and duration of non-operative treatment for adhesive small bowel obstruction. Aust N Z J Surg 1993;63(5):367–71.
62. Jeong WK, Lim SB, Choi HS, et al. Conservative management of adhesive small bowel obstructions in patients previously operated on for primary colorectal cancer. J Gastrointest Surg 2008;12(5):926–32.
63. Bilderback PA, Massman JD 3rd, Smith RK, et al. Small bowel obstruction is a surgical disease: patients with adhesive small bowel obstruction requiring operation have more cost-effective care when admitted to a surgical service. J Am Coll Surg 2015;221(1):7–13.
64. Malangoni MA, Times ML, Kozik D, et al. Admitting service influences the outcomes of patients with small bowel obstruction. Surgery 2001;130(4):706–11 [discussion: 11–3].
65. Schwab DP, Blackhurst DW, Sticca RP. Operative acute small bowel obstruction: admitting service impacts outcome. Am surg 2001;67(11):1034–8 [discussion: 8–40].
66. Oyasiji T, Angelo S, Kyriakides TC, et al. Small bowel obstruction: outcome and cost implications of admitting service. Am surg 2010;76(7):687–91.
67. Schmocker RK, Vang X, Cherney Stafford LM, et al. Involvement of a surgical service improves patient satisfaction in patients admitted with small bowel obstruction. Am J Surg 2015;210(2):252–7.

68. Musiienko AM, Shakerian R, Gorelik A, et al. Impact of introduction of an acute surgical unit on management and outcomes of small bowel obstruction. ANZ J Surg 2016;86(10):831–5.
69. Scrima A, Lubner MG, King S, et al. Value of MDCT and clinical and laboratory data for predicting the need for surgical intervention in suspected small-bowel obstruction. AJR Am J Roentgenol 2017;208(4):785–93.
70. Baghdadi YMK, Morris DS, Choudhry AJ, et al. Validation of the anatomic severity score developed by the American Association for the Surgery of Trauma in small bowel obstruction. J Surg Res 2016;204(2):428–34.
71. Barkan H, Webster S, Ozeran S. Factors predicting the recurrence of adhesive small-bowel obstruction. Am J Surg 1995;170(4):361–5.
72. Williams SB, Greenspon J, Young HA, et al. Small bowel obstruction: conservative vs. surgical management. Dis Colon Rectum 2005;48(6):1140–6.
73. Meier RP, de Saussure WO, Orci LA, et al. Clinical outcome in acute small bowel obstruction after surgical or conservative management. World J Surg 2014; 38(12):3082–8.
74. Bauer J, Keeley B, Krieger B, et al. Adhesive small bowel obstruction: early operative versus observational management. Am surg 2015;81(6):614–20.
75. Schraufnagel D, Rajaee S, Millham FH. How many sunsets? Timing of surgery in adhesive small bowel obstruction: a study of the nationwide inpatient sample. J Trauma Acute Care Surg 2013;74(1):181–7 [discussion: 7–9].
76. Keenan JE, Turley RS, McCoy CC, et al. Trials of nonoperative management exceeding 3 days are associated with increased morbidity in patients undergoing surgery for uncomplicated adhesive small bowel obstruction. J Trauma Acute Care Surg 2014;76(6):1367–72.
77. Baghdadi YM, Choudhry AJ, Goussous N, et al. Long-term outcomes of gastrografin in small bowel obstruction. J Surg Res 2016;202(1):43–8.
78. Yao S, Tanaka E, Ikeda A, et al. Outcomes of laparoscopic management of acute small bowel obstruction: a 7-year experience of 110 consecutive cases with various etiologies. Surg Today 2017;47(4):432–9.
79. Suh SW, Choi YS. Laparoscopy for Small Bowel Obstruction Caused by Single Adhesive Band. JSLS 2016;20(3) [pii:e2016.00048].
80. Siow SL, Mahendran HA. A case series of adult intussusception managed laparoscopically. Surg Laparosc Endosc Percutan Tech 2014;24(4):327–31.
81. Sajid MS, Khawaja AH, Sains P, et al. A systematic review comparing laparoscopic vs open adhesiolysis in patients with adhesional small bowel obstruction. Am J Surg 2016;212(1):138–50.
82. Kelly KN, Iannuzzi JC, Rickles AS, et al. Laparotomy for small-bowel obstruction: first choice or last resort for adhesiolysis? A laparoscopic approach for small-bowel obstruction reduces 30-day complications. Surg Endosc 2014;28(1): 65–73.
83. Wiggins T, Markar SR, Harris A. Laparoscopic adhesiolysis for acute small bowel obstruction: systematic review and pooled analysis. Surg Endosc 2015; 29(12):3432–42.
84. Vettoretto N, Carrara A, Corradi A, et al. Laparoscopic adhesiolysis: consensus conference guidelines. Colorectal Dis 2012;14(5):e208–15.
85. Behman R, Nathens AB, Byrne JP, et al. Laparoscopic surgery for adhesive small bowel obstruction is associated with a higher risk of bowel injury: a population-based analysis of 8584 patients. Ann Surg 2017;266(3):489–98.

86. Fevang BT, Fevang J, Stangeland L, et al. Complications and death after surgical treatment of small bowel obstruction: a 35-year institutional experience. Ann Surg 2000;231(4):529–37.
87. Springer JE, Bailey JG, Davis PJ, et al. Management and outcomes of small bowel obstruction in older adult patients: a prospective cohort study. Can J Surg 2014;57(6):379–84.
88. Krause WR, Webb TP. Geriatric small bowel obstruction: an analysis of treatment and outcomes compared with a younger cohort. Am J Surg 2015; 209(2):347–51.
89. Webster PJ, Bailey MA, Wilson J, et al. Small bowel obstruction in pregnancy is a complex surgical problem with a high risk of fetal loss. Ann R Coll Surg Engl 2015;97(5):339–44.
90. ACR-SPR practice parameter for imaging pregnant or potentially pregnant adolescents and women with ionizing radiation. 2013. Available at: https://www.acr.org/-/media/ACR/Files/Practice-Parameters/pregnant-pts.pdf2013; https://www.acr.org/-/media/ACR/Files/Practice-Parameters/pregnant-pts.pdf. Accessed December 17, 2017.
91. ACR Committee on Drugs and Contrast Media. ACR Manual on contrast media. 2017. Available at: https://www.acr.org/-/media/ACR/Files/Clinical-Resources/Contrast_Media.pdf2017. Accessed December 17, 2017.
92. Tavangari FR, Batech M, Collins JC, et al. Small bowel obstructions in a virgin abdomen: is an operation mandatory? Am surg 2016;82(10):1038–42.
93. Beardsley C, Furtado R, Mosse C, et al. Small bowel obstruction in the virgin abdomen: the need for a mandatory laparotomy explored. Am J Surg 2014; 208(2):243–8.
94. Won Y, Lee HW, Ku YM, et al. Multidetector-row computed tomography (MDCT) features of small bowel obstruction (SBO) caused by Meckel's diverticulum. Diagn Interv Imaging 2016;97(2):227–32.
95. Miller G, Boman J, Shrier I, et al. Readmission for small-bowel obstruction in the early postoperative period: etiology and outcome. Can J Surg 2002;45(4):255–8.
96. Goussous N, Kemp KM, Bannon MP, et al. Early postoperative small bowel obstruction: open vs laparoscopic. Am J Surg 2015;209(2):385–90.
97. Ferguson HJ, Ferguson CI, Speakman J, et al. Management of intestinal obstruction in advanced malignancy. Ann Med Surg (Lond) 2015;4(3):264–70.
98. Francescutti V, Miller A, Satchidanand Y, et al. Management of bowel obstruction in patients with stage IV cancer: predictors of outcome after surgery. Ann Surg Oncol 2013;20(3):707–14.
99. Pujara D, Chiang YJ, Cormier JN, et al. Selective approach for patients with advanced malignancy and gastrointestinal obstruction. J Am Coll Surg 2017; 225(1):53–9.
100. Henry JC, Pouly S, Sullivan R, et al. A scoring system for the prognosis and treatment of malignant bowel obstruction. Surgery 2012;152(4):747–56 [discussion: 56–7].
101. Mercadante S, Porzio G. Octreotide for malignant bowel obstruction: twenty years after. Crit Rev Oncol Hematol 2012;83(3):388–92.
102. Mangili G, Aletti G, Frigerio L, et al. Palliative care for intestinal obstruction in recurrent ovarian cancer: a multivariate analysis. Int J Gynecol Cancer 2005; 15(5):830–5.
103. Cousins SE, Tempest E, Feuer DJ. Surgery for the resolution of symptoms in malignant bowel obstruction in advanced gynaecological and gastrointestinal cancer. Cochrane Database Syst Rev 2016;(1):CD002764.

104. Zucchi E, Fornasarig M, Martella L, et al. Decompressive percutaneous endoscopic gastrostomy in advanced cancer patients with small-bowel obstruction is feasible and effective: a large prospective study. Support Care Cancer 2016;24(7):2877–82.
105. Laval G, Marcelin-Benazech B, Guirimand F, et al. Recommendations for bowel obstruction with peritoneal carcinomatosis. J Pain Symptom Manage 2014; 48(1):75–91.
106. Peng X, Wang P, Li S, et al. Randomized clinical trial comparing octreotide and scopolamine butylbromide in symptom control of patients with inoperable bowel obstruction due to advanced ovarian cancer. World J Surg Oncol 2015;13:50.
107. Ripamonti CI, Easson AM, Gerdes H. Management of malignant bowel obstruction. Eur J Cancer 2008;44(8):1105–15.
108. Davis MP, Furste A. Glycopyrrolate: a useful drug in the palliation of mechanical bowel obstruction. J Pain Symptom Manage 1999;18(3):153–4.
109. Girvent M, Carlson GL, Anderson I, et al. Intestinal failure after surgery for complicated radiation enteritis. Ann R Coll Surg Engl 2000;82(3):198–201.
110. Sekhon S. Chronic radiation enteritis: women's food tolerances after radiation treatment for gynecologic cancer. J Am Diet Assoc 2000;100(8):941–3.
111. Jain G, Scolapio J, Wasserman E, et al. Chronic radiation enteritis: a ten-year follow-up. J Clin Gastroenterol 2002;35(3):214–7.
112. Galland RB, Spencer J. Surgical management of radiation enteritis. Surgery 1986;99(2):133–9.
113. Lillemoe KD, Brigham RA, Harmon JW, et al. Surgical management of small-bowel radiation enteritis. Arch Surg 1983;118(8):905–7.
114. Laws HL, Aldrete JS. Small-bowel obstruction: a review of 465 cases. South Med J 1976;69(6):733–4.
115. Stewardson RH, Bombeck CT, Nyhus LM. Critical operative management of small bowel obstruction. Ann Surg 1978;187(2):189–93.
116. Loukas M, Pellerin M, Kimball Z, et al. Intussusception: an anatomical perspective with review of the literature. Clin Anat 2011;24(5):552–61.
117. Azar T, Berger DL. Adult intussusception. Ann Surg 1997;226(2):134–8.
118. Yakan S, Caliskan C, Makay O, et al. Intussusception in adults: clinical characteristics, diagnosis and operative strategies. World J Gastroenterol 2009;15(16): 1985–9.
119. Croome KP, Colquhoun PH. Intussusception in adults. Can J Surg 2007;50(6): E13–4.
120. Horton KM, Fishman EK. MDCT and 3D imaging in transient enteroenteric intussusception: clinical observations and review of the literature. AJR Am J Roentgenol 2008;191(3):736–42.
121. Palanivelu C, Rangarajan M, Senthilkumar R, et al. Minimal access surgery for adult intussusception with subacute intestinal obstruction: a single center's decade-long experience. Surg Laparosc Endosc Percutan Tech 2007;17(6): 487–91.
122. Markogiannakis H, Messaris E, Dardamanis D, et al. Acute mechanical bowel obstruction: clinical presentation, etiology, management and outcome. World J Gastroenterol 2007;13(3):432–7.
123. Burger JW, Luijendijk RW, Hop WC, et al. Long-term follow-up of a randomized controlled trial of suture versus mesh repair of incisional hernia. Ann Surg 2004; 240(4):578–83 [discussion: 83–5].
124. Kalaba S, Gerhard E, Winder JS, et al. Design strategies and applications of biomaterials and devices for hernia repair. Bioact Mater 2016;1(1):2–17.

125. Bessa SS, Abdel-fattah MR, Al-Sayes IA, et al. Results of prosthetic mesh repair in the emergency management of the acutely incarcerated and/or strangulated groin hernias: a 10-year study. Hernia 2015;19(6):909–14.
126. Emile SH, Elgendy H, Sakr A, et al. Outcomes following repair of incarcerated and strangulated ventral hernias with or without synthetic mesh. World J Emerg Surg 2017;12:31.
127. Warren JA, Beffa LR, Carbonell AM, et al. Prophylactic placement of permanent synthetic mesh at the time of ostomy closure prevents formation of incisional hernias. Surgery 2017. https://doi.org/10.1016/j.surg.2017.09.041.
128. Fischer JP, Basta MN, Mirzabeigi MN, et al. A comparison of outcomes and cost in VHWG grade II hernias between Rives-Stoppa synthetic mesh hernia repair versus underlay biologic mesh repair. Hernia 2014;18(6):781–9.
129. Rosen MJ, Bauer JJ, Harmaty M, et al. Multicenter, prospective, longitudinal study of the recurrence, surgical site infection, and quality of life after contaminated ventral hernia repair using biosynthetic absorbable mesh: the COBRA study. Ann Surg 2017;265(1):205–11.
130. Stenberg E, Szabo E, Agren G, et al. Closure of mesenteric defects in laparoscopic gastric bypass: a multicentre, randomised, parallel, open-label trial. Lancet 2016;387(10026):1397–404.
131. Brolin RE, Kella VN. Impact of complete mesenteric closure on small bowel obstruction and internal mesenteric hernia after laparoscopic Roux-en-Y gastric bypass. Surg Obes Relat Dis 2013;9(6):850–4.
132. Elms L, Moon RC, Varnadore S, et al. Causes of small bowel obstruction after Roux-en-Y gastric bypass: a review of 2,395 cases at a single institution. Surg Endosc 2014;28(5):1624–8.
133. Iannuccilli JD, Grand D, Murphy BL, et al. Sensitivity and specificity of eight CT signs in the preoperative diagnosis of internal mesenteric hernia following Roux-en-Y gastric bypass surgery. Clin Radiol 2009;64(4):373–80.
134. Patel RY, Baer JW, Texeira J, et al. Internal hernia complications of gastric bypass surgery in the acute setting: spectrum of imaging findings. Emerg Radiol 2009;16(4):283–9.
135. Park J, Chung M, Teixeira J, et al. Computed tomography findings of internal hernia after gastric bypass that may precede small bowel obstruction. Hernia 2016;20(3):471–7.
136. Spector D, Perry Z, Shah S, et al. Roux-en-Y gastric bypass: hyperamylasemia is associated with small bowel obstruction. Surg Obes Relat Dis 2015;11(1):38–43.
137. Shimizu H, Maia M, Kroh M, et al. Surgical management of early small bowel obstruction after laparoscopic Roux-en-Y gastric bypass. Surg Obes Relat Dis 2013;9(5):718–24.
138. Martin MJ, Beekley AC, Sebesta JA. Bowel obstruction in bariatric and nonbariatric patients: major differences in management strategies and outcome. Surg Obes Relat Dis 2011;7(3):263–9.
139. Varban O, Ardestani A, Azagury D, et al. Resection or reduction? The dilemma of managing retrograde intussusception after Roux-en-Y gastric bypass. Surg Obes Relat Dis 2013;9(5):725–30.
140. Miller G, Boman J, Shrier I, et al. Etiology of small bowel obstruction. Am J Surg 2000;180(1):33–6.
141. Zissin R, Hertz M, Paran H, et al. Small bowel obstruction secondary to Crohn disease: CT findings. Abdom Imaging 2004;29(3):320–5.

142. Berg DF, Bahadursingh AM, Kaminski DL, et al. Acute surgical emergencies in inflammatory bowel disease. Am J Surg 2002;184(1):45–51.
143. Yamamoto T, Fazio VW, Tekkis PP. Safety and efficacy of strictureplasty for Crohn's disease: a systematic review and meta-analysis. Dis Colon Rectum 2007;50(11):1968–86.
144. Michelassi F, Taschieri A, Tonelli F, et al. An international, multicenter, prospective, observational study of the side-to-side isoperistaltic strictureplasty in Crohn's disease. Dis Colon Rectum 2007;50(3):277–84.
145. Nguyen DL, Nguyen ET, Bechtold ML. Outcomes of initial medical compared with surgical strategies in the management of intra-abdominal abscesses in patients with Crohn's disease: a meta-analysis. Eur J Gastroenterol Hepatol 2015; 27(3):235–41.
146. MacLean AR, Cohen Z, MacRae HM, et al. Risk of small bowel obstruction after the ileal pouch-anal anastomosis. Ann Surg 2002;235(2):200–6.
147. Marcello PW, Roberts PL, Schoetz DJ Jr, et al. Long-term results of the ileoanal pouch procedure. Arch Surg 1993;128(5):500–3 [discussion: 3–4].

Volvulus

Zachary M. Bauman, DO, MHA*, Charity H. Evans, MD, MHCM

KEYWORDS

• Volvulus • Small bowel • Sigmoid • Cecum • Gastric • Ischemia • Intestine

KEY POINTS

- Intestinal volvulus is a rare disease process but has a high morbidity/mortality if not diagnosed in a timely fashion.
- Most patients with intestinal volvulus require some form of surgical intervention whether emergent or in a delayed fashion.
- High suspicion for intestinal volvulus is required given its rare nature and often vague symptoms to limit intestinal necrosis and prevent perforation because this carries the highest risk of mortality.
- The goals with any intestinal volvulus surgical management are as follows: reduction of the volvulus, removal of a septic source, restoration of bowel continuity if possible, and prevention of recurrence. Because every patient and situation are different, it is important to understand the various surgical options to accomplish these goals and provide good patient outcomes.

INTRODUCTION

The term volvulus is derived from the Latin word "volvere," which means "to roll or twist."[1] This twisting or torsion of a segment of the alimentary tract was first described around BC 1550 in the Papyrus Ebers, where the natural course of the disease led to "rotting" of the intestines.[2] Hippocrates also studied this disease, describing perhaps the first treatment with the insertion of a suppository 10 digits long, or approximately 22 cm in length. Coincidently, modern proctoscopic decompression requires similar instrument length.[1]

It was not until 1841 when von Rokitansky first described volvulus in Western literature, describing it as a cause of intestinal strangulation.[1] Modern Western therapy began to evolve with Gay's publication of transanal volvulus reduction on the cadaver of a patient with sigmoid volvulus.[1,2] Furthermore, Atherton described the first laparotomy and adhesiolysis for treatment of volvulus in 1883.[1,3–5] By the mid-20th century,

Disclosure: The authors have nothing to disclose.

Division of Trauma, Emergency General Surgery and Critical Care Surgery, Department of General Surgery, University of Nebraska Medical Center, 983280 Nebraska Medical Center, Omaha, NE 68198-3280, USA
* Corresponding author.
E-mail address: Zachary.bauman@unmc.edu

Surg Clin N Am 98 (2018) 973–993
https://doi.org/10.1016/j.suc.2018.06.005

surgical management of volvulus had become the mainstay of volvulus treatment with three surgical techniques: (1) detorsion and plication of the mesentery, (2) bowel resection with anastomosis, and (3) the Hartmann procedure for colonic volvulus (CV).[1]

Volvulus remains a rare disease process in the United States affecting 2 to 3 out of 100,000 individuals per year.[6] A volvulus is defined as a loop of intestine that twists around itself and the mesentery that supports it.[6] This often results in an obstructive pathophysiology. If the mesentery is further twisted tight enough or the bowel dilation is excessive, blood flow to the involved intestine can become compromised resulting in ischemia. The mortality related to volvulus is highest in cases that have progressed to necrosis, putting emphasis on the surgeon's ability to quickly identify the disease and intervene.

The small bowel, stomach, and colon are all subject to volvulus. There are a variety of reasons that can cause a volvulus to develop including anatomically variations, medications, lifestyle, changes in physiology, and just bad luck. The various forms of volvulus are discussed in greater detail in the remainder of this article including epidemiology, diagnostic work-up, presentation, and management for these assorted disease processes.

SMALL BOWEL VOLVULUS

Epidemiology

Defined as the torsion of the small bowel around its mesenteric axis, small bowel volvulus (SBV) is typically thought to be a diagnosis in newborns. Approximately 1 in 500 live births have intestinal malrotation with roughly 80% of these patients presenting with SBV within the first month of life.[7–9] As a result, SBV secondary to intestinal malrotation is most common in children and young adults.[10] Adult patients, however, present with either primary SBV (no predisposing anatomic abnormalities) or secondary SBV (precipitated by underlying anatomic abnormalities).[7,11] Patients presenting with small bowel obstruction secondary to SBV tend to be older (>65 year old) and are more commonly female (56%).[10] Examples of anatomic abnormalities causing secondary SBV include adhesions, tumors, previous stoma, pregnancy, Meckel or other small bowel diverticula, and complications following laparoscopic surgery.[11–14] Given the rare nature of SBV in the adult population, limited studies have been completed examining the epidemiologic nature of this disease process. Studies over the last several decades suggest the annual incidence of SBV is 1.7 to 5.7 per 100,000 adults in Western countries and 24 to 60 per 100,000 adults in Africa, Middle East, and Asia.[10,15–17] The large discrepancy in incidence between Western countries and these regions is associated with fiber-rich and serotonin-rich diets and increased fasting in Africa, Middle East, and Asia comparatively.[16]

A recent study by Coe and colleagues[10] examined the US Nationwide Inpatient Sample database from 1998 to 2010 and found that of the 10.33 million hospital admissions for adult small bowel obstruction, only 1% was attributable to SBV. Furthermore, of this 1% with SBV, 0.82% were patients presenting with SBV and intestinal malrotation.[10] This further demonstrates the rarity of this disease process, especially within the United States. Despite the rare nature of this disease, SBV must be kept in the differential diagnosis of all patients with bowel obstruction to appropriately manage these individuals. This is important because the mortality from small bowel obstruction is significantly higher in the SBV patient population (7.92%) compared with the non-SBV patient population (5.61%), making timely recognition of the disease all that more imperative.[10] Although the exact rationale behind this statistic is not yet known, it is thought that because patients with SBV often present more emergently than patients without SBV bowel obstruction, the pathophysiology behind SBV and resultant vascular compromise produces a more advanced bowel ischemia at the time of presentation.[10]

Presentation and Work-up

Given the rare nature of the disease, the diagnosis of SBV in adults is challenging because of its intermittent and vague symptoms, which are mistaken for irritable bowel syndrome, peptic ulcer disease, biliary disease, pancreatic disease, and psychiatric disease.[11,18] If the symptoms are less vague, they usually resemble that of a small bowel obstruction including nausea, vomiting, abdominal distention and pain, and a decrease in flatus production. Stool production should not rule out the possibility of a SBV, however, because stool is stored in the colon for days before defecation. Patients with SBV are more likely to present emergently (89% of the time) with acute vascular insufficiency and peritonitis, therefore high suspicion for SBV must be applied in these individuals because this emergent presentation is directly associated with a higher overall mortality.[10]

Work-up for a presumed SBV should consist of routine laboratory studies, including a lactic acid level. Increased lactic acid levels are associated with strangulated bowel; however, they can lag behind by up to 8 hours.[19] Given this lag time, the diagnosis of SBV should not be based solely on the lactic acid level, but rather the overall presentation and hemodynamic status of the patient. Various imaging modalities are used to establish the diagnosis of SBV and to rule out other causes of abdominal pain and bowel obstruction. Plain abdominal radiographs are not useful because they are often normal appearing or may reveal some evidence of bowel distention.[11,18] Abdominal ultrasonography is sensitive in infants to identify obstruction from SBV; however, it is not as sensitive in the adult population usually because of its dependence on ultrasonography operator experience.[11,20,21] If it is used and successful, it demonstrates either a "whirlpool" sign or classic "barber-pole" sign.[11,21] Furthermore, an upper gastrointestinal series with small bowel follow-though is helpful at depicting a "corkscrew" appearance of the small bowel; however, this test is time consuming and often poorly tolerated by someone with an SBV.[11,22] Computed tomography (CT) is the most reliable imaging modality often revealing the characteristic whirlpool pattern of the mesentery encircling the superior mesenteric artery (**Fig. 1**).[11,23] CT scan also reveals

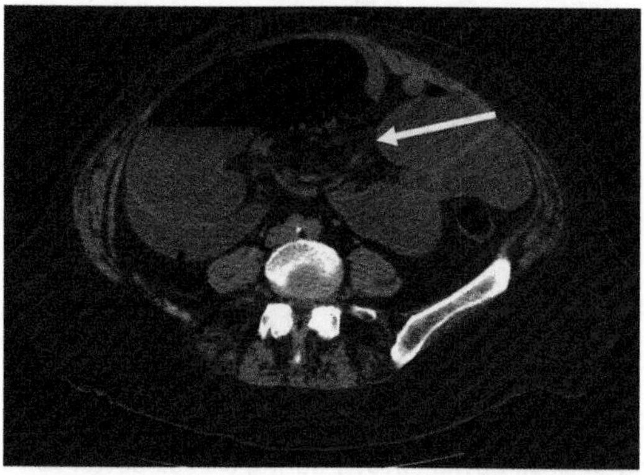

Fig. 1. CT scan demonstrating the "whirlpool" sign of the mesentery (*arrow*) seen in small bowel volvulus.

evidence of bowel ischemia and/or infarction, pneumatosis, bowel wall thickening, intra-abdominal ascites, and any other serious intra-abdominal diseases that may be present.[11] CT imaging may also provide prognostic indicators for the need for surgical intervention. Kulvatunyou and colleagues[24] found that patients with the triad of a high-grade bowel obstruction, presence of free fluid on CT, and absence of flatus on clinical examination have a higher likelihood of needing early surgical intervention compared with patients lacking these three predictors.

Management

Management of a SBV should begin with appropriate fluid resuscitation, placement of a nasogastric tube for bowel decompression because of the obstructive process, and placement of a Foley catheter for accurate urine output monitoring. If the patient is hypotensive or with signs of shock, a central venous catheter and/or arterial catheter may be required for appropriate hemodynamic monitoring and resuscitation. Furthermore, these patients likely require surgical intensive care unit admission.

Most of these patients (65.2%) require surgical intervention for correction and relief of their SBV.[10] In fact, mortality rates are higher for patients undergoing nonoperative management compared with patients undergoing operative management for SBV (11.65% vs 5.94%, respectively).[10] The question remains as to the timing of surgical intervention. If the patient presents emergently with signs and symptoms consistent with peritonitis or acute vascular insufficiency (89.2%), the patient needs emergent surgical intervention (**Fig. 2**).[10] However, if the patient presents without peritonitis or signs and symptoms of an acute abdomen, a nonoperative approach can be initiated. Approximately 90% of nonemergent SBV related to adhesions is resolved with simple gastric decompression and bowel rest.[25,26] The difficulty remains as to when to take the patient to surgery if nonoperative management is unsuccessful at resolution of the obstruction. A recent study by Thornblade and colleagues[27] demonstrated a wide variety in practices among surgeons where patients without peritonitis were taken to the operating room anywhere from 1 to 7 days after presentation for unsuccessful nonoperative management of small bowel obstruction. This study revealed there has been a paradigm shift in surgeon decision-making and patient preferences when it comes to more emergent surgery for small bowel obstruction.[27] Unfortunately, this is a direct

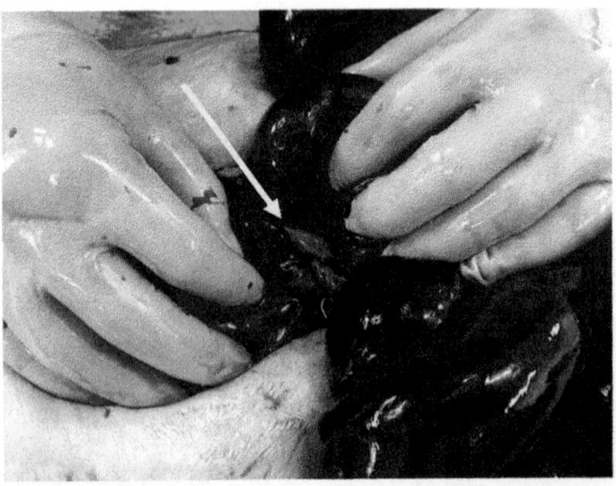

Fig. 2. Tight twisting of small bowel (*arrow*) during a small bowel volvulus surgery. Notice the necrotic bowel from the significant vascular compromise. This patient required emergent surgery for peritonitis on presentation.

result of the lack of evidence in managing patients with a small bowel obstruction secondary to a SBV.[27]

Although exploratory laparotomy is the mainstay surgical management, laparoscopic surgery for SBV has been gaining popularity as more surgeons have become familiar with the technique.[10] Most operative intervention for SBV involves some form of adhesiolysis (32.4%).[10] Small bowel resection or manipulation may be required for nonviable bowel or enterotomies caused by the adhesiolysis, accounting for 46.1% of SBV surgeries.[10] In 23.9% of patients with SBV, the cause is congenital intestinal malrotation.[10] These cases require a Ladd procedure with untwisting of the small bowel in a counterclockwise fashion, division of Ladd bands, widening of the base of the mesentery, appendectomy, and placing viable bowel in a position of nonrotation with small bowel on the right and colon on the left.[28] It is important to manage every patient with SBV individually because the need for bowel resection or other intervention may not truly be known until in the operating room. Furthermore, adherence to good surgical technique is mandatory because missed bowel injuries from adhesiolysis or bowel manipulation can result in intra-abdominal abscess formation, sepsis, and possible enterocutaneous fistula formation.[29]

GASTRIC VOLVULUS

Epidemiology

Gastric volvulus (GV), although rare, is recognized to be a life-threatening condition, thus prompt diagnosis and treatment is imperative.[30,31] It is defined as abnormal rotation of the stomach by more than 180°.[30,32] The exact prevalence of GV is unfortunately unknown in current literature.[33] Peak age group of incidence is in the fifth decade of life comprising 10% to 20% of cases.[30] No association with either sex or race has been identified.[30,34,35] Risk factors for GV in adults include: age greater than 50, diaphragmatic abnormalities, diaphragm eventration, phrenic nerve paralysis, other anatomic gastrointestinal or splenic abnormalities and kyphoscoliosis.[30] Acute GV is a surgical emergency, with mortality rates ranging anywhere from 30% to 50%.[34,36–39] This is often caused by strangulation of the stomach resulting in necrosis, perforation, and septic shock.[30] Because of this increased mortality rate, a high index of suspicion for GV with early diagnosis is essential for a good outcome for these patients.

Presentation and Work-up

GV is classified by its cause and axis of rotation. It can either be primary or secondary. Primary GV is the result of either neoplasm, adhesions, or abnormalities in the attachment of the stomach.[30,35,40] The stomach is normally fixed by four ligaments: (1) gastrocolic, (2) gastrohepatic, (3) gastrophrenic, and (4) gastrosplenic.[30] These ligaments along with the pylorus and gastroesophageal junction keep the stomach from rotating.[30] However, if these ligaments are congenitally absent, or become disrupted or elongated, this may predispose the patient to developing GV.[30,41,42] Secondary GV, however, is related to disorders of gastric anatomy or function or abnormalities of adjacent organs, such as the spleen and/or diaphragm.[30] In adults, secondary GV is most commonly associated with paraesophageal hernias.[30,42] GV is more likely to be secondary to another cause with only 30% of GV occurring as the primary event.[30,34,36]

GV can also be classified according to its axis of rotation. Organoaxial volvulus is most common with an incidence of 60%.[30,35,40–43] It is associated most commonly with paraesophageal hernias and diaphragmatic eventration.[30,35,42] The rotation occurs around an axis adjoining the gastroesophageal junction and the pylorus (long axis).[30] This results in the greater curvature of the stomach resting superior to the lesser curvature causing an inverted stomach.[30,33,44] The distinguishing feature of this rotation is that the stomach is actually laying in the horizontal plane when viewed on radiography.[30,33,35,42] Mesenteroaxial volvulus is less common and characterized by rotation of the stomach along an axis perpendicular to its longitudinal axis, also known as the short axis.[30,33,35,40] In this position, the stomach lies in the vertical plane with displacement of the antrum and pylorus above the gastroesophageal junction.[30,33,35,40] Lastly, and most rare, GV may occur by the stomach rotating about both the organoaxial and mesenteroaxial axes.[30,33]

Clinical presentation of GV depends on the speed of onset, type of volvulus, and degree of obstruction.[30] Pain is common in the upper abdomen and/or lower chest. Borchardt triad, which is present in 70% of patients with acute GV, is the combination of upper abdominal pain, severe retching, and inability to pass a nasogastric tube.[30,34] Hematemesis may also be present because mucosal sloughing may result from gastric mucosal ischemia or a mucosal tear from retching.[30,35,40] Chronic presentation may include vague symptoms, such as mild upper abdominal pain, dysphagia, bloating, and pyrosis.[30,35] Because of the vague nature of these symptoms, they can often be overlooked or attributed to other gastrointestinal disorders, such as peptic ulcer disease and gastroenteritis. GV is more likely to be primary in cause, although a secondary cause can occur.[30,35]

Given its rare nature, GV is seldom considered when a patient initially presents with upper abdominal pain or lower chest pain. Because of this, diagnosis is often difficult and often achieved with conventional radiography.[30,33–35] Although chest radiographs can demonstrate a retrocardiac, air-filled mass and plain abdominal films can show a distended, fluid-filled stomach, these features may not be present in the case of acute or intermittent obstruction.[30,43] Therefore, additional radiographic studies are required. Upper gastrointestinal barium studies are highly sensitive for GV; however, they are usually not obtained given the rarity of clinical suspect on patient presentation.[33,36,45,46] Because of the ease and usefulness of CT, images are often obtained for patients presenting to the emergency department with abdominal pain.[30,33] A recent study by Millet and colleagues[33] demonstrated CT scan has a high sensitivity and specificity for the diagnosis of GV, reaching 100% in the presence of an antropyloric transition point without any abnormality at the transition zone and an abnormally located antrum at the same level or higher than the gastric fundus (**Figs. 3** and **4**). A swirl sign, in which the esophagus and stomach rotate around each other on transverse plane images, may also be evident.[47] CT may also show other anatomic abnormalities that predispose the individual to GV. CT is sensitive for detecting small amounts of free air, free fluid in the abdomen or gastric pneumatosis, which can be a sign of necrosis. Unfortunately, there is no radiologic modality, including CT, which correlates well with stomach ischemia, therefore a high clinical suspicion needs to be maintained during the work-up of this disease.[33] A review of imaging findings in GV is shown in **Table 1**.[48]

Management

Management of GV has changed in recent years showing successful results with surgical and nonsurgical interventions.[30,36,40] On diagnosis, a nasogastric tube should be placed if possible to help with decompression.[30,35,43] Nasogastric tube decompression not only helps with the symptoms of upper abdominal pain and retching, but may also allow the stomach to spontaneously derotate. By resolving gastric distention, tension in the stomach wall is reduced and perfusion improved, thereby

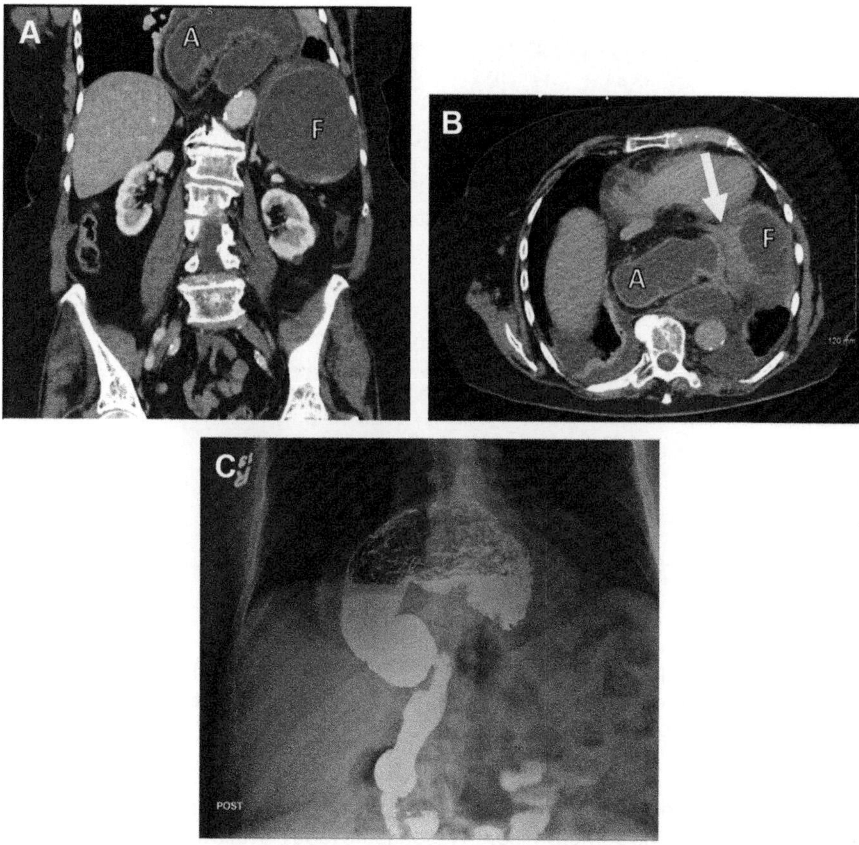

Fig. 3. Organoaxial volvulus of the stomach. (*A*) Coronal view shows the fundus (F) at a lower level than the antrum (A). (*B*) Axial slice shows the twist of the stomach (*arrow*) with bowel wall thickening and the antrum (A) above the fundus (F). (*C*) Upper gastrointestinal barium study showing the "inverted" stomach.

decreasing the risk for gastric ischemia and necrosis. Additionally, placing the patient prone if possible can further help with gastric decompression and placement of the nasogastric tube.[30,35,43] If a nasogastric tube cannot be passed blindly, endoscopy is used to guide the tube into the volvulized stomach. A repeat abdominal film ensures proper position of the tube and effective decompression of the stomach. Early intensive care involvement for invasive hemodynamic monitoring and resuscitation is important, especially if the patient presents with shock or suspected intrathoracic gastric perforation.[32] Large paraesophageal hernias resulting in GV can cause cardiac compression, compromising cardiac output, or arrhythmias.[32] Furthermore, large hernias can result in significant respiratory compromise, which may result in the need for ventilator support.[32] Immediate surgical consultation should be obtained in the case of acute GV because of the risk of vascular compromise and overall patient mortality.[30,41,49] For a significant portion of patients with GV, operative intervention is necessary. However, not all patients are good surgical candidates and with the advent of less invasive techniques to manage this disorder, each patient needs to be evaluated on a case-by-case basis with the type and timing of intervention based on patient presentation and index of suspicion for stomach vascular compromise.[30]

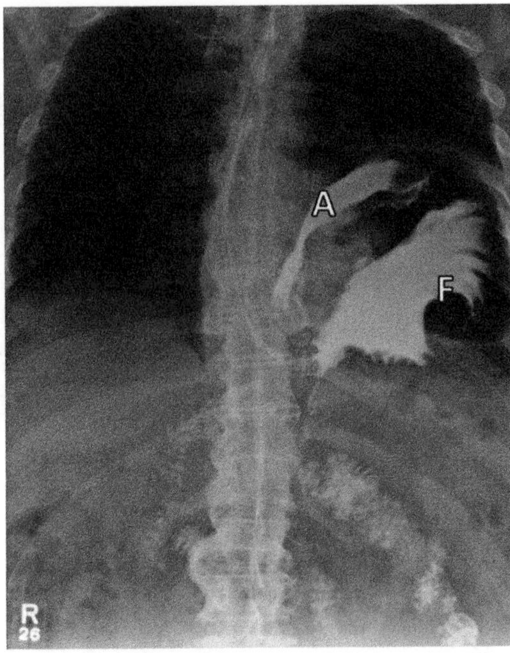

Fig. 4. Mesenteroaxial volvulus. Upper gastrointestinal barium study showing the stomach fundus (F) in the vertical plane rotated along the "short axis" with the antrum (A) and pylorus above the gastroesophageal junction.

Nonoperative management is considered in patients who have no clinical or radiologic evidence of gastric compromise.[32] Nasogastric tube can allow for decompression of the stomach and actual reduction of the GV. However, given the fact that most GV is related to a diaphragmatic defect, the likelihood of repeat volvulus is high.[32] Endoscopy can also play a role in the management of GV. It is used diagnostically and therapeutically.[32] The viability of the gastric mucosa can be assessed and like a sigmoid volvulus, distention of the stomach can lead to unfolding of the GV.[32] Because endoscopy is less invasive than surgery, it may be better tolerated than surgery, especially in those patients with multiple medical comorbidities. One intervention that has gained popularity over the past decade consists of endoscopic detorsion and gastric fixation, without repair of the anatomic defect.[34–36,39] If endoscopic detorsion is successful, a percutaneous endoscopic gastrostomy tube is placed, allowing for the stomach to be secured to the anterior abdominal wall.[50,51] This same approach can also be used for the rare patient who presents with acute primary GV. However, if endoscopic detorsion is unsuccessful, surgery is necessary to complete this process. It is important to remember that this intervention does not address the anatomic defect potentially causing the GV, therefore it may be less optimal for patients with secondary volvulus.

If surgical intervention is indicated, the goal is always the same regardless of whether it is emergent or elective: reduction of the volvulus; resection/repair of nonviable or injured stomach to control the sepsis source; nutrition; and prevention of recurrence by repair of any predisposing factors to GV, such as diaphragmatic hernias.[30,32,37,39,49,52] With this principle in mind, several operative strategies should be used in the operating room. Surgery should start with reduction of the volvulus. If there is a diaphragmatic hernia, the hernia sac should be excised if possible because

Table 1
Imaging findings for gastric volvulus

Imaging Type	Findings
Plain radiograph	Chest radiograph • Intrathoracic; upside-down stomach • Retrocardiac fluid level Abdominal radiograph (performed with the patient upright) • Double air-fluid level • Distended stomach • Collapsed small bowel
Upper gastrointestinal barium study	• Distended stomach in the left upper quadrant extending into thorax • Inversion of stomach • Volvulus with >180° twist causing luminal obstruction • Incomplete or absent entrance of contrast material into and/or out of stomach is indicative of acute obstructive volvulus • "Beaking" may be demonstrated at point of twist • Mesenteroaxial: antrum and pylorus lie above gastric fundus
Computed tomography	• Appearance depends on points of torsion, extent of gastric herniation, and final positioning of stomach • Linear septum visible within the gastric lumen corresponds to the site of torsion • Entire stomach may be herniated or only part of it resulting in twisting of stomach. ○ Ischemia may be represented by lack of contrast enhancement of gastric wall or pneumotosis

Data from Vandendries C, Jullès MC, Boulay-Coletta I, et al. Diagnosis of colonic volvulus: findings on multidetector CT with three-dimensional reconstructions. Br J Radiol 2010;83(995):983–90.

it can significantly reduce recurrence.[32,46] Because diaphragmatic hernia is the leading cause of GV, it should be repaired either primarily by reapproximating the crura or placement of a mesh.[30,32,35,36] In most of these patients, diaphragmatic hernia repair is achievable.[32] For patients who are unable to tolerate a more prolonged surgery, simply reducing the stomach with fixation via the anterior abdominal wall and diaphragmatic gastropexy without hiatal hernia repair is a viable option significantly reducing operative time.[32] As Tam and colleagues[53] demonstrated in a recent series, long-term symptomology and recurrence rates were no different between patients with and without mesh placement for paraesophageal hernias. Given these findings, it should be up to the discretion of the operating surgeon whether or not to place mesh. Of note, it is not recommended to repair the diaphragmatic hernia with mesh in the face of a contaminated surgical field.[32]

Once the GV is reduced and the hernia repaired, the other tenant of GV surgery originally described by Tanner is that of gastropexy.[30,32,36,54] Tanner's original description included division of the gastrocolic ligament/omentum along with gastropexy to reduce traction on the greater curvature of the stomach therefore avoiding recurrence.[32,54] Over the years since Tanner first described the operation, an anterior gastropexy has been favored for its technical ease, showing favorable results with comparable recurrence rates.[32,55,56] In addition to gastropexy, fundoplication has also been used in GV repair to prevent recurrence with good outcomes demonstrated.[32] In the case of GV, fundoplication is used primarily for fixation rather than reflux; therefore, loose anterior 180° wraps are preferred.[32] Currently, literature supports either method (gastropexy vs fundoplication) for stomach fixation with good outcomes for both; therefore, which method to use should be based on surgeon preference and the overall clinical picture of the patient.[32]

Gastric necrosis often accompanies the diagnosis of GV especially when it is an acute presentation.[32] Most gastric necrosis occurs at the fundus, which is a favorable anatomic location for access.[32] Because of this location, a perforation or necrosis can either be repaired primarily or excised, often with a sleeve resection.[32] It is important to consider nutrition when operating on these patients. If the stomach is viable and the patient is likely to maintain appropriate calorie intake orally, a gastropexy is performed without feeding tube. However, if there is concern for decreased oral intake or prolonged ventilation, gastrostomy tube is placed at the time of surgery, actually serving as the gastropexy.[32,35,36] If a large amount of stomach has to be excised secondary to necrosis, then a jejunostomy feeding tube should be considered.[30] Lastly, whether or not to proceed with laparoscopic surgery or open surgery is left up to the discretion and skill set of the operating surgeon. Outcomes from either approach are similar and all the tenets of operative intervention for GV are obtained from either approach.[30,32] Whether or not to perform the surgery laparoscopically is also determined by the patient's hemodynamic status. **Fig. 5** demonstrates an algorithm for the management of GV.[57]

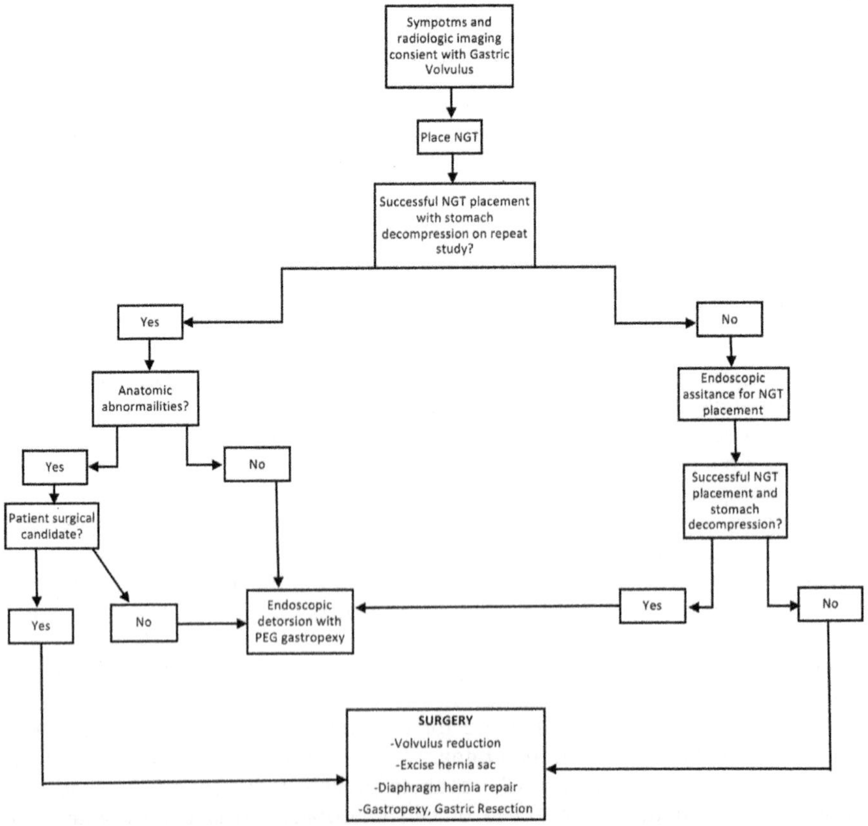

Fig. 5. Algorithm for management of gastric volvulus. NGT, nasogastric tube; PEG, percutaneous endoscopic gastrostomy tube. (*Data from* Refs.[30,32,34–37,39–41,43,46,49,51,52,54–58])

COLONIC VOLVULUS

Epidemiology

CV is the third leading cause of colonic obstruction in the world, following colorectal cancer and complicated sigmoid diverticulitis.[58,59] The condition typically occurs in a long redundant colonic segment that has elongated mesentery with a narrow base.[60–62] CV is rare, representing less than 5% of all bowel obstructions in the United States.[58,60] However, 13% to 42% of all intestinal obstructions in the so-called "volvulus belt," which includes Africa, South America, Russia, Eastern Europe, the Middle East, India, and Brazil, are caused by CV.[58,60,63,64] It has been shown that this difference is likely caused by anatomic differences and differences in diet, altitude, cultural factors, and endemic infections.[60,65–68] CV is most commonly present in the sigmoid colon (60%–75% of all cases), followed by the cecum (25%–40% of all cases), and rarely in the transverse colon (1%–4% of all cases) and splenic flexure (1% incidence).[58,59,69,70]

Sigmoid volvulus preferentially affects elderly men (age > 70 years), which vastly contrasts countries in the "volvulus belt" in which sigmoid volvulus is more common in younger men (fourth decade of life) at a male to female ratio of 4:1.[58,60] The fact that it is not as common in females is anatomically explained by their capacious pelvis and lax abdominal musculature allowing for the untwisting of a floppy sigmoid colon.[60,71] Furthermore, there is also a higher incidence of sigmoid volvulus in African Americans.[60] Cecal volvulus, however, is a disease more commonly affecting younger women (age ≤60).[58,60] This has been linked to pregnancy, because the gravid uterus can elongate the cecal mesentery, and hysterectomies, because pelvic surgery may create a more mobile cecum or create adhesions to which the cecum can rotate.[60,72–76] In the last few years, the incidence of cecal volvulus has been growing more rapidly than that of sigmoid volvulus despite the aging population.[60]

Presentation and Work-up

In sigmoid volvulus, mesosigmoid twisting of up to 180° is considered physiologic.[58,59] It is torsion beyond 180° that leads to complications of colonic obstruction, ischemia, or necrosis with perforation.[58] The most commonly cited predisposing factor for sigmoid volvulus is an elongated sigmoid colon with a narrow mesenteric base.[58,62] Other risk factors that must be kept in mind when working up patients with sigmoid volvulus include diabetes, neuropsychiatric history leading to reduced autonomy, institutional placement, prolonged bedrest, and in younger patients, megacolon caused by Hirschsprung or Chagas disease.[1,58] For unknown reasons, the twist of the sigmoid colon preferentially favors a counterclockwise direction (70% of the time).[77] Once the volvulus occurs, this results in colonic distention, which further results in decreased capillary perfusion and the onset of ischemia.[58,78] The onset of ischemia promotes bacterial translocation and bacterial gas production, further increasing colonic distention and the toxic phenomena.[58] If this disease process is not reversed in a timely fashion, a vicious toxic circle ensues.[58]

Cecal volvulus, however, is likely linked to anatomic predispositions secondary to failure of parietal fixation of the ileocecal region during embryologic development.[58,59] Although common to all CV cases, chronic constipation, high-fiber diet, frequent laxative use, and history of laparotomy may result in slightly high rates of cecal volvulus.[58] Other risk factors for cecal volvulus include pregnancy, pelvic surgery, colonoscopy, and previous laparoscopy.[58,79] There are two distinct anatomic types of cecal volvulus: clockwise axial rotation of the ileocecal region around its mesentery and anterior-superior folding of the cecum without axial rotation, often known as cecal bascule.[1,58] The axial rotation type of cecal volvulus is more common, occurring 80% of the time, whereas the cecal bascule only occurs 5% to 20% of the time.[80,81] Although cecal bascule is rare, it is the more favorable type because it causes less vascular compromise as there is no true mesenteric torsion.[58,82] A summary of risk factors for CV is presented in **Table 2**.

It does not matter the location of the CV; the clinical symptoms are nonspecific and therefore a high index of suspicion is necessary. Sigmoid volvulus often presents with a clinical triad of abdominal distention, low abdominal crampy pain, with constipation and vomiting.[1,58] The classic patient is elderly, institutionalized, and taking psychotropic medications that cause constipation.[58] A total of 30% to 40% of patients with sigmoid volvulus have a history of previous abdominal distention or sigmoid volvulus.[1,58] Cecal volvulus also presents with intermittent episodes of abdominal distention, crampy abdominal pain, constipation, nausea, and vomiting, but in someone with "mobile cecum syndrome," these episodes may spontaneously resolve.[58,83] CV can present with acute vascular compromise resulting in colonic necrosis and perforation. In cases where the individual presents with peritonitis and shock, colonic necrosis and perforation have likely already occurred, resulting in a worse prognosis.[58,84] Laboratory tests, although important, do not point to the diagnosis but rather are a reflection of bowel obstruction, bowel necrosis, and/or sepsis.[58] They should help guide treatment of the patient, increasing the diagnostic suspicion for CV and the overall severity of the patient's disease process.

In addition to clinical examination and laboratory studies, radiographic imaging is important in the work-up of these patients. Plain abdominal radiographs and water-soluble contrast enemas used to be the key diagnostic imagining modalities for CV.[58] However, these two modalities have been almost completely abandoned in favor of CT scans.[58] This makes sense, nonetheless, because CT scan confirm the diagnosis of CV with almost 100% sensitivity and greater than 90% specificity.[58,85,86] Because of its volume acquisition, CT allows multiplanar reconstruction that further facilitates definitive diagnosis.[58] Furthermore, a CT scan can demonstrate indirect signs, such as dilated proximal intestine and colon when the ileocecal valve is incompetent, absence of air in the distal colon and rectum, and it can identify the transition zone between dilated and empty intestine.[58] Lastly, a crucial benefit of CT scan is its ability to detect signs of gravity, which may modify the therapeutic management of the patient.[58] Gravity allows for detection of the degree of colonic distention, direct signs of intestinal ischemia through pneumatosis intestinalis (arterial ischemia) and bowel wall thickening (venous ischemia), indirect signs of intestinal ischemia through free peritoneal fluid or portal venous gas, mesenteric injury with hyperemia or mesenteric

Table 2
Risk factors for colonic volvulus development

Sigmoid Volvulus	Cecal Volvulus
• Chronic constipation	• Chronic constipation
• Recurrent obstipation	• High-fiber diet
• Laxative dependency	• Frequent laxative use
• Hirschsprung disease	• History of laparoscopy/laparotomy
• Diabetes	• Failure of fetal parietal fixation of ileocecal region
• Neuropsychiatric history	• Pregnancy
• Prolonged bedrest	• Pelvic surgery
• Chagas disease	• Colonoscopy
• Institutional placement	

hematoma, and pneumoperitoneum suggesting perforation.[58] A review of imaging findings for CV is presented in **Table 3**.[48] Radiographic images of CV are seen in **Figs. 6** and **7**.

Management of Acute Colonic Volvulus with Ischemia or Perforation

Whatever the location of the CV, criteria for clinical severity and/or radiologic evidence of colonic ischemia or perforation requires emergent surgical intervention. In these situations, aggressive fluid resuscitation must be initiated in a timely fashion, especially if the patient is in shock. Electrolytes and coagulopathies should also be corrected rapidly as to allow this patient to move to the operating room as quickly as possible for definitive source control. Early intensive care involvement is imperative, hastening the resuscitation process and placement of central venous and atrial catheters for better hemodynamic status monitoring. Colonic necrosis and peritonitis are the two main risk factors that increase the risk of mortality with approximately 61% of CV resulting in colonic necrosis.[60,68,87,88] Necrosis can lead to perforation and stool spillage, so obtaining source control in a timely fashion is extremely important.[89] Surgery in this emergent setting should consist of a midline laparotomy with reduction of volvulus and resection of any necrotic bowel.[58]

Whether or not the patient's bowel is placed in continuity is at the surgeon's discretion based on the clinical stability of the patient.[58] If the patient is too unstable, damage control laparotomy is completed to allow for additional resuscitation in the intensive care unit until that patient is able to return to the operating room for definitive surgery.[90] For cecal volvulus, immediate restoration of intestinal continuity is performed with ease by a side-to-side stapled anastomosis as long as there is minimal

Table 3
Radiographic imaging signs for sigmoid and cecal volvulus

Imaging Type	Sigmoid Volvulus	Cecal Volvulus
Plain radiograph	• Large, dilated loop of the colon, often with a few air-fluid levels • "Coffee bean" sign (colon shaped like a coffee bean) • Absence of rectal gas	• Marked distention of a loop of large bowel with its long axis extending from the right lower quadrant to the epigastrium or left upper quadrant • One air-fluid level
Enema study	• Uncommonly performed • A water-soluble contrast enema shows a beak sign	• Uncommonly performed • Nondilated distal colon to the point of the twist
CT	• Large gas-filled loop of colon lacking haustra • "Whirl" sign: twisting of the mesentery and mesenteric vessels • "Bird's beak" sign • "X-marks-the-spot" sign: crossing loops of bowel at the site of the transition • "Split wall" sign: mesenteric fat seen indenting or invaginating the wall of the bowel	• Severe dilatation of the cecum • Rounded focal collection of air-distended bowel with haustral creases in the upper left quadrant • "Bird's beak" sign • "Whirl" sign • "X-marks-the-spot" sign, referring to the crossing loops of bowel at the site of the transition

Data from Vandendries C, Jullès MC, Boulay-Coletta I, et al. Diagnosis of colonic volvulus: findings on multidetector CT with three-dimensional reconstructions. Br J Radiol 2010;83(995):983–90.

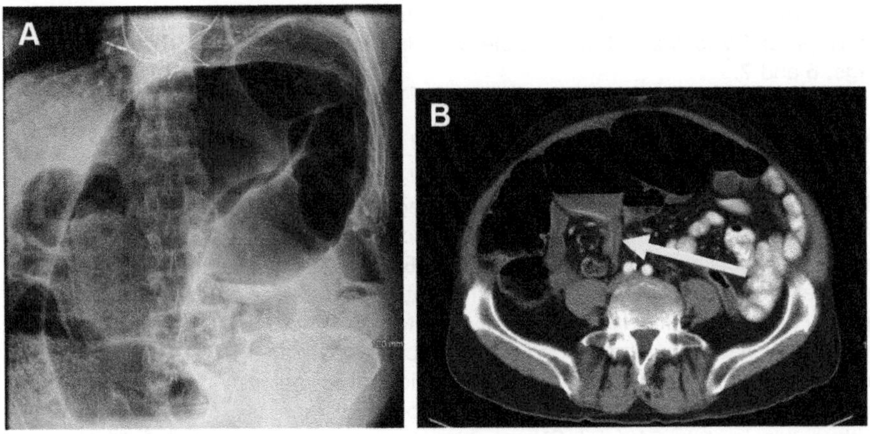

Fig. 6. Sigmoid volvulus. (*A*) Plain radiograph showing severely dilated colon and "coffee bean" sign. (*B*) CT scan showing "swirl" and "bird's beak" sign (*arrow*).

peritoneal contamination.[58,91] This is different in sigmoid volvulus because restoration of continuity is still controversial even in the absence of peritoneal contamination.[1,58] Some studies favor restoration of continuity in the absence of peritoneal contamination demonstrating no difference in mortality between Hartmann's procedure (22%) versus resection with anastomosis (19%).[92] Caution still is the rule and it is wise to proceed with creation of a colostomy if there are adverse local or systemic conditions ongoing.[58] As damage control laparotomy has gained more popularity over the last decade, it is also a viable option that may allow the patient to avoid colostomy at the initial surgery and return to the operating room after resuscitation to undergo restoration of bowel continuity.[90] Damage control laparotomy should not be forgotten when caring for these severely ill individuals.

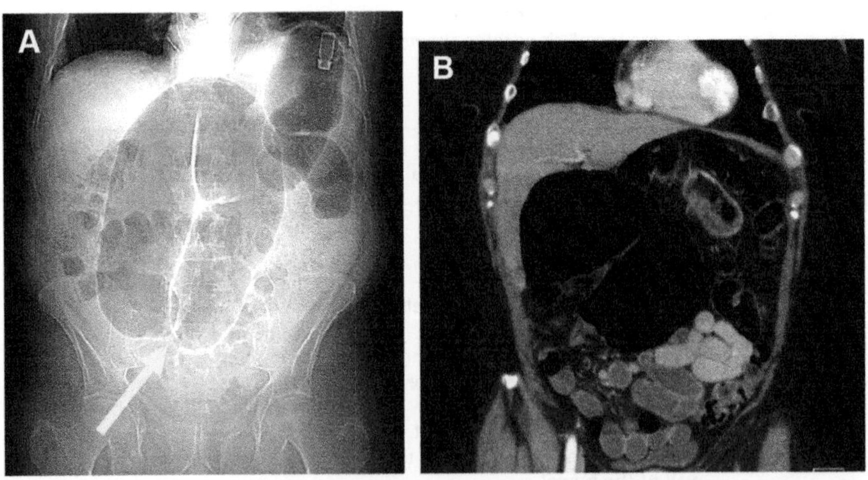

Fig. 7. Cecal volvulus. (*A*) Plain radiograph showing severely dilated cecum and "coffee bean" sign directed toward the left diaphragm. Also note the "X-marks-the-spot" sign where the obstruction is located (*arrow*). (*B*) CT scan showing cecal volvulus.

Management of Uncomplicated Colonic Volvulus

The management of uncomplicated sigmoid volvulus starts with sigmoidoscopy because it is used as a diagnostic tool and as a treatment.[58] Sigmoidoscopy allows the investigator to not only examine the viability of the sigmoid colon, but also to achieve detorsion of the volvulus.[58] If the sigmoid colon appears necrotic, the patient needs to undergo immediate surgery. However, if there is no necrosis and detorsion is obtained, it now turns an urgent situation into an elective one.[58] Colonic detorsion is associated with a 70% to 95% success rate with 4% morbidity and 3% mortality, making it a fairly safe and effective, minimally invasive procedure.[87,92,93] As technology continues to advance, flexible endoscopy is now favored over rigid endoscopy because it has been shown to have superior diagnostic performance.[93] A recent Turkish study demonstrated that although there was a fairly high rate of successful decompression using barium enema (69%), it also had a high rate of morbidity (23%), mortality (8%), and recurrence (11%) compared with flexible endoscopy, which had a decompression rate of 76% and morbidity, mortality, and recurrence rates of 25%, 0.3%, and 6%, respectively.[58,85] Given these findings, barium enema should no longer be considered for decompression of sigmoid volvulus because of its poor safety profile.[58] After endoscopic decompression, a rectal tube is left in place for up to 72 hours to continue the decompression process and prevent further twisting of the sigmoid mesentery.[58] Of note, complete colonoscopy is not necessary in these individuals unless additional pathology is suspected in the more proximal colon.

Nonoperative management after endoscopic detorsion of sigmoid volvulus is fraught with recurrent sigmoid volvulus ranging anywhere from 45% to 71% in current literature.[87,94–97] Furthermore, mortality from nonoperative management ranges anywhere from 9% to 36%.[87,94–97] Given these findings and the fact that there is no randomized controlled trial, the current consensus is to perform colonic resection with 2 to 5 days following endoscopic detorsion.[58,98] Another new option that is used, especially for the multiple comorbidity or institutionalized patients, is that of percutaneous endoscopic colostomy.[58,99–101] Given its minimally invasive approach, it is an attractive approach for patients who likely will not tolerate surgery well.[58,99–101] Despite several authors reporting on its feasibility and low morbidity and mortality, these patient samples were extremely small so these results must be interpreted with caution at this time.[58,99–101] Although a tool available in the management of sigmoid volvulus, percutaneous endoscopic colostomy should not be considered standard of care at this time.

In the absence of a randomized study, the type of surgical treatment of sigmoid volvulus remains controversial.[58] Several alternatives exist, which include detorsion without resection, colopexy, colostomy, and resection with restoration of bowel continuity.[58] Despite these several options, colonic resection with restoration of continuity is the standard of treatment in most of the literature.[1,58,60,102] With a 44% recurrence rate after detorsion alone, 30% recurrence after detorsion with colopexy, and a 13% mortality rate after sigmoidostomy,[60] colonic resection with restoration of bowel continuity has emerged as the superior surgical option with less than 10% recurrence[103] and 9% mortality[60] for uncomplicated sigmoid volvulus.

Cecal volvulus, however, is much easier to manage. Colonoscopy should be avoided because of its low efficacy of only 30%.[91,104] For most cases of cecal volvulus, it should be considered a surgical emergency, consisting of a nononcologic surgical resection of the cecum with a side-to-side stapled anastomosis because this ideally accommodates the luminal size disparity between the ileum and right colon.[58] Furthermore, detorsion and colopexy without resection should also be avoided because it is associated with significant morbidity and mortality.[58]

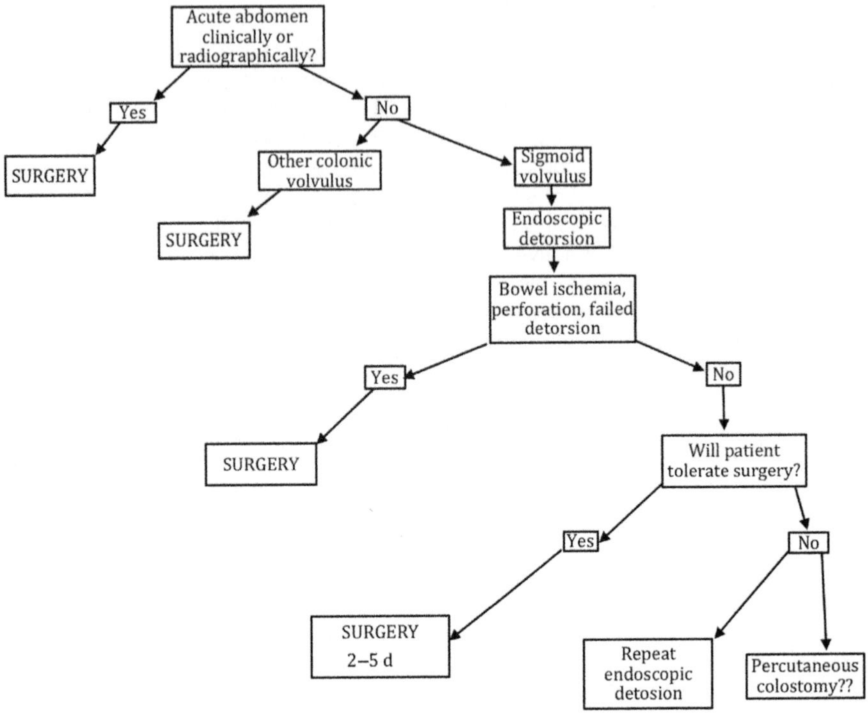

Fig. 8. Decisional algorithm for colonic volvulus management. (*Adapted from* Perrot L, Fohlen A, Alves A, et al. Management of the colonic volvulus in 2016. J Visc Surg 2016;153:189; with permission.)

With the growing popularity of laparoscopic surgery, it can be considered for surgery involving sigmoid volvulus because the outcomes, although limited, have been similar to that of patients undergoing laparotomy.[105] However, laparoscopic surgery is not advised and technically impractical for cecal volvulus given the significant distention of the volvulized loop and proximal intestine.[58] **Fig. 8** provides a CV surgical decision algorithm.[58]

SUMMARY

Intestinal volvulus, regardless of location, is a rare disease process, but one that requires high suspicion and timely diagnosis given the high incidence of intestinal necrosis and potential mortality. Once the diagnosis of intestinal volvulus is made, appropriate and adequate resuscitation is required but most patients with intestinal volvulus require some form of surgical intervention. Recognizing the need for emergent versus more elective surgery is imperative because this can surely change the morbidity and mortality for the individual patient. Furthermore, knowing the appropriate surgical options for the given location of the intestinal volvulus can help guide the operative intervention and prevent future recurrences, which can also affect the overall morbidity and mortality. Because of the rare nature of this disease process, surgeon comfort levels managing intestinal volvulus certainly vary. However, damage control surgery with removal of the septic source is always a viable option that can save a life and allow for additional preparation to definitive surgery. Through early recognition and development of a thorough, individualized care plan, intestinal volvulus is managed with good outcomes.

REFERENCES

1. Gingold D, Murrell Z. Management of colonic volvulus. Clin Colon Rectal Surg 2012;25(4):236–44.
2. Ballantyne GH. Review of sigmoid volvulus: history and results of treatment. Dis Colon Rectum 1982;25(5):494–501.
3. Case by Dr. Atherton. Boston Med Surg J 1883;CVIII(24):553.
4. Peterson MA. Chapter 95: disorders of the large intestine. In: John AM, Hockberger RS, Walls RM, editors. Rosen's emergency medicine – concepts and clinical practice. 8th edition. Philadelphia: Elsevier; 2014. p. 1261–75.
5. Nivatvongs S. Chapter 29: volvulus of the colon. In: Gordon PH, Nivatvongs S, editors. Principles and practice of surgery for the colon, rectum and anus. 3rd edition. Boca Raton (FL): CRC Press; 2007. p. 971–86.
6. National Institute of Diabetes and Digestive and Kidney Diseases. Anatomic problems of the lower GI tract. Bethesda (MD): National Digestive Diseases Information Clearinghouse; 2011. No. 12-5120.
7. Welch GH, Anderson JR. Volvulus of the small intestine in adults. World J Surg 1986;10:496–500.
8. Strouse PJ. Disorders of intestinal rotation and fixation ("malrotation"). Pediatr Radiol 2004;34:837–51.
9. Torres AM, Ziegler MM. Malrotation of the intestine. World J Surg 1993;17: 326–31.
10. Coe TM, Chang DC, Sicklick JK. Small bowel volvulus in the adult populace of the United States: results from a population-based study. Am J Surg 2015;210: 201–10.
11. Huang JC, Shin JS, Huang YT, et al. Small bowel volvulus among adults. J Gastroenterol Hepatol 2005;20:1906–12.
12. Vaez-Zadeh K, Dutz W, Nowrooz-Zadeh M. Volvulus of the small intestine in adults: a study of predisposing factors. Ann Surg 1969;169:265–71.
13. Lay PS, Tsang TK, Caprini J, et al. Volvulus of the small bowel: an uncommon complication after laparoscopic cholecystectomy. J Laparoendosc Adv Surg Tech A 1997;7:59–62.
14. Hu JL, Chen WZ. Midgut volvulus due to jejunal diverticula: a case report. World J Gastroenterol 2012;18(40):5826–9.
15. Cathcart RS 3rd, Williamson B, Gregorie HS Jr, et al. Surgical treatment of midgut nonrotation in the adult patient. Surg Gynecol Obstet 1981;152:207–10.
16. Gulati SM, Grover NK, Tagore NK, et al. Volvulus of the small intestine in India. Am J Surg 1973;126:661–4.
17. Iwuagwu O, Deans GT. Small bowel volvulus: a review. J R Coll Surg Edinb 1999;44:150–5.
18. Fukuya T, Brown BP, Lu CC. Midgut volvulus as a complication of intestinal malrotation in adults. Dig Dis Sci 1993;38:438–44.
19. Tanaka K, Hashimoto H, Ohki T. Lactate levels in bowel strangulation with experimental animal model. Int Surg 2015;100:240–3.
20. Hayden CK Jr, Boulden TF, Swischuk LE, et al. Sonographic demonstration of duodenal obstruction with midgut volvulus. AJR Am J Roentgenol 1984;143: 9–10.

21. Nichols DM. The ultrasonic barberpole: midgut volvulus and malrotation in a young adult. Clin Radiol 2000;55:400–2.
22. Pracros JP, Sann L, Genin G, et al. Ultrasound diagnosis of midgut volvulus: the "whirlpool" sign. Pediatr Radiol 1992;22:18–20.
23. Fisher JK. Computed tomographic diagnosis of volvulus in intestinal malrotation. Radiology 1981;140:145–6.
24. Kulvatunyou N, Pandit V, Moutamn S, et al. A multi-institutional prospective observational study of small bowel obstruction: clinical and computerized tomography predictors of which patients may require early surgery. J Trauma Acute Care Surg 2015;79(3):393–8.
25. Cantena F, Di Saverio S, Coccolini F, et al. Adhesive small bowel adhesions obstruction: evolutions in diagnosis, management and prevention. World J Gastrointest Surg 2016;8(3):222–31.
26. Farid M, Fikry A, El Nakeeb A, et al. Clinical impacts of oral gastrografin follow-through in adhesive small bowel obstruction (SBO). J Surg Res 2010;162:170–6.
27. Thornblade LW, Truitt AR, Davidson GH, et al. Surgeon attitudes and practice patterns in managing small bowel obstruction: a qualitative analysis. J Surg Res 2017;219:347–53.
28. Warner BW. Chapter 71: pediatric surgery. In: Townsend CM Jr, Beauchamp RD, Evers BM, et al, editors. Sabiston textbook of surgery. 18th edition. Philadelphia: Saunders-Elsevier; 2008. p. 2060–2.
29. Bauman ZM, Lineen EB, Lopez PP. Chapter 46: Enterocutaneous fistulas. In: Cohn SM, Dolich MO, Inaba K, editors. Acute care surgery and trauma evidence-based practice. Boca Raton (FL): CRC Press; 2016. p. 383–90.
30. Rashid F, Thangarajah T, Mulvey D, et al. A review article on gastric volvulus: a challenge to diagnosis and management. Int J Surg 2010;8:18–24.
31. Flanagan NM, McAloon J. Gastric volvulus complicating cerebral palsy with kyphoscoliosis. Ulster Med J 2003;72:118–20.
32. Light D, Links D, Griffin M. The threatened stomach: management of the acute gastric volvulus. Surg Endosc 2016;30:1847–52.
33. Millet I, Orliac C, Alili C, et al. Computed tomography findings of acute gastric volvulus. Eur Radiol 2014;24:3115–22.
34. Chau B, Dufel S. Gastric volvulus. Emerg Med J 2007;24:446–7.
35. McElreath DP, Olden KW, Aduli F. Hiccups: a subtle sign in the clinical diagnosis of gastric volvulus and a review of the literature. Dig Dis Sci 2008;53:3033–6.
36. Teague WJ, Ackroyd R, Watson DI, et al. Changing patterns in the management of gastric volvulus over 14 years. Br J Surg 2000;87:358–61.
37. Godshall D, Mossallam U, Rosenbaum R. Gastric volvulus: case report and review of the literature. J Emerg Med 1999;17:837–40.
38. Al-Salem AH. Acute and chronic gastric volvulus in infants and children: who should be treated surgically? Pediatr Surg Int 2007;23:1095–9.
39. Channer LT, Squires GT, Price PD. Laparoscopic repair of gastric volvulus. JSLS 2000;4:225–30.
40. Cribbs RK, Gow KW, Wulkan ML. Gastric volvulus in infants and children. Pediatrics 2008;122:e752–62.
41. Darani A, Mendoza-Sagon M, Reinberg O. Gastric volvulus in children. J Pediatr Surg 2005;40:855–8.
42. Shivanand G, Seema S, Srivastava DN, et al. Gastric volvulus: acute and chronic presentation. Clin Imaging 2003;27:265–8.
43. Karande TP, Oak SN, Karmarkar SJ, et al. Gastric volvulus in childhood. J Postgrad Med 1997;43:46–7.

44. Peterson CM, Anderson JS, Hara AK, et al. Volvulus of the gastrointestinal tract: appearances at multimodality imaging. Radiographics 2009;29:1281–93.
45. Carter R, Brewer LA 3rd, Hinshaw DB. Acute gastric volvulus: a study of 25 cases. Am J Surg 1980;140:99–106.
46. Gourgiotis S, Vougas V, Germanos S, et al. Acute gastric volvulus: diagnosis and management over 10 years. Dig Surg 2006;23:169–72.
47. Oh SK, Han BK, Levin TL, et al. Gastric volvulus in children: the twists and turns of an unusual entity. Pediatr Radiol 2008;38:297.
48. Vandendries C, Jullès MC, Boulay-Coletta I, et al. Diagnosis of colonic volvulus: findings on multidetector CT with three-dimensional reconstructions. Br J Radiol 2010;83(995):983–90.
49. Kotobi H, Auber F, Otta E, et al. Acute mesenteroaxial gastric volvulus and congenital diaphragmatic hernia. Pediatr Surg Int 2005;21:674–6.
50. Eckhauser ML, Ferron JP. The use of dual percutaneous endoscopic gastrostomy (DPEG) in the management of chronic intermittent gastric volvulus. Gastrointest Endosc 1985;31(5):340–2.
51. Baudet JS, Armengol-Miro JR, Medina C, et al. Percutaneous endoscopic gastrostomy as a treatment for chronic gastric volvulus. Endoscopy 1997;29(2):147.
52. Mangray H, Latchmanan NP, Govindasamy V, et al. Grey's Ghimenton gastropexy: an anatomic make-up for management of gastric volvulus. J Am Coll Surg 2008;206:195–8.
53. Tam V, Luketich JD, Levy RM, et al. Mesh cruroplasty in laparoscopic repair of paraesophageal hernias is not associated with better long-term outcomes compared to primary repair. Am J Surg 2017;214(4):651–6.
54. Tanner NC. Chronic and recurrent volvulus of the stomach. Am J Surg 1968;115:105–9.
55. Koger K, Stone J. Laparoscopic reduction of acute gastric volvulus. Am Surg 1993;59:325–8.
56. Siu WT, Leong HT, Li MK. Laparoscopic gastropexy for chronic gastric volvulus. Surg Endosc 1998;12:1356–7.
57. Wee JO. Gastric volvulus in adults. 2017. Available at: https://www.uptodate.com/contents/gastric-volvulus-in-adults. Accessed Janurary 25, 2018.
58. Perrot L, Fohlen A, Alves A, et al. Management of the colonic volvulus in 2016. J Visc Surg 2016;153:183–92.
59. Ballantyne GH, Brander MD, Beart RW, et al. Volvulus of the colon: incidence and mortality. Ann Surg 1985;202:83–92.
60. Halabi WJ, Jafari MD, Kang CY, et al. Colonic volvulus in the United States: trends, outcomes, and predictors of mortality. Ann Surg 2014;259(2):293–301.
61. Brothers TE, Strodel WE, Eckhauser FE. Endoscopy in colonic volvulus. Ann Surg 1987;206:1–4.
62. Akinkuotu A, Samuel JC, Msiska N, et al. The role of the anatomy of the sigmoid colon in developing sigmoid volvulus: a case-control study. Clin Anat 2011;24:634–7.
63. Pahlman L, Enblad P, Rudberg C, et al. Volvulus of the colon: a review of 93 cases and current aspects of treatment. Acta Chir Scand 1989;155:53–6.
64. Oncu M, Piskin B, Calik A, et al. Volvulus of the sigmoid colon. S Afr J Surg 1991;29:48–9.
65. Samuel JC, Msiska N, Muyco AP, et al. An observational study addressing the anatomic basis of mesosigmoidopexy as a rational treatment of non-gangrenous sigmoid volvulus. Trop Doct 2012;42:44–5.

66. Madiba TE, Haffajee MR. Sigmoid colon morphology in the population groups of Durban, South Africa, with special reference to sigmoid volvulus. Clin Anat 2011; 24:441–53.
67. Gama AH, Haddad J, Simonsen O, et al. Volvulus of the sigmoid colon in Brazil: a report of 230 cases. Dis Colon Rectum 1976;19:314–20.
68. Raveenthiran V, Madiba TE, Atamanalp SS, et al. Volvulus of the sigmoid colon. Colorectal Dis 2010;12:e1–17.
69. Hiltunen KM, Syrja H, Matikainen M. Colonic volvulus: diagnosis and results of treatment in 82 patients. Eur J Surg 1992;158:607–11.
70. Merono Carajosa EA, Menarguez Pina FJ, Morales Calderon M, et al. Current management of colonic volvulus: results of a treatment protocol. Rev Esp Enferm Dig 1998;90:863–9.
71. Bruusgaard C. Volvulus of the sigmoid colon and its treatment. Surgery 1947;22: 466–78.
72. Pal A, Corbett E, Mahadevan N. Caecal volvulus secondary to malrotation presenting after caesarean section. J Obstet Gynaecol 2005;25:805–6.
73. Kosmidis C, Efthimidis C, Anthimidis G, et al. Cecal volvulus after twin gestation: laparoscopic approach. Tech Coloproctol 2011;15(suppl 1):S101–3.
74. Whiteman MK, Hillis SD, Jamieson DJ, et al. Inpatient hysterectomy surveillance in the United States, 2000-2004. Am J Obstet Gynecol 2008;198:34.e31-e37.
75. Habre J, Sautot-Vial N, Marcotte C, et al. Caecal volvulus. Am J Surg 2008;1996: e48–9.
76. Pulvirenti E, Palmieri L, Toro A, et al. Is laparotomy the unavoidable step to diagnose caecal volvulus? Ann R Coll Surg Engl 2010;92:W27–9.
77. Shepard JJ. The epidemiology and clinical presentation of sigmoid volvulus. Br J Surg 1969;56:353–9.
78. Altarac S, Glavas M, Drazinic I, et al. Experimental and clinical study in the treatment of sigmoid volvulus. Acta Med Croatica 2001;55:67–71.
79. Chung Y, Eu K, Nyam D, et al. Minimizing recurrence after sigmoid volvulus. Br J Surg 1999;86:231–3.
80. Lung BE, Yelika SB, Murthy AS, et al. Cecal bascule: a systemic review of the literature. Tech Coloproctol 2018;22(2):75–80.
81. Haskin PH, Teplick SK, Teplick JG, et al. Volvulus of the cecum and right colon. J Am Med Assoc 1981;245(23):2433–5.
82. Hasbahceci M, Basak F, Alimoglu O. Cecal volvulus. Indian J Surg 2012;74: 476–9.
83. Rogers RL, Harford FJ. Mobile cecum syndrome. Dis Colon Rectum 1984;27: 399–402.
84. Shepard JJ. Treatment of volvulus of sigmoid colon: a review of 425 cases. Br Med J 1968;1:280–3.
85. Atamanalp SS. Treatment of sigmoid volvulus: a single-center experience of 952 patient over 46.5 years. Tech Coloproctol 2013;17:561–9.
86. Atamanalp SS, Ozturk G. Sigmoid volvulus in the elderly: outcomes of a 43-year, 454-patient experience. Surg Today 2011;41:514–9.
87. Grossmann EM, Longo WE, Stratton MD, et al. Sigmoid volvulus in Department of Veteran Affairs medical centers. Dis Colon Rectum 2000;43:414–8.
88. Kuzu MA, Aslar AK, Soran A, et al. Emergent resection for acute sigmoid volvulus: result of 106 consecutive cases. Dis Colon Rectum 2002;45:1085–90.
89. Atamanalp SS, Kisaoglu A, Ozogul B. Factors affecting bowel gangrene development in patients with sigmoid volvulus. Ann Saudi Med 2013;33:144–8.

90. Becher RD, Peitzman AB, Sperry JL, et al. Damage control operations in non-trauma patients: defining criteria for the staged rapid source control laparotomy in emergency general surgery. World J Emerg Surg 2016;11:10.
91. Consorti ET, Liu TH. Diagnosis and treatment of caecal volvulus. Postgrad Med J 2005;81:772–6.
92. Oren D, Atamanalp SS, Aydinli B, et al. An algorithm for the management of sigmoid colon volvulus and the safety of primary resection: experience with 827 cases. Dis Colon Rectum 2007;50:489–97.
93. Turan M, Sen M, Karadayi A, et al. Our sigmoid colon volvulus experience and benefits of colonoscope in detorsion process. Rev Esp Enferm Dig 2004;96: 32–5.
94. Larkin JO, Thekiso TB, Waldron R, et al. Recurrent sigmoid volvulus-early resection may obviate later emergency surgery and reduce morbidity and mortality. Ann R Coll Surg Engl 2009;91:205–9.
95. Mulas C, Bruna M, Garcia-Armengol J, et al. Management of colonic volvulus: experience in 75 patients. Rev Esp Enferm Dig 2010;102:239–48.
96. Swenson BR, Kwaan MR, Burkart NE, et al. Colonic volvulus: presentation and management in metropolitan Minnesota, United States. Dis Colon Rectum 2012; 55:444–9.
97. Tan KK, Chong CS, Sim R. Management of acute sigmoid volvulus: an institution's experience over 9 years. World J Surg 2010;83:74–8.
98. Tsai MS, Lin MT, Chang KJ, et al. Optimal interval from decompression to semi-elective operation in sigmoid volvulus. Hepatogastroenterology 2006;53:354–6.
99. Baraza IR, Brown S, McAlindon M, et al. Prospective analysis of percutaneous endoscopic colostomy at a tertiary referral centre. Br J Surg 2007;94:1415–20.
100. Cowlam S, Watson C, Elltringham M, et al. Percutaneous endoscopic colostomy of the left side of the colon. Gastrointest Endosc 2007;65:1007–14.
101. Dabiels IR, Lamparelli MJ, Chave H, et al. Recurrent sigmoid volvulus treated by percutaneous endoscopic colostomy. Br J Surg 2007;87:1419.
102. Kasten K, Marcello P, Roberts P, et al. What are the results of colon volvulus surgery. Dis Colon Rectum 2015;58:502–7.
103. Bruzzi M, Lefèbre JH, Desaint B, et al. Management of acute sigmoid volvulus: short and long-term results. Colorectal Dis 2015;17(10):922–8.
104. Renzulli P, Maurer CA, Netzer P, et al. Preoperative colonoscopic derotation is beneficial in acute colonic volvulus. Dig Surg 2002;19:223–9.
105. Basato S, Lin Sun Fui S, Pautrat K, et al. Comparison of two surgical techniques for resection of uncomplicated sigmoid volvulus: laparoscopy or open surgical approach? J Visc Surg 2014;151:444–8.

Acute Gut Ischemia

Bryan A. Ehlert, MD

KEYWORDS

• Acute mesenteric ischemia • Mesenteric arterial occlusion • Mesenteric thrombosis • Mesenteric embolectomy • Mesenteric bypass • Catheter-directed thrombolysis • Retrograde open mesenteric stenting

KEY POINTS

- Acute mesenteric ischemia is a surgical emergency with high mortalities. Common causes include emboli from a cardiac origin and thrombosis of a mesenteric plaque.
- Prompt diagnosis, fluid resuscitation, systemic anticoagulation, and mesenteric revascularization are critical for successful outcomes.
- Revascularization options include open embolectomy or mesenteric bypass, catheter-directed therapies or a hybrid approach of the 2, retrograde open mesenteric stenting.
- Despite technological advances, mortalities have not improved over the past decades, and, although endovascular therapies have improved outcomes, a selection bias exists. Revascularization modality should be chosen on a case-by-case basis.

INTRODUCTION

Acute mesenteric ischemia (AMI) remains a dreaded surgical emergency that continues to be fraught with elevated morbidity and mortality rates. Despite advances in imaging modalities and laboratory techniques, the diagnosis and management of AMI are difficult secondary to nonspecific symptoms at presentation and coexisting comorbidities. Although the advent of endovascular techniques has allowed for minimally invasive therapies, patient outcomes have only seen subtle improvements over the past few decades. This article aims to review the cause, clinical presentation and diagnosis, treatments, and outcomes for patients who present with AMI. The emphasis is aimed at AMI resulting from mesenteric arterial occlusion as a result of embolus and thrombosis, because these conditions most commonly require emergent surgical intervention and revascularization compared with mesenteric venous thrombosis or nonocclusive mesenteric ischemia.

Disclosure: The author has nothing to disclose.
Department of Cardiovascular Sciences, East Carolina University Brody School of Medicine, 115 Heart Drive, Mail Stop 651, Greenville, NC 27834, USA
E-mail address: ehlertb@ecu.edu

Surg Clin N Am 98 (2018) 995–1004
https://doi.org/10.1016/j.suc.2018.06.002 surgical.theclinics.com

CAUSE

Insufficient perfusion that fails to meet the metabolic demands of the bowel results in the underlying pathophysiology in AMI.[1,2] Arterial obstruction is the underlying cause of AMI and can be the result of embolization from a more proximal source or thrombosis of a preexisting lesion. The incidence of embolization versus thrombosis varies depending on the series and institution; however, thrombosis is often found to be the most common cause, accounting for 50% to 70% of cases.[3–6]

Embolization

Emboli originate from a cardiac source in upwards of 90% of cases, with atrial fibrillation and ventricular thrombus following myocardial infarction being common pathologic conditions. Less likely origins include thoracic and abdominal aortic atheromas or aneurysms.[1,7–10] Emboli have a predilection to enter and obstruct the superior mesenteric artery (SMA) due to its size and the angle of origin as it comes off the aorta.[1,11] Furthermore, these emboli frequently become lodged distal to the jejunal branches and middle colic artery, subsequently sparing the proximal bowel and causing distal small bowel and colonic ischemia.[11] The remaining mesenteric arteries are unlikely to be affected by emboli, and involvement of the hypogastric arteries is unlikely to cause clinically significant ischemia given the robust pelvic collateral pathways.[11]

Thrombosis

Chronic proximal atherosclerotic plaques are the common underlying cause of SMA thrombosis, whereas other pathologic conditions, such as vasculitis, aneurysms, and dissections, are rare sources.[1,11] Patients incurring SMA thrombosis often present with a spectrum of symptoms and varying degrees of ischemia dependent on preexisting collateral pathways that have developed over time. This population will often have a history of prior chronic mesenteric ischemia symptoms with the triad of postprandial pain, food fear, and weight loss.[1] With the onset of acute on chronic ischemia, they not only may express symptoms of vague postprandial pain consistent with chronic mesenteric ischemia but also can exhibit sudden, intense pain equal to that of embolic phenomenon.[12] Furthermore, the distribution of intestinal ischemia will vary contingent on the collaterals that have been formed before complete thrombosis. Another distinction between embolus and thrombosis is the anatomic location, wherein thrombosis typically occurs flush with the SMA origin arising off the aorta.[1,11]

CLINICAL PRESENTATION AND DIAGNOSIS

Clinical Presentation

Patients presenting with AMI are usually in their 60s or 70s.[4,6,8,10,13] Women are up to 3 times more prone to suffer AMI compared with men.[14] Almost all patients present with abdominal pain as their chief complaint.[10,12] As mentioned previously, the characterization of the pain may vary depending on the cause of the arterial obstruction. In most cases, symptoms have been present for greater than 24 hours at the time of presentation.[5,10,15] A high index of suspicion is imperative when making the diagnosis, because AMI can be misdiagnosed as pancreatitis, hepatobiliary disease, diverticulitis, appendicitis, or bowel obstruction.[14] The classic description of AMI is severe, constant pain that is out of proportion to physical examination, and patients may experience emesis with the onset of pain.[12] The delay of physical examination findings such as rebound and guarding results from the progression of ischemia from the mucosal layer to the seromuscular layers, and then eventually full-thickness necrosis.

Only when there is full-thickness necrosis does peritoneal irritation occur that translates to classical physical examination features of peritonitis.[1] Other symptoms that may be present on initial evaluation include nausea and diarrhea (30%–40%), hypotension (30%), and blood per rectum (16%).[3,5,10] AMI patients resulting from embolization will often have associated arrhythmias on presentation because atrial fibrillation is the most common cardiac source[1,2] For those whereby thrombosis of the SMA has occurred, they will often describe a history of postprandial pain, weight loss, and food fearing in the weeks to months preceding the acute event.[12]

Diagnosis

As mentioned above, the diagnosis of AMI can be difficult and requires a high index of suspicion.[5,7,10,14,16,17] Reasons for this include the often subtle physical examination findings and the lack of any specific laboratory values.[1,12,14] Although some markers are helpful in raising the concern for the diagnosis, such as leukocytosis, lactic acidosis, elevated creatinine, and elevated pancreatic enzymes, these findings are nonspecific and can occur late in the acute process.[1,2,12] Furthermore, these laboratory findings oftentimes result in providers focusing on other etiologies as causes for abdominal pain, for instance, pancreatitis, appendicitis, or diverticulitis. Although commonly used as a marker for AMI, because of the ability of the liver to clear lactate, lactic acidosis is a late finding that oftentimes represents the presence of bowel infarction.[12] All patients presenting with acute onset abdominal pain with a profound leukocytosis should have AMI included in the differential diagnosis.[12]

Diagnostic imaging plays a pivotal role in confirming a suspected diagnosis of AMI. Traditionally, diagnostic angiography was used for evaluation of the mesenteric vessels; however, this methodology was not always readily available, and the results may be provided hours following the examination.[7] With the advances of computed tomography (CT) imaging, including CT angiography, this has now become the gold standard for mesenteric vessel imaging. AMI can be diagnosed with either standard axial or angiography imaging and is almost universally available with immediate results in most medical centers and all tertiary care centers.[5,14,18] Additional advantages to CT angiography include the ability to evaluate for compromised bowel (bowel wall thickening, free fluid, or pneumatosis intestinalis), cause of AMI (thrombosed plaque vs embolus), and can aid in revascularization planning.[3,12,14] Studies evaluating the accuracy and utility of CT imaging have found this modality to have a sensitivity and specificity of 100% and 89%, respectively, with, positive and negative predictive values 100% and 96%, respectively.[19,20] Although CT imaging has become more efficient and accessible, patients presenting with hemodynamic compromise, gross evidence of peritonitis, and/or severe acidosis do not require imaging and should proceed immediately to the operating room for exploratory laparotomy and possible revascularization.[5,10]

TREATMENT

AMI should be treated as a surgical emergency, and therapy should begin immediately following confirmation of the diagnosis and while awaiting operative intervention. Patients should be resuscitated with isotonic crystalloid infusion; electrolyte imbalances should be corrected (particularly hyperkalemia, if present), and broad-spectrum antibiotics covering enteric organisms should be initiated to protect against bacterial translocation.[2,14] In the absence of contraindications, therapeutic anticoagulation should be obtained with a heparin bolus and continuous infusion, titrated to an activated thromboplastin time 2 times the normal value.[2,14] Vasopressors may also be necessary for patients arriving in distributive shock; however, initiation of these agents should be withheld until appropriate volume resuscitation has occurred so as not to worsen bowel ischemia from exacerbation of visceral vasospasm.[14] Aims of surgical management consist of resection of infarcted bowel and revascularization of the SMA. Whenever possible, revascularization should be performed first so that the viability of the threatened bowel can be assessed before resection. One caveat is the finding of frank bowel necrosis with perforation and peritoneal contamination. In this setting, source control should be obtained with resection of the affected bowel and the bowel left in discontinuity pending mesenteric revascularization.[2,12,14]

Revascularization options include open thromboembolectomy with or without endarterectomy, mesenteric bypass, endovascular therapies such as catheter-directed thrombolysis (CDT) with or without percutaneous transluminal angioplasty (PTA) and stent placement, or a hybrid approach that includes laparotomy with retrograde open mesenteric stenting (ROMS). When planning SMA revascularization, 3 criteria should be considered when determining whether to proceed with an immediate surgical approach versus endovascular therapy:

1. Duration and severity of bowel ischemia
2. Cause and nature of the inciting lesion
3. Availability and capabilities of endovascular interventionalists.[12]

After considering these factors, one of the operative interventions detailed in later discussion should be chosen.

Open Surgical Revascularization

In scenarios where there are clinical or diagnostic concerns for bowel infarction and necrosis, patients should be taken for emergent exploratory laparotomy and for an attempt at revascularization.[3,15] The cause of AMI will impact the operative decision making. In cases of embolic SMA occlusion, most of the emboli will have originated from the heart and be too organized for attempts at thrombolysis. Furthermore, lysis of these clots may result in showering of the material in the distal branches of the SMA, resulting in segmental bowel infarction and need for resection.[12] Thromboembolectomy of the SMA is the standard treatment in this scenario.[1–3,10,14] While continuing systemic anticoagulation with a continuous heparin infusion, SMA thromboembolectomy is performed through a generous midline laparotomy where the transverse colon is retracted cephalad and the small bowel contents are retracted to the patient's right. As mentioned above, only grossly necrotic and perforated bowel should be resected before revascularization. At the base of the transverse colon mesentery, a horizontal opening is made and the SMA and superior mesenteric vein (SMV) can be dissected out. The SMV is usually encountered first, and small branches and tributaries will need to be ligated and divided to reach the SMA. The SMA will be encountered to the left of the SMV. A segment of the SMA, usually between the middle and right colic branches, is circumferentially dissected free and proximal and distal control obtained with silastic vessel loops. At this time, it should be confirmed with the anesthesia team that the patient has remained anticoagulated, and if not appropriately anticoagulated, a heparin bolus of 5000 units should be given. Most embolic occlusions occur from a cardiac source and lodge in a relatively normal vessel. If the dissection portion of the SMA is soft, a transverse arteriotomy is made and extended with Potts scissors if necessary (**Fig. 1**). Balloon-tipped embolectomy catheters are then passed proximally until all clot burden has been retrieved and there is return of normal pulsatile inflow. Next, a smaller catheter should be passed distally to ensure removal of any fragmented or synchronous embolus. Care should be taken during

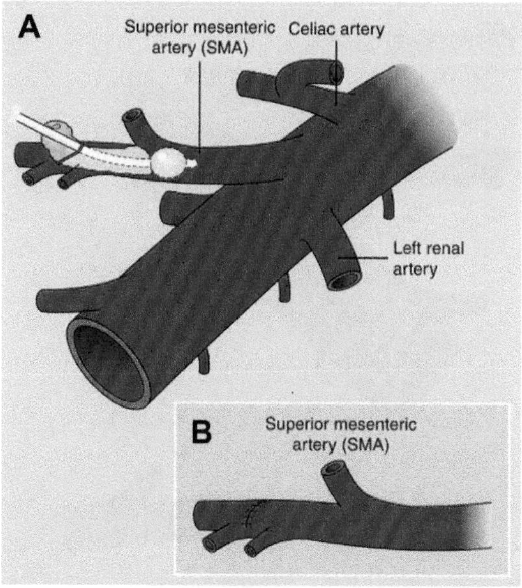

Fig. 1. Surgical technique for open thromboembolectomy of the SMA. (*A*) Following dissection and control of the SMA, an arteriotomy is performed and a balloon-tipped embolectomy catheter is used to retrieve the embolus to restore normal arterial inflow. (*B*) In a healthy SMA, a transverse arteriotomy can be closed primarily with interrupted polypropylene suture. (*From* Bower TC, Oderich GS. Acute and chronic mesenteric ischemia. In: Hallet JW, editor. Comprehensive vascular and endovascular surgery. 2nd edition. Philadelphia: Mosby Elsevier; 2009. p. 339–50; with permission.)

passage of the catheter distally, because the distal SMA and its branches are fragile and prone to dissection or perforation. Following retrieval of all clot burden and return of normal inflow, the artery should be flushed with heparinized saline and the arteriotomy can then be closed primarily with interrupted polypropylene suture. In patients with a calcified or diseased SMA, the same dissection is carried out; however, a longitudinal arteriotomy with patch angioplasty may be necessary to prevent narrowing of the SMA (**Fig. 2**). Options for a patch include saphenous or gonadal vein, bovine pericardium, or prosthetic patches. Prosthetic patches should be avoided in the setting of gross peritoneal contamination.

Surgical bypass is oftentimes necessary in the presence of a thrombosed SMA plaque.[2,11,14] Attempts at thromboembolectomy can be made; however, sufficient inflow to adequately perfuse the ischemic bowel is difficult to maintain. Surgical bypass may be constructed in an antegrade fashion from the supraceliac aorta or retrograde from the infrarenal aorta or iliac artery. Dissection of the supraceliac aorta may be time consuming and proximal control tedious, with the added hemodynamic effects of an aortic cross-clamp. As such, a retrograde bypass is often preferred for efficiency.[12,14,21] The infrarenal aorta or common iliac arteries are exposed by dividing the peritoneum overlying them. If using the infrarenal aorta for inflow, care should be taken to not injure or avulse the lumbar arteries or veins. For the iliac arteries, the neighboring iliac vein can easily be injured if meticulous dissection is not performed. The saphenous or femoral vein can be used for conduit in the presence of gross peritoneal contamination; however, prosthetic grafts are thought to be less prone to kink or buckle.[21] The graft is fashioned in a C-loop configuration to help

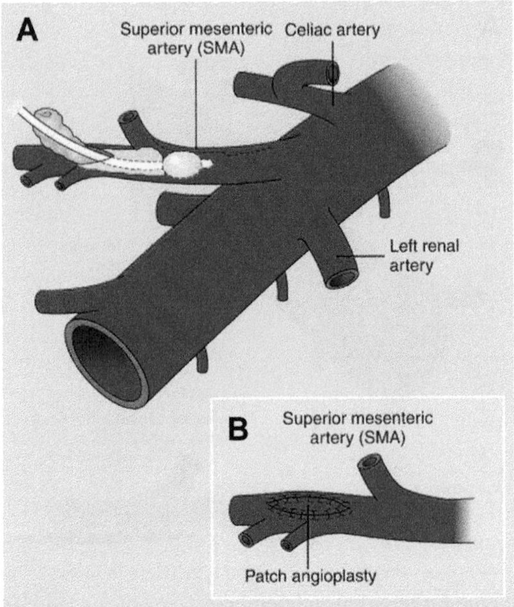

Fig. 2. Surgical technique for open thromboembolectomy of the SMA with patch angioplasty closure. (*A*) Again, an arteriotomy is performed and a balloon-tipped embolectomy catheter is used to retrieve the embolus to restore normal arterial inflow. In a diseased SMA, the arteriotomy may need to be extended longitudinally and limited endarterectomy performed depending on severity of disease present. (*B*) The longitudinal arteriotomy is closed with a patch angioplasty. (*From* Bower TC, Oderich GS. Acute and chronic mesenteric ischemia. In: Hallet JW, editor. Comprehensive vascular and endovascular surgery. 2nd edition. Philadelphia: Mosby Elsevier; 2009. p. 339–50; with permission.)

prevent kinking or buckling of the graft, and this also allows for the distal anastomosis to the SMA to be constructed in an antegrade fashion. With the presentation of a thrombosed SMA plaque, there is likely to be multivessel disease that also includes the celiac artery. In the acute setting, only revascularization of the SMA is necessary.[14,21] Before completion of the distal anastomosis, flushing maneuvers should be performed to clear out any residual thrombus, debris, or air from the graft and native vessels.

Following completion of the revascularization, hemostasis is achieved and the abdomen is irrigated. The bowel contents are then returned to their normal configuration in the abdomen. Approximately 20 to 30 minutes should be given for the bowel to reperfuse before assessing for viability.[1,12,14] A host of adjuncts in conjunction with clinical assessment is available for assessing bowel viability and has been described, including Doppler flow in the antimesenteric border, palpable pulse in the distal mesenteric arcades, return of peristalsis, and uptake of intravenous fluorescein.[2,14,22,23] Most contemporary series advocate for a second-look laparotomy, even in the absence of gross bowel infarction at the initial laparotomy, because mucosal infarction may progress to full-thickness necrosis despite revascularization.[3,12,14]

Endovascular Techniques

In medical centers with access to either Interventional Radiology or Vascular Surgery services, a variety of endovascular techniques have been described in the management of acute on chronic mesenteric ischemia, with first reports in the mid-1980s.[6,24–29] Most patients being treated with endovascular techniques are the result of a thrombosed preexisting SMA plaque.[1,6,12] Different therapies include CDT, mechanical thrombectomy, and PTA with or without stent. Treatment of AMI with thrombolysis and adjunctive PTA/stent is most suitable for patients presenting without evidence of peritonitis, hemodynamic lability, or large thrombus burden.[5,24,25,29,30] In a large retrospective review of the National Inpatient Sample database, patients undergoing endovascular treatment of AMI are less likely to present with significant lactic acidosis or other signs of shock, such as acute respiratory distress syndrome.[31] The role of thrombolytic agents such as urokinase and streptokinase to treat AMI has been described as early as the mid 1990s.[24,25] Patients undergoing CDT should be monitored closely, and, if there is no improvement in patient condition or worsening of clinical status, thrombolytic therapy should be discontinued and emergent exploratory laparotomy performed.[1] Contemporary series show that between 37.5% and 100% of patients initiated on thrombolytic therapy will ultimately require exploratory laparotomy.[5,6,28,30,32] Some have advocated for the use of laparoscopy in conjunction with catheter-directed therapies for the assessment of bowel viability; however, this combination of treatment has not been widely accepted because of the risk of unrecognized nonviable bowel.[33] The inability to assess bowel viability has prevented endovascular treatment of AMI to be as widely accepted compared with other vascular surgery emergencies.[14]

Retrograde Open Mesenteric Stenting

In 2004, a case report illustrated a hybrid approach to the treatment of AMI that combined the principles of an open exploration and minimally invasive endovascular techniques.[34] ROMS was further described a few years later in a case series whereby, following traditional exploratory laparotomy and bowel viability assessment, the distal SMA is dissected and accessed, and then revascularization performed with retrograde PTA and stenting of the SMA occlusion.[35] In 6 patients, technical success was 100%, including 5 patients in which previous attempts at percutaneous antegrade therapy had failed. Although this was a small sample size, perioperative mortality was only 17% compared with 80% in the open bypass cohort. More contemporary studies have demonstrated similar findings in regards to technical success and patient mortality.[27,36,37] Recurrent stenosis rates are similar to those of other stenting procedures; however, repeated interventions are a viable, safe option. Many patients will remain poor operative candidates secondary to poor life expectancy and preexisting comorbidities, although, in patients with acceptable recovery and appropriate for surgery, ROMS may serve as a bridge to more definitive, elective mesenteric bypass in a sterile operative field.[5,38] Others have used ROMS in patients with significant aortoiliac occlusive disease prohibiting appropriate inflow for a retrograde mesenteric bypass.[39] Similar to other endovascular therapies, ROMS should only be attempted in clinical settings with interventional capabilities. The literature is void of any randomized, prospective trials comparing ROMS to other revascularization techniques; however, initial results suggest this to be a viable option in the setting of acute on chronic mesenteric ischemia where other techniques are not thought to be appropriate.

OUTCOMES

Despite advances in diagnostic and therapeutic modalities, mortality from AMI remains high even in more contemporary series, ranging between 26% and 81%.[3–5,10,13,15,40,41] Studies investigating patient outcomes over different decades have unfortunately found no significant improvements in overall mortality.[4,13] Factors found to be associated with poor patient survival include bowel infarction and hypotension on presentation, markers of atherosclerosis, age greater than 60 years, renal insufficiency, metabolic acidosis, and bowel resection required at second-look laparotomy.[3–5,10] Furthermore, delays in diagnosis have been associated with drastic increases in patient mortality.[3,7,8] There does not appear to be any impact on mortality depending on the occlusive cause in AMI.[3,5,10]

As with many other vascular surgery populations, use of endovascular techniques in AMI has increased over the years.[4,31] Perioperative mortality following endovascular treatment of AMI has been found to be lower than traditional open revascularization, ranging from 9% to 39%.[6,26,30–32] Theoretic advantages include prevention of secondary injury incurred from an exploratory laparotomy following the initial ischemic event (pulmonary and renal failure), potentially faster restoration of bowel perfusion, and decreased length of bowel resection.[6] Studies comparing outcomes in patients undergoing endovascular treatment versus traditional open revascularization have suggested improved morbidity and mortality.[6,31,32] However, to date, all studies performed have been retrospective in nature with no randomized controlled prospective trials. A selection bias also exists, as Schoots and colleagues[30] found on a review of 20 case reports and 7 small case series, totaling 48 patients, that only one-third of all patients treated with endovascular methods were found to have total or near-total SMA occlusion. Furthermore, as referenced above, patients undergoing catheter-directed therapies were more likely to present without evidence of shock or peritonitis on arrival. For these reasons, endovascular therapies should not be considered the initial treatment of choice for AMI. In patients diagnosed with AMI, each one should be evaluated expeditiously and a treatment plan developed on a case-by-case basis depending on history and physical examination, diagnostic findings, hemodynamic status, and medical center resources.

SUMMARY

AMI continues to be a lethal surgical emergency, despite technological advances that have helped to improve delays in diagnosis and expand therapeutic options. Patients presenting with acute onset, sharp abdominal pain should have AMI included on the differential diagnosis. Common causes include embolic phenomena from a cardiac source or thrombotic occlusion of a preexisting atherosclerotic plaque. Prompt diagnosis, fluid resuscitation, systemic anticoagulation, and mesenteric revascularization are pivotal in providing optimal patient care and improving patient outcomes. Revascularization options include open surgical embolectomy or mesenteric bypass, catheter-directed endovascular techniques, or a hybrid approach of these, ROMS. The method chosen depends on many factors, including patient history and physical examination, diagnostic findings, hemodynamic status, and medical center resources.

REFERENCES

1. McKinsey JF, Gewertz BL. Acute mesenteric ischemia. Surg Clin North Am 1997;77(2):307–18.
2. Oldenburg WA, Lau LL, Rodenberg TJ, et al. Acute mesenteric ischemia: a clinical review. Arch Intern Med 2004;164(10):1054–62.
3. Kougias P, Lau D, El Sayed HF, et al. Determinants of mortality and treatment outcome following surgical interventions for acute mesenteric ischemia. J Vasc Surg 2007;46(3):467–74.

4. Ryer EJ, Kalra M, Oderich GS, et al. Revascularization for acute mesenteric ischemia. J Vasc Surg 2012;55(6):1682–9.
5. Park WM, Gloviczki P, Cherry KJ, et al. Contemporary management of acute mesenteric ischemia: Factors associated with survival. J Vasc Surg 2002;35(3): 445–52.
6. Arthurs ZM, Titus J, Bannazadeh M, et al. A comparison of endovascular revascularization with traditional therapy for the treatment of acute mesenteric ischemia. J Vasc Surg 2011;53(3):698–705.
7. Boley SJ, Feinstein FR, Sammartano R, et al. New concepts in the management of emboli of the superior mesenteric artery. Surg Gynecol Obstet 1981;153(4): 561–9.
8. Batellier J, Kieny R. Superior mesenteric artery embolism: eighty-two cases. Ann Vasc Surg 1990;4(2):112–6.
9. Lazaro T, Sierra L, Gesto R, et al. Embolization of the mesenteric arteries: surgical treatment in twenty-three consecutive cases. Ann Vasc Surg 1986;1(3):311–5.
10. Edwards MS, Cherr GS, Craven TE, et al. Acute occlusive mesenteric ischemia: surgical management and outcomes. Ann Vasc Surg 2003;17(1):72–9.
11. Moore WS. Visceral ischemic syndromes. In: vascular and endovascular surgery. 7th edition. New York: Saunders; 2005.
12. Sise MJ. Acute mesenteric ischemia. Surg Clin North Am 2014;94(1):165–81.
13. Mamode N, Pickford I, Leiberman P. Failure to improve outcome in acute mesenteric ischaemia: seven-year review. Eur J Surg 1999;165(3):203–8.
14. Wyers MC. Acute Mesenteric ischemia: diagnostic approach and surgical treatment. Semin Vasc Surg 2010;23(1):9–20.
15. Endean ED, Barnes SL, Kwolek CJ, et al. Surgical management of thrombotic acute intestinal ischemia. Ann Surg 2001;233(6):801–8.
16. Smith JS, Patterson LT. Acute mesenteric infarction. Am Surg 1976;42(8):562–7.
17. Stoney RJ, Cunningham CG. Acute mesenteric ischemia. Surgery 1993;114(3): 489–90.
18. Czerny M, Trubel W, Claeys L, et al. Acute mesenteric ischemia. Zentralbl Chir 1997;122(7):538–44 [in German].
19. Kirkpatrick IDC, Kroeker MA, Greenberg HM. Biphasic CT with mesenteric CT angiography in the evaluation of acute mesenteric ischemia: initial experience. Radiology 2003;229(1):91–8.
20. Aschoff AJ, Stuber G, Becker BW, et al. Evaluation of acute mesenteric ischemia: accuracy of biphasic mesenteric multi-detector CT angiography. Abdom Imaging 2009;34(3):345–57.
21. Foley MI, Moneta GL, Abou-Zamzam AM, et al. Revascularization of the superior mesenteric artery alone for treatment of intestinal ischemia. J Vasc Surg 2000; 32(1):37–47.
22. Ballard JL, Stone WM, Hallett JW, et al. A critical analysis of adjuvant techniques used to assess bowel viability in acute mesenteric ischemia. Am Surg 1993;59(5): 309–11.
23. Bergman RT, Gloviczki P, Welch TJ, et al. The role of intravenous fluorescein in the detection of colon ischemia during aortic reconstruction. Ann Vasc Surg 1992; 6(1):74–9.
24. Gallego AM, Ramírez P, Rodríguez JM, et al. Role of urokinase in the superior mesenteric artery embolism. Surgery 1996;120(1):111–3.
25. McBride KD, Gaines PA. Thrombolysis of a partially occluding superior mesenteric artery thromboembolus by infusion of streptokinase. Cardiovasc Intervent Radiol 1994;17(3):164–6.

26. Jia Z, Jiang G, Tian F, et al. Early endovascular treatment of superior mesenteric occlusion secondary to thromboemboli. Eur J Vasc Endovasc Surg 2014;47(2): 196–203.
27. Moyes LH, McCarter DHA, Vass DG, et al. Intraoperative retrograde mesenteric angioplasty for acute occlusive mesenteric ischaemia: a case series. Eur J Vasc Endovasc Surg 2008;36(2):203–6.
28. Resch TA, Acosta S, Sonesson B. Endovascular techniques in acute arterial mesenteric ischemia. Semin Vasc Surg 2010;23(1):29–35.
29. VanDeinse WH, Zawacki JK, Phillips D. Treatment of acute mesenteric ischemia by percutaneous transluminal angioplasty. Gastroenterology 1986;91(2):475–8.
30. Schoots IG, Levi MM, Reekers JA, et al. Thrombolytic therapy for acute superior mesenteric artery occlusion. J Vasc Interv Radiol 2005;16(3):317–29.
31. Beaulieu RJ, Arnaoutakis KD, Abularrage CJ, et al. Comparison of open and endovascular treatment of acute mesenteric ischemia. J Vasc Surg 2014;59(1): 159–64.
32. Block TA, Acosta S, Björck M. Endovascular and open surgery for acute occlusion of the superior mesenteric artery. J Vasc Surg 2010;52(4):959–66.
33. Sauerland S, Agresta F, Bergamaschi R, et al. Laparoscopy for abdominal emergencies. Surg Endosc 2006;20(1):14–29.
34. Milner R, Woo EY, Carpenter JP. Superior mesenteric artery angioplasty and stenting via a retrograde approach in a patient with bowel ischemia: a case report. Vasc Endovascular Surg 2004;38(1):89–91.
35. Wyers MC, Powell RJ, Nolan BW, et al. Retrograde mesenteric stenting during laparotomy for acute occlusive mesenteric ischemia. J Vasc Surg 2007;45(2): 269–75.
36. Blauw JTM, Meerwaldt R, Brusse-Keizer M, et al. Retrograde open mesenteric stenting for acute mesenteric ischemia. J Vasc Surg 2014;60(3):726–34.
37. Stout CL, Messerschmidt CA, Leake AE, et al. Retrograde open mesenteric stenting for acute mesenteric ischemia is a viable alternative for emergent revascularization. Vasc Endovascular Surg 2010;44(5):368–71.
38. Biebl M, Oldenburg WA, Paz-Fumagalli R, et al. Endovascular treatment as a bridge to successful surgical revascularization for chronic mesenteric ischemia. Am Surg 2004;70(11):994–8.
39. Pisimisis GT, Oderich GS. Technique of hybrid retrograde superior mesenteric artery stent placement for acute-on-chronic mesenteric ischemia. Ann Vasc Surg 2011;25(1):132.e7-11.
40. Char DJ, Cuadra SA, Hines GL, et al. Surgical intervention for acute intestinal ischemia: experience in a community teaching hospital. Vasc Endovascular Surg 2003;37(4):245–52.
41. Acosta-Merida MA, Marchena-Gomez J, Hemmersbach-Miller M, et al. Identification of risk factors for perioperative mortality in acute mesenteric ischemia. World J Surg 2006;30(8):1579–85.

Evolution and Current Trends in the Management of Acute Appendicitis

Michel Wagner, MD[a,b,*], Dustin John Tubre, MD[c],
Juan A. Asensio, MD, FCCM, FRCS (England), KM[d]

KEYWORDS

- Acute appendicitis • Alvarado score
- Nonoperative management of acute appendicitis
- Medical imaging in acute appendicitis • Epidemiology of acute appendicitis

KEY POINTS

- Since the first surgical appendectomy in the 18th century the treatment of appendicitis has changed.
- The use of scoring systems has helped refine the diagnosis of acute appendicitis.
- Medical imaging techniques, such as ultrasound, CT scans, and MRI, have assisted in the diagnosis of acute appendicitis.
- Nonoperative management is being investigated and may prove to be acceptable in most cases of acute appendicitis.
- The microbiome of the appendix is being investigated and may prove to have a role in the development of acute appendicitis; treatment in the future may focus on modifying the microbiome.

INTRODUCTION

The appendix is a vestigial organ of dubious utility; its function and normal physiology remain unclear. The appendix is notable in medicine because appendicitis (the inflammatory state of this organ) is the most common indication for emergent surgery

Disclosure Statement: The authors have nothing to disclose.
[a] Division of Trauma Surgery and Surgical Critical Care, Department of Surgery, Creighton University School of Medicine, Creighton University Medical Center, 7710 Mercy Road #2000, Omaha, NE 68124, USA; [b] Department of Translational Science, Creighton University School of Medicine, Creighton University Medical Center, 7500 Mercy Road, Omaha, NE 68124, USA; [c] General Surgery, Creighton University School of Medicine, Omaha, NE, USA; [d] Department of Translational Science, Creighton University School of Medicine, Uniformed Services University of the Health Sciences, F. Edward Hébert School of Medicine, Walter Reed National Military Medical Center, Bethesda, MD, USA
* Corresponding author. Department of Translational Science, Creighton University School of Medicine, Creighton University Medical Center, 7500 Mercy Road, Suite 2871, Omaha, NE 68124.
E-mail addresses: michel.wagner@alegent.org; michelwagner@creighton.edu

Surg Clin N Am 98 (2018) 1005–1023
https://doi.org/10.1016/j.suc.2018.05.006 surgical.theclinics.com

worldwide[1]; it is the most common nonobstetric surgical emergency during pregnancy[2,3] and it is the most common surgical emergency in childhood.[4] A small organ located at the base of the cecum, the appendix has a unique position in history, is a medical oddity, and is even the subject of a beloved children's book.

A 27-year-old Leonid Rogozov performed an autoappendectomy on April 30, 1961, while isolated with a team of Soviets on an expedition to the Antarctic.[5] As medical officer, meteorologist, and driver he was the only one qualified to perform this surgical procedure. After a brief therapeutic attempt at unsuccessful nonoperative management he realized that his survival depended on a surgical intervention. Using his teammates as his surgical team, he directed them to carefully sterilize the instruments required, perform an appropriate surgical wash, and then assist him as he performed his own open appendectomy under local anesthetic. When asked to comment about this in later years Dr. Rogozov is recorded to have replied, "A job like any other, a life like any other."

In 1939, Ludwig Bemelmans published the first in his series of *Madeline* books, a favorite of children, describing the heroine's travails with acute appendicitis.[6] An additional oddity, Dr Jeffrey Sedlack founded a virtual online museum of the appendix and appendicitis (www.appendicitis.pro).[7] Because of the prevalence of acute appendicitis, Sir Alexander Cope, in his classic treatise *Early Diagnosis of the Acute Abdomen*,[8] stated that "appendicitis should never be lower than second" when considering the differential diagnosis of abdominal pain.

Since the first documented appendectomy in 1735 by Claudius Amyand there have been many changes in the management of the appendix and its surgical pathology. The appendectomy performed by Amyand was on an 11-year-old boy with a fecal fistula through an inguinal hernia. After surgical intervention it was noted that the boy had an inguinal hernia that contained the appendix. He had swallowed a pin, and this led to the fistula formation. The eponymous Amyand hernia now defines the condition of an appendix in the inguinal canal.[9] The French physician, Mestier is credited with performing the first appendectomy for acute appendicitis in 1759.[10,11]

Although the works of Charles McBurney[12–14] and Reginald Fitz[15] are frequently quoted when discussing the history of acute appendicitis, perhaps the most famous case of acute appendicitis is the case of King Edward of England. King Edward developed symptoms of abdominal pain in late May 1902, a short time before his scheduled coronation on June 16, 1902. Tended by Sir Frederick Treves, Sir Joseph Lister, and other eminent surgeons of the era, the future King is said to have refused surgical intervention initially. He waxed and waned clinically and eventually underwent an incision and drainage of a large periappendicieal abscess by Treves just 2 days before his scheduled coronation. The coronation was delayed and eventually the King was crowned on August 8, 1902.[7,16]

EPIDEMIOLOGY

Inquiries as to the distribution of this pathology within the population have produced similar results globally.[17–25] These assessments are limited by their retrospective nature and because there is little or no controlled prospective evaluations. Additionally, there is a question as to the detail of the databases that are used to collect the data because these are often administrative databases.[24] Certain studies focus on limited populations, such as active duty or reserve military[18] or children.[21] The lifetime risk has been estimated to range from 8.6% to 12% in males and 6.7% to 23.1% in females.[1,19] When analyzed by age, the greatest frequency of appendicitis is seen in the age range of 10 to 19 years of age.[19,20,22,24] However, Andreu-Ballester and colleagues,[23] in a large study from Spain, found that the highest incidence was in the 1 to

4 years of age group. Seasonal variation has also been noted in multiple studies; the incidence of acute appendicitis is more prevalent in the summer months.[20,22] Cases of perforated appendicitis have decreased over time, although no rational was given for the cause.[26] Not surprisingly, cases of perforated appendicitis have a hospital length of stay that was much longer and a cost that was almost double cases of nonperforated appendicitis.[26]

ANATOMY

The vermiform or "wormlike" appendix is an antimesenteric luminal outpouching found at the base of the cecum where the three bands of colonic longitudinal smooth muscle or taeniae coli coalesce. The size of the appendix varies but averages 10 cm in length. Its histology resembles that of other luminal abdominal structures in that it is composed of mucosal, submucosal, muscular, and serosal layers; however, it is distinct in that it contains lymphoid aggregates and a subepithelial neurosecretory layer. It contains the polymicrobial flora of bacterial species seen in the colon, such as *Escherichia coli*, *Bacteroides*, *Enterococcus*, and *Pseudomonas*. The vascular supply is from the appendiceal artery, a branch of the ileocolic artery arising from the distal superior mesenteric artery. Venous and lymphatic drainage follow that of the arterial supply. It receives autonomic parasympathetic innervation from fibers of the vagus nerve that passes through the superior celiac plexus. Sympathetic fibers arise from the thoracic spinal cord as splanchnic nerve fibers. The vessels, lymphatics, and nerves enter the appendix through its mesentery or mesoappendix to which it is adherent to the mesentery of the adjacent ileum. In its normal position, it is an entirely intraperitoneal structure with the overlying peritoneum in close relation, lying deep in the right pelvis. However, its location varies greatly and has been described as located in almost any location in the abdomen.[8] The anatomy and embryology are relevant to explain the typical clinical findings seen during an acute episode of appendicitis.

Pathophysiology of Appendicitis

Acute appendicitis has been thought of as a sequence of events with an initial enticing event and natural progression, keeping in mind that patients presenting at different points in time present with different clinical pictures. Appendicitis is thought to begin with outflow obstruction of the lumen. Fecaliths (a hard mass of stool also known as appendicoliths when originating in the appendix) have often been cited as a cause for appendicitis and common teaching is to look for a fecalith in the abdominal radiograph; however, there is no clear-cut evidence that this is the case.[27] Other proposed causes include lymphoid hyperplasia preceded by a viral illness or a bacterial enteritis. Most cases occur without a known cause and is rarely of clinical significance. One exception is middle-aged to elderly patients with appendicitis, because an obstructing tumor is not an uncommon cause of obstruction in this group.

The mucosal and secretory function of the inflamed appendix continues, and without a patent lumen, this causes increased intraluminal pressure, leading to bowel wall distention. This is transmitted as visceral pain, via afferent sympathetic autonomic nerve fibers of the splanchnic origin to the dorsal root ganglion of the thoracic spinal cord segments that are shared with the other abdominal organs of midgut embryologic origin. This is manifested as the earliest symptom: poorly localized midabdominal pain. This point in time is considered early acute appendicitis. With ongoing luminal obstruction and stasis of intraluminal contents, enteric bacterial overgrowth ensues simultaneously as venous outflow ceases followed by loss of arterial inflow. The culmination of these events leads to initiation of the systemic acute inflammatory response, with cytokine release and leukocyte activation, causing neutrophil migration to the site of inflammation. The combination of these events results in acute transmural inflammation of the appendiceal wall and the overlying parietal peritoneum. Irritation of the peritoneum, which is under somatic sensory innervation, causes localized pain in the right lower abdomen and corresponding point tenderness to palpation. The systemic inflammatory response gives rise to the fever, leukocytosis, and anorexia seen at this stage, which is considered as late acute appendicitis. Gross examination of the appendix reveals a purulent or suppurative appendix, caused by neutrophil response to infection. Without arterial supply, the appendicular wall becomes ischemic, gangrenous, until free wall perforation occurs. This late presentation is considered complicated appendicitis and typically occurs 2 to 3 days after symptom onset. Appendiceal wall perforation can progress into abscess formation or gross intraperitoneal spillage with peritonitis. The latter results in inflammation of the entire peritoneum causing the severe diffuse abdominal pain of peritonitis. Untreated, this ultimately leads to transmigration of enteric bacteria into the bloodstream, septic shock, circulatory collapse, and death. More commonly, perforation leads to abscess formation with persistent right lower quadrant pain and ongoing signs and symptoms of systemic inflammation.

DIAGNOSIS

History

The presentation of acute appendicitis generally follows a typical sequence of events: the sudden or gradual onset of vague periumbilical or epigastric pain followed by anorexia, nausea, and vomiting. Often, there is a preceding history of bowel distress, either in the form of diarrhea or constipation. The initial onset of periumbilical or epigastric pain is postulated to be the result of hyperperistalsis of the appendix to overcome luminal obstruction and to be visceral in origin. At times the initial pain may be felt all over the abdomen. Nausea and anorexia (with or without emesis) are the next symptoms to follow, a consequence of bowel wall distention. Many clinicians consider a lack of appetite as the most consistent symptom, so much so that its absence should give rise to alternative diagnoses; however, this claim is unsupported by evidence.

About 24 hours after the onset of symptoms, the pain often shifts and is localized to the right lower quadrant with accompanying tenderness to palpation. Because the anatomic position of the appendix varies, the localization and character of pain also varies. Three anatomic positions that are well described include the ascending appendix, iliac appendix, and pelvic appendix. When located in the retrocecal position, localizing symptoms are often mild or even absent. Pelvic appendices may give rise to suprapubic pain and urinary symptoms, or symptoms of painful defecation when in proximity to the rectum. Patients often describe exacerbation of the pain on the car ride to hospital, especially when going over bumps.

Fever and anorexia follow as the infection progresses from a localized to a systemic inflammatory process. The disease may progress to perforation and peritonitis within 2 to 3 days of symptoms onset. If perforation happens to occur in an area of the abdomen that is contained within other loops of bowel, mesentery, or omentum, the infection remains localized to the right lower quadrant, causing continued right lower quadrant pain without signs and symptoms of peritonitis, and occasionally a mass is palpated.

Physical

Fever is a consistent finding but may be absent at early onset of symptoms. Tachycardia may present because of sympathetic response to abdominal pain; however, persistent tachycardia despite pain control in conjunction with hypotension may be caused by the systemic inflammatory response or sepsis. Abdominal examination reveals tenderness, most often in the right lower quadrant near the iliac fossa; this is known as McBurney point after Charles McBurney, who initially described this clinical finding.[12,14] The exact point of maximal tenderness varies and is affected by the position of appendix in relation to surrounding structures. Rebound tenderness, elicited either by gentle percussion or rapid release of pressure from the abdomen, indicates inflammatory irritation of the parietal peritoneum. A useful technique in children includes having them hop or cough (Dunphy sign), or shaking the bed. Involuntary guarding may also be present with peritoneal irritation and Rovsing sign, right-sided abdominal pain elicited with left-sided abdominal palpation. When the appendix is located near the psoas or obturator internus muscles, inducing contraction of these muscles by hip flexion or external rotation, respectively, causes severe pain (the so-called psoas sign). Similarly, in women, cervical motion tenderness during pelvic examination occurs when the cervix and other pelvic organs are brought into contact with an inflamed appendix. Rectal examination may elicit pain when palpation of an inflamed pelvic appendix in proximity to the rectum occurs.

Laboratory

Laboratory studies classically include a basic or comprehensive metabolic panel, a complete blood count, and urinalysis. Coagulation parameters should be obtained if the patient has a history of bleeding dyscrasia or is currently on antiplatelet or anticoagulation medications. These studies can help determine if the patient has electrolyte disturbances, is dehydrated, or has a leukocytosis, all elements that can help rule in or out acute appendicitis or other pathology. The urinalysis may also help in determining if the complaints and findings on clinical examination are of urologic origin. Females should also have a pregnancy test.

Markers

It would be ideal and facilitate the diagnosis of acute appendicitis if the appendix had a unique biochemical marker that would be highly diagnostic of acute appendicitis if positive. Unfortunately, this is not the case. Multiple studies have looked at various markers independently and jointly to help in the diagnosis of acute appendicitis. Although the white blood cell count remains the most common laboratory marker, other markers, such as C-reactive protein, bilirubin, granulocyte colony–stimulating factor, fibrinogen, interleukin, procalcitonin, the APPY1 test, and calprotectin, have been investigated.[28–41] An industry-sponsored study claims 97% sensitivity for a biomarker produced by the sponsor.[34,36,37]

Thuijls and coworkers[39] reported that lactoferrin and calprotectin are significantly elevated in cases of acute appendicitis. Kwan and Nager[38] concluded that elevated C-reactive protein, in conjunction with a leukocytosis, increased the likelihood of appendicitis; D-lactate was not useful. Bilirubin may be a marker to consider; a prospective study showed hyperbilirunemia had a high specificity for acute appendicitis, especially when the appendix is perforated.[33] A meta-analysis proposed that an elevated bilirubin along with clinical signs of acute appendicitis should be considered for early appendectomy because there was a greater chance of appendiceal perforation.[35] Fibrinogen has also been proposed as a marker of perforated appendicitis.[30] The recent World Society of Emergency Surgery Jerusalem Guidelines for Diagnosis and Treatment of Acute Appendicitis makes no recommendation for use of any of these markers.[42]

Scores

Since its earliest description, appendicitis has remained a diagnostic challenge for clinicians. A negative appendectomy rate has been used as a quality measure; this has been a moving target as diagnostic technology has improved. History and physical examination have been the most important modalities in the evaluation of a patient with suspected appendicitis. The addition of routine laboratory values further aides in the diagnosis. The Alvarado score, first described in 1986,[43] uses eight predictive factors from history, physical examination, and laboratory studies, to categorize suspected appendicitis into probability groups. Factors include (in order of strongest predictive value) localized right lower quadrant abdominal tenderness, new-onset leukocytosis, pain migration, left shift, fever, nausea/vomiting, anorexia, and direct rebound pain. A prospective clinical trial by Owen and coworkers[44] validated the Alvarado score in 215 patients, reducing the negative appendectomy rate without increasing morbidity or mortality. Since its description, clinicians have adopted its use with varying degrees of success in reliably predicting appendicitis. Rodrigues and colleagues[45] came to a similar conclusion while performing a prospective assessment of the Alvarado score concluding that a score of 7 to 10 "virtually confirmed the diagnosis" and that patients with score one to four can be "discharged unless otherwise indicated." However, as use of computed topographic imaging became more readily available with improved imaging quality, clinicians have become less reliant on thorough clinical judgment. As evidence of the association with radiation and the increased lifetime risk of cancer began to surface, attention again turned to scoring systems, such as the Alvarado score, to help stratify when computed tomography (CT) scan was necessary and which patients could be spared from radiation. In 2008, the Appendicitis Inflammatory Response Score proposed by Andersson and Andersson[46] was shown to outperform the Alvarado score in predicting advanced and all appendicitis.[47] A recent prospective evaluation concluded that the use of the Appendicitis Inflammatory Response Score would reduce the use of diagnostic imaging.[48] This score used similar factors from the history and physical examination, such as pain, rebound, guarding, leukocytosis, fever, vomiting, and left shift, but with the addition of C-reactive protein.

In 2014 Sammalkorpi and coworkers[1] published results from a prospective study of 829 patients using a New Adult Appendicitis Score that showed further predictive accuracy by incorporating duration and timing of symptoms. Similar to the Alvarado score, the Pediatric Appendicitis Score[49] uses a simple 10-point scale, specifically designed for children. This was later validated by Goldman[50] in a prospective evaluation, who determined that 61% of patients with a score of greater than or equal to seven had acute appendicitis. The RIPASA (from the Raja Isteri Pengiran Anak Saleha Hospital in Brunei Darussalam) score was developed in 2010 to address the poor sensitivity and specificity of the other scores when applied to Middle Eastern and Asian populations.[51] **Table 1** compares the components of each of these scores.

Apisarnthanarak and coworkers[52] performed a retrospective study comparing reliability of the Alvarado score with CT scans. The conclusion was that the Alvarado score was not as reliable as CT scans because almost 50% of the patients in the study with documented acute appendicitis had low or equivocal Alvarado scores.

Imaging Studies

As part of the work-up of acute abdominal pain, classically an obstructive series has been performed of the abdomen. Although rarely helpful, the presence of a fecalith in the right lower quadrant, and there suspected in the appendix, was supportive of the working diagnosis of acute appendicitis. It is probably most useful in ruling out other

Table 1
A comparison of different scoring systems in acute appendicitis

Finding	Alvarado	PAS[49]	RIPASA[51]	New Score		AIRS[46]	
RLQ pain	1	—	0.5	—		1	
Gender	—	—	—	—		—	
Male			1.0				
Female			1.5				
Age	—	—	—	—		—	
<40			0.5				
>40			1.0				
Migration of pain (relocation)	—	1	0.5	2		—	
Nausea/vomiting	1	1	1.0	—		1	
Duration, h	—	—	—	—		—	
<48			1.0				
>48			0.5				
Anorexia	1	1	1.0	—		—	
Guarding	—	—	2.0	—	Pts	—	
				Mild	2		
				Moderate/severe	4		
RLQ tenderness	2	1	1.0	3/1[a]		—	
Rebound	1	1	1.0	—		Light	1
						Medium	2
						Strong	3
Rovsing sign	—	—	2.0	—		—	
Exacerbation with hopping/cough/percussion	—	1	—	—		—	
Fever	1	1	1.0	—		—	
Leukocytosis	2	1	1.0	—	Pts	—	Pts
WBC ($\times 10^9$)				7.2–10.9	1	10–14.9	1
				10.9–14.0	2	>15	2
				>14	3		
CRP, mg/dL	—	—	—	<48-h symptoms	Pts	—	Pts
				4–11	2	1–4.9	1
				11–25	3	>5	2
				25–83	5		
				>83	1		
	—	—	—	>48-h symptoms	Pts	—	
				12–53	2		
				53–152	2		
				>152	1		
Negative urinalysis	—	—	1.0	—		—	
Left shift	1	1	—	%	Pts	%	Pts
				62–75	2	70–84	1
PMN, %				75–83	3	>85	2
				>83	4		
Sum total	10	10	16.5	—		12	
Low-probability group	5–6	<5	—	<16		0–4	
Intermediate group	7–8	5	—	16–18		5–8	
High-probability group	9–10	6–10	—	>18		9–12	

The Alvarado score[43]: 8 factors with the resultant score being characterized as low probability, moderate probability, and high probability.

New Appendicitis Score.[1]

Abbreviations: AIRS, Appendicitis Inflammatory Response Score; CRP, C-reactive protein; PAS, Pediatric Appendicitis Score; PMN, polymorphonuclear leukocytes; RIPASA, from the Raja Isteri Pengiran Anak Saleha Hospital in Brunei Darussalam; RLQ, right lower quadrant; WBC, white blood count.

[a] New score age: men and women age 50+/women age 16–49.

causes of abdominal pain, such as free air in the case of a perforated viscus, or a small bowel obstruction.

Other medical imaging technologies are also helpful in the assessment of the acute abdomen. The most commonly used modalities used are ultrasonography (UC), CT scan, and MRI. Each of these has advantages and disadvantages, such as sensitivity, specificity, costs, and exposure to ionizing radiation. Although UC is inexpensive and has no exposure to ionizing radiation, it is operator dependent and only has a specificity of 83% and a sensitivity of 78%. CT scans have a specificity of 90% and a sensitivity of 94%, but is more costly and exposes the patient to nonnegligible ionizing radiation.[53,54] CTs have not been demonstrated to be reliable at determining if there is appendiceal perforation.[55]

The diagnostic accuracy of MRI is comparable with CT and better than US.[56] MRI has a sensitivity of 97% and a specificity of 97% but without the ionizing radiation; however, there is increased cost relative to CT.[57,58] Reddy and coworkers[59] proposed a combined US-Alvarado score could reduce the need for CT scans in patients suspected of having appendicitis.

SURGICAL APPROACHES

Open Surgery

Open appendectomies are now rarely performed as the initial operation, and many surgical residents now complete their training having never performed one. However, familiarity with this approach is important because it may be necessary when contraindications to laparoscopy or difficult adhesions are encountered or in austere environments where laparoscopy is not available. In 1894 Charles McBurney described the oblique right lower quadrant incision and muscle-splitting approach, which continued to be used until the late 20th century (before this, surgeons typically used a midline laparotomy approach). A Rockey-Davis or transverse right lower quadrant incision just lateral to the rectus muscle and through McBurney point is thought to provide a better cosmetic outcome and more access to the pelvis. After incising the skin and sharply incising the aponeurosis of the external oblique muscle, the three layers of the abdominal wall lateral to the rectus are bluntly dissected and retracted to gain access to the peritoneum. On entering the peritoneal cavity, the appendix is identified at the base of the cecum. Tracing the taeniae coli of the ascending colon proximally can facilitate identification. The appendiceal artery is identified as a branch of the mesentery of the appendix and ligated. The base of the appendix is then ligated with suture and removed. Inversion of the appendiceal stump into the cecum, historically thought to decrease risk of fistula, has now largely been abandoned after multiple studies proved no significant difference in outcomes[60,61] The peritoneal cavity is then irrigated with saline solution, and the muscle, fascia, and skin are closed separately in layers.

Laparoscopic Surgery

Semm, a German gynecologist and pioneer of laparoscopic surgery, performed the first laparoscopic appendectomy in 1980, which had previously been used mainly as a diagnostic tool in gynecologic surgery. His attempts to bring this new technique to mainstream surgery were met by a great deal of skepticism and backlash from the surgical community. Over the next several years, his efforts to promote laparoscopic surgery ultimately brought about the "laparoscopic revolution" leading to its widespread adoption in not only appendectomy but also cholecystectomy.[62] Several advances in technique and instrumentation have evolved, and numerous studies have solidified laparoscopic appendectomy as the current gold standard treatment of appendicitis with improved outcomes compared with the open approach.

Comparison of Open Versus Laparoscopic

Numerous studies of level I evidence have compared open and laparoscopic appendectomies. A meta-analysis of 33 prospective randomized controlled trials, accounting for more than 3500 patients, showed that laparoscopic appendectomy in adults had a statistically significant decrease in incidence of wound infection, length of hospitalization, and postoperative complication, and an earlier returned to work. This conclusion did not apply to the pediatric population.[63]

Single Incision Laparoscopic Surgery

Single incision laparoscopic surgery (SILS) has been described since 1997 for cholecystectomy.[64] This technique uses one incision to access the peritoneal cavity, placing multiple operative ports through this incision. The primary motive to this procedure is cosmesis.[65] Multiple studies have demonstrated the feasibility of this technique.[65–70] However, SILS has a longer operative time[65,67] and is more expensive.[70] In addition, at least one study has found that SILS patients had more postoperative pain.[65]

Natural Orifice Transluminal Surgery

Natural orifice transluminal surgery (NOTES) is a procedure whereby the peritoneal cavity is accessed via a natural orifice: the stomach via the mouth, the vagina in women, or the rectum. Once the peritoneal cavity is accessed in this fashion the surgical procedure is performed. First described in 2007 it has been used to perform appendectomies and even colon resections. Additional acronyms for this procedure exist: transgastric appendectomy (TGAE) and transvaginal appendectomy (TVAE). In 2008 the German Society of General and Visceral Surgery formed the German NOTES Registry (GNR) to track and follow NOTES surgery performed in Germany.[71]

In 2014, a total of 13 cases were described with successful outcomes. These cases were part of the GNR.[72] An analysis of the first 217 appendectomies entered into the GNR was published recently.[71] The hybrid NOTES nomenclature is used for cases where additional transabdominal trocars are used. There were 181 TVAE performed with a median time of 35 minutes duration, without any conversions to laparotomy. The median postoperative hospital stay was 3 days. Only one center was designated as a TGAE center, performing 36 of these procedures. The median duration of this procedure was 96 minutes, with two conversions to laparotomy, and a median postoperative hospital stay of 3 days. Complications occurred in 6.5% of the patients and included pouch of Douglas abscesses, other intra-abdominal infections, intra-abdominal bleeding, and a case of gastric leak of the gastric clip closure.

The overall conversion rate for both procedures was conversion to laparoscopy of 2.8% and a conversion rate to laparotomy of 0.9%, the latter two cases from the TGAE group. The purported advantage of NOTES is to decrease the risk of wound infections, trocar hernias, and neuropathic scar pain.

Endoluminal Surgery

Recently, an endoluminal appendectomy was performed in Brazil.[73] The patient, a 67-year-old man with a history of a transverse colostomy, presented with abdominal discomfort. After ultrasonography demonstrated an enlarged appendix the patient underwent an endoluminal appendectomy: a modified colonoscope was passed, the appendiceal lumen was cannulated with a shark tooth grasping forceps, and the appendix was inverted. An endoloop was placed at the base of the appendix, the appendiceal base was then transected with a snare loop. Hemostatic clips were then used to reinforce the closure of the appendiceal lumen.

Nonoperative Management

In 1902 Ochsner wrote in his *Handbook of Appendicitis*,[74] "I say this because I am confident that with proper non-operative treatment almost all of the cases which are diagnosed reasonably early may be carried through any acute attack, no matter what its character may be." Stengel[75] also wrote at the beginning of the twentieth century, "Treated in a purely medical or tentative manner, the great majority of patients with appendicitis recover." Coldrey[76,77] was a proponent of nonoperative management in the 1950s, but this never caught on. Buckley and coworkers[68] state "During the course of over 30 years of surgery, a good deal of which has been emergency surgery, I have gradually been tending more and more to conservative treatment in cases of advanced appendicitis. For many years I have believed it best to treat appendix abscesses conservatively. For more than 4 years I have believed it best to treat all cases of acute appendicitis over 24 hours old conservatively. It is probably wise to treat all cases of acute appendicitis under 24 hours old by an emergency appendicectomy, and this is our usual custom. One sometimes wonders whether it would not be a sound procedure to treat all cases of acute appendicitis conservatively. They seem to settle down quite nicely, and some never seem to have any further trouble: the appendix has wizened. We should then be left with appendicectomy for recurrent acute appendicitis, and for chronic appendicitis-the 'grumblers' with fecaliths in the appendix, with kinks, and with adhesions. Looking into the future, one cannot help feeling that our successors will be more conservative in their outlook in this matter, and may look back on us as having been too 'appendicectomy-minded'."[68]

Nonoperative management of acute appendicitis has regained more popularity recently and has been supported by several studies. Nonoperative management terminology includes nonoperative management (the concept of not performing an appendectomy on a patient with a diagnosis of acute appendicitis), treatment failure (wherein the patient's symptoms worsen and requires a surgical intervention while still under nonoperative therapy), and recurrence (when the patient develops appendicitis after successful completion of a course of nonoperative management).

The Appendectomy vs Antibiotics in the Treatment of Acute Uncomplicated Appendicitis (APPAC) study,[78,79] a randomized, prospective controlled study, assessed nonoperative management versus surgery using ertapenem as antibiotic of choice initially, followed by levofloxacin with metronidazole. Of those patients managed nonoperatively almost 73% did not require surgical appendectomy within the first year of their enrollment. This study was later followed up with an economic assessment.[80] Not surprisingly, surgical intervention cost was 1.6 times greater than nonoperative management; surgical patients required more sick leave, leading the authors to conclude surgical intervention has greater societal costs.

DiSaverio and coworkers,[81] in the Non-Operative Treatment for Acute Appendicitis (NOTA) study, prospectively followed 159 patients with suspected acute appendicitis based on clinical assessment. The patients were treated with amoxicillin/clavulanate for up to 7 days. Treatment failure was 12%. The recurrence rate was an additional 14%, but these patients were all treated successfully with antibiotics.

Additional reviews and meta-analyses have shown that nonoperative management is successful in upward of 70% of patients.[82,83] There is some evidence that appendicitis should be stratified into noncomplicated and complicated, and that those cases that are complicated should undergo a surgical intervention.[84] In this study complicated appendicitis was defined as "patients with evidence of perforation, peri-appendiceal abscess, or phlegmon, or duration of symptoms greater than 48 h prior to admission to the Emergency Department."[84]

A recent World Wide Web–based survey of almost 2000 persons found that those surveyed predominantly favored laparoscopic appendectomy for themselves and their children; the survey was unbalanced, however, with a preponderance of females (70.9% of respondents) and non-Hispanic white (90.5%) respondents.[85] More recently, the Comparison of Outcomes of Antibiotic Drugs and Appendectomy (CODA) trial[86] was initiated in the United States with a goal to recruit 1500 patients. This study is currently enrolling patients.

Bacteriology

The microbiome of the appendix in normal state and in acute appendicitis has been analyzed as a possible factor in acute appendicitis. One of the classic theories of the development of acute appendicitis has been luminal occlusion of the appendix by either a fecalith or hypertrophic lymphoid tissue.[87] Subsequently, this blind pouch becomes a breeding ground for bacteria, leading to acute appendicitis. Although some of the original studies did not demonstrate a difference in the microbiome in patients with acute appendicitis confirmed by pathology versus normal appendix as confirmed by pathology,[88] it was suspected that a higher preponderance of anaerobic bacteria was present in the appendix and ileum in patients with acute appendicitis.[89]

Technological advances, such as gene sequence analysis, have allowed for better assessment of the microbiome and better quantification and qualification of the microbiome has become possible. With these differences, the hypothesis that a shift in the appendiceal microbiome may play a key role in the pathophysiology of acute appendicitis was postulated.[90,91] Further investigation shows that *Fusobacterium* is more predominant in patients with acute appendicitis with a concomitant decrease in the *Bacteroides* population.[87,91–93]

The inferences of these studies are challenged by small numbers of patients studied to make some of the conclusions put forth; for example, Salö and coworkers[92] documents a nonstatistical increase in *Fusobacterium* and an associated decrease in *Bacteroides* in phlegmonous appendicitis and perforated appendicitis compared with control subjects. However, he found that the microbiome is similar in gangrenous appendicitis and control subjects. These conclusions were made after studying only 22 patients.

These findings support the hypothesis that appendicitis is actually a disease of inflammation and changes in immune function.[87] This concept still needs refinement; support for this is the fact that appendicitis has some cultural findings, with appendicitis remaining stable in industrialized countries, but rapidly increasing in newly industrialized countries.[25] This knowledge can be used to drive antibiotic management in cases of nonoperative management.

SPECIAL CIRCUMSTANCES

Interval Appendectomy

Patients may present late in the natural course of the appendicitis, after perforation has occurred. If the perforation is contained, an intra-abdominal abscess or phlegmon forms within 5 days. This causes persistent right lower quadrant pain and tenderness, sometimes associated with a palpable mass and is typically diagnosed with CT scan or US. Percutaneous drainage along with antibiotic therapy is currently the standard of care. Immediate surgical intervention in setting of an abscess or phlegmon carries an increased risk of adjacent bowel injury, potentially requiring more extensive resection, such as a right hemicolectomy or ileocecectomy.[94] There has been much debate and research in the pediatric and adult population regarding outcomes, cost, morbidity, and recurrence rates for each of these options. In the pediatric population, percutaneous drainage and antibiotics with interval appendectomy compared with immediate appendectomy resulted in no difference regarding cost, length of hospitalization, or abscess recurrence rate.[95] Initial nonoperative management may also have negative psychosocial impact on the family, decreasing the quality of life because of a delay in definitive treatment.[96]

After successful nonoperative management of appendicitis or an appendiceal abscess, an interval appendectomy may be performed. Proponents of interval appendectomy justify this based on a reported recurrence rate ranging from 6% to 20%, with most recurrences within the first 6 months.[97] Interval appendectomy is most often performed in the pediatric population, who are believed to have higher recurrence rates and lower surgical complication rates.[98,99] A larger retrospective study combining adult and pediatric populations showed recurrence of 5% within 4 years, with the authors concluding that the practice of interval appendectomy should be abandoned.[100] Multiple factors should be considered in deciding when to do an interval appendectomy. Very young children and elderly adults are more likely to present after perforation, because of inability to independently seek medical attention and communicate effectively. Elderly patients are also less likely to tolerate a second episode of acute appendicitis and are more apt to progress to sepsis because of weakened immune system and comorbid conditions. There is also a higher likelihood of associated malignancy or undiagnosed inflammatory bowel disease in those 40 years of age and older.[94]

For these reasons, interval appendectomy should be strongly considered in these select populations. Healthy adolescents and young adults are least likely to have serious sequelae from an appendicitis recurrence. Routine interval appendectomy is not recommended in this population.

Pregnancy

Acute appendicitis is the most common nonobstetric surgical emergency during pregnancy with a prevalence of 1 in 500 pregnancies.[2,3] The diagnosis is somewhat challenging because some of the diagnostic modalities used to diagnose acute appendicitis in the nongravid patient are often confounded by the gravid state. The physical examination is altered because of displacement of the appendix. The state of pregnancy tends to leukocytosis and therefore the use of leukocytosis to help make the diagnosis of acute appendicitis is challenged. Imaging adjuncts to help with the diagnosis are also affected. US may not locate the pathologic appendix as easily. Although a CT scan has good sensitivity and specificity, it is preferred to not expose the fetus to a high level of radiation. MRI has not been known to affect the fetus.[101] The American College of Radiology has created appropriateness criteria with frequent revisions. Under the rubric of "Right Lower Quadrant Pain – Suspected Appendicitis," the latest revision, dated 2013, has four variants.[102] The third variant, specifically addressing the pregnant patient, rates the MRI of the abdomen and pelvis without intravenous contrast a seven of a maximum nine. Abdominal US received the highest rating with a rating of eight. The specificity of MRI is 98%, sensitivity of 97%, positive predictive value of 92.4%, and negative predictive value of 99%, challenged by the fact that the nonvisualization may be high.[2,3,57] Although limited by this, MRI should be considered the choice imaging modality for assessing the pregnant patient suspected of acute appendicitis.[2] However, because of the cost of MRIs, many authors recommend an US as the first step in the work-up of the pregnant patient with a follow-up MRI if the results of the US are not conclusive.[2,101] Unfortunately, not all hospitals have an MRI machine or the radiologists trained to read the images.

Rapid and accurate diagnosis of acute appendicitis in pregnancy is paramount because of the effect that untreated acute appendicitis can have on the outcome of the pregnancy. Surgery can either be open or laparoscopic depending on surgeon comfort.[2]

Other Possible Diagnoses

In the differential diagnosis consideration must be given to alternative pathologies that may present in a fashion similar to acute appendicitis. Gynecologic pathology, such as ovarian torsion, ectopic pregnancy, and pelvic inflammatory disease, must be considered the differential diagnosis. In the elderly, concern that this may be an initial presentation of a neoplastic disease must be entertained. In addition, this may be the initial presentation of inflammatory bowel disease; in one study 0.3% of pediatric appendectomies were later found to have Crohn disease.[103] Parasites have also been known to cause or contribute to acute appendicitis,[104–106] as has tuberculosis.[107]

SUMMARY

Appendicitis continues to be a frequent cause of emergency surgery because of its high prevalence in society. Diagnosis continues to remain a challenge and adjuncts, such as new biomarkers and advanced imaging technology, are being used to help facilitate this diagnosis. Although the new biomarkers may hold some promise, additional work needs to be done. Advanced imaging technology, such as CT and MRI, have high sensitivity and specificity but are costly and, in the case of CT scans, subject the patient to significant ionizing radiation. Nonoperative management continues to be investigated and as a better understanding of the true pathophysiology of acute appendicitis matures this will have a significant effect on the number of surgical interventions for acute appendicitis.

Clinical equipoise is still mandatory in the assessment of the patient who presents to the emergency department with right lower quadrant pain suspicious of appendicitis. Clinical scores, biomarkers, and advanced imaging technology help facilitate this challenging diagnosis.

Historically, nonoperative management has been underappreciated but is now seeing a resurgence in academic support and may be more cost effective. The future may see a new approach combining a more detailed physical examination and better usage of laboratory studies and medical imaging, leading to more nonoperative management being safely justified.

REFERENCES

1. Sammalkorpi HE, Mentula P, Leppaniemi A. A new adult appendicitis score improves diagnostic accuracy of acute appendicitis: a prospective study. BMC Gastroenterol 2014;14:114.
2. Flexer SM, Tabib N, Peter MB. Suspected appendicitis in pregnancy. Surgeon 2014;12(2):82–6.
3. Burke LM, Bashir MR, Miller FH, et al. Magnetic resonance imaging of acute appendicitis in pregnancy: a 5-year multiinstitutional study. Am J Obstet Gynecol 2015;213(5):693.e1-6.
4. Rautio M, Saxen H, Siitonen A, et al. Bacteriology of histopathologically defined appendicitis in children. Pediatr Infect Dis J 2000;19(11):1078–83.
5. Rogozov V, Bermel N. Auto-appendectomy in the Antarctic: case report. BMJ 2009;339:b4965.

6. Madeline (book) - Wikipedia. 2017. Available at: https://en.wikipedia.org/wiki/Madeline_(book)#References. Accessed December 06, 2017.
7. The appendicitis museum is open! | Welcome to appendicitis.pro. 2017. http://www.appendicitis.pro/. Accessed December 06, 2017.
8. Silen W. Cope's early diagnosis of the acute abdomen, 21st edition. New York: Oxford University Press; 2005.
9. Hutchinson R. Amyand's hernia. J R Soc Med 1993;86(2):104–5.
10. Douneff NM. Contribution à l'étude de la pérityphlite et de l'appendicite. Geneva (Switzerland): University of Geneva; 1893.
11. Edebohl GM. A review of the history and the literature of appendicitis. New York: Medical Record; 1899.
12. McBurney C. Experience with early operative interference in cases of disease of the vermiform appendix. N Y State J Med 1889;50:676–84.
13. McBurney C II. The indications for early laparotomy in appendicitis. Ann Surg 1891;13(4):233–54.
14. McBurney C IV. The incision made in the abdominal wall in cases of appendicitis, with a description of a new method of operating. Ann Surg 1894;20(1):38–43.
15. Fitz RH. Perforating inflammation of the vermiform appendix: with special reference to its early diagnosis and treatment, vol. 1. Philadelphia: Dornan; 1886.
16. Mirilas P, Skandalakis JE. Not just an appendix: Sir Frederick Treves. Arch Dis Child 2003;88(6):549–52.
17. Appendicitis and appendectomies among non-service member beneficiaries of the Military Health System, 2002-2011. MSMR 2012;19(12):13–6.
18. Appendicitis and appendectomies, active and reserve components, U.S. Armed Forces, 2002-2011. MSMR 2012;19(12):7–12.
19. Addiss DG, Shaffer N, Fowler BS, et al. The epidemiology of appendicitis and appendectomy in the United States. Am J Epidemiol 1990;132(5):910–25.
20. Al-Omran M, Mamdani M, McLeod RS. Epidemiologic features of acute appendicitis in Ontario, Canada. Can J Surg 2003;46(4):263–8.
21. Andersen SB, Paerregaard A, Larsen K. Changes in the epidemiology of acute appendicitis and appendectomy in Danish children 1996-2004. Eur J Pediatr Surg 2009;19(5):286–9.
22. Anderson JE, Bickler SW, Chang DC, et al. Examining a common disease with unknown etiology: trends in epidemiology and surgical management of appendicitis in California, 1995-2009. World J Surg 2012;36(12):2787–94.
23. Andreu-Ballester JC, Gonzalez-Sanchez A, Ballester F, et al. Epidemiology of appendectomy and appendicitis in the Valencian community (Spain), 1998-2007. Dig Surg 2009;26(5):406–12.
24. Buckius MT, McGrath B, Monk J, et al. Changing epidemiology of acute appendicitis in the United States: study period 1993-2008. J Surg Res 2012;175(2):185–90.
25. Ferris M, Quan S, Kaplan BS, et al. The global incidence of appendicitis: a systematic review of population-based studies. Ann Surg 2017;266(2):237–41.
26. Barrett ML, Hines AL, Andrews RM. Trends in rates of perforated appendix, 2001-2010: statistical brief #159. In: Healthcare Cost and Utilization Project (HCUP) statistical briefs. Rockville (MD): Agency for Healthcare Research and Quality (US); 2006.
27. Singh J, Mariadason J. Role of the faecolith in modern-day appendicitis. Ann R Coll Surg Engl 2013;95(1):48–51.

28. Al-Abed YA, Alobaid NK, Myint F. Diagnostic markers in acute appendicitis. Am J Surg 2015;209(6):1043–7.
29. Allister L, Bachur R, Glickman J, et al. Serum markers in acute appendicitis. J Surg Res 2011;168(1):70–5.
30. Alvarez-Alvarez FA, Maciel-Gutierrez VM, Rocha-Muñoz AD, et al. Diagnostic value of serum fibrinogen as a predictive factor for complicated appendicitis (perforated). A cross-sectional study. Int J Surg 2016;25(Supplement C):109–13.
31. Andersson M, Rubér M, Ekerfelt C, et al. Can new inflammatory markers improve the diagnosis of acute appendicitis? World J Surg 2014;38(11):2777–83.
32. Benito J, Acedo Y, Medrano L, et al. Usefulness of new and traditional serum biomarkers in children with suspected appendicitis. Am J Emerg Med 2016;34(5):871–6.
33. D'Souza N, Karim D, Sunthareswaran R. Bilirubin; a diagnostic marker for appendicitis. Int J Surg 2013;11(10):1114–7.
34. Depinet H, Copeland K, Gogain J, et al. Addition of a biomarker panel to a clinical score to identify patients at low risk for appendicitis. Am J Emerg Med 2016;34(12):2266–71.
35. Giordano S, Paakkonen M, Salminen P, et al. Elevated serum bilirubin in assessing the likelihood of perforation in acute appendicitis: a diagnostic meta-analysis. Int J Surg 2013;11(9):795–800.
36. Huckins DS, Simon HK, Copeland K, et al. Prospective validation of a biomarker panel to identify pediatric ED patients with abdominal pain who are at low risk for acute appendicitis. Am J Emerg Med 2016;34(8):1373–82.
37. Huckins DS, Simon HK, Copeland K, et al. A novel biomarker panel to rule out acute appendicitis in pediatric patients with abdominal pain. Am J Emerg Med 2013;31(9):1368–75.
38. Kwan KY, Nager AL. Diagnosing pediatric appendicitis: usefulness of laboratory markers. Am J Emerg Med 2010;28(9):1009–15.
39. Thuijls G, Derikx JPM, Prakken FJ, et al. A pilot study on potential new plasma markers for diagnosis of acute appendicitis. Am J Emerg Med 2011;29(3):256–60.
40. Wu H-P, Chen C-Y, Kuo I-T, et al. Diagnostic values of a single serum biomarker at different time points compared with Alvarado score and imaging examinations in pediatric appendicitis. J Surg Res 2012;174(2):272–7.
41. Ozan E, Atac GK, Alisar K, et al. Role of inflammatory markers in decreasing negative appendectomy rate: a study based on computed tomography findings. Ulus Travma Acil Cerrahi Derg 2017;23(6):477–82.
42. Di Saverio S, Birindelli A, Kelly MD, et al. WSES Jerusalem guidelines for diagnosis and treatment of acute appendicitis. World J Emerg Surg 2016;11:34.
43. Alvarado A. A practical score for the early diagnosis of acute appendicitis. Ann Emerg Med 1986;15(5):557–64.
44. Owen T, Williams H, Stiff G, et al. Evaluation of the Alvarado score in acute appendicitis. J R Soc Med 1992;85(2):87–8.
45. Rodrigues G, Rao A, Khan SA. Evaluation of Alvarado score in acute appendicitis: a prospective study. Int J Surg 2006;9(1):1–5.
46. Andersson M, Andersson RE. The appendicitis inflammatory response score: a tool for the diagnosis of acute appendicitis that outperforms the Alvarado score. World J Surg 2008;32(8):1843–9.

47. Kollar D, McCartan DP, Bourke M, et al. Predicting acute appendicitis? A comparison of the Alvarado score, the Appendicitis Inflammatory Response Score and clinical assessment. World J Surg 2015;39(1):104–9.
48. Andersson M, Kolodziej B, Andersson RE. Randomized clinical trial of Appendicitis Inflammatory Response Score-based management of patients with suspected appendicitis. Br J Surg 2017;104(11):1451–61.
49. Samuel M. Pediatric appendicitis score. J Pediatr Surg 2002;37(6):877–81.
50. Goldman RD. Prospective validation of the pediatric appendicitis score. The Journal of Pediatrics 2008;153(2):278–82.
51. Chong CF, Adi MI, Thien A, et al. Development of the RIPASA score: a new appendicitis scoring system for the diagnosis of acute appendicitis. Singapore Med J 2010;51(3):220–5.
52. Apisarnthanarak P, Suvannarerg V, Pattaranutaporn P, et al. Alvarado score: can it reduce unnecessary CT scans for evaluation of acute appendicitis? Am J Emerg Med 2015;33(2):266–70.
53. Rosen MP, Ding A, Blake MA, et al. ACR Appropriateness Criteria(R) right lower quadrant pain–suspected appendicitis. J Am Coll Radiol 2011;8(11):749–55.
54. Doria AS. Optimizing the role of imaging in appendicitis. Pediatr Radiol 2009; 39(2):S144–8.
55. Gaskill CE, Simianu VV, Carnell J, et al. Use of computed tomography to determine perforation in patients with acute appendicitis. Curr Probl Diagn Radiol 2018;47(1):6–9.
56. Kinner S, Pickhardt PJ, Riedesel EL, et al. Diagnostic accuracy of MRI versus CT for the evaluation of acute appendicitis in children and young adults. AJR Am J Roentgenol 2017;209(4):911–9.
57. Kulaylat AN, Moore MM, Engbrecht BW, et al. An implemented MRI program to eliminate radiation from the evaluation of pediatric appendicitis. J Pediatr Surg 2015;50(8):1359–63.
58. Orth RC, Guillerman RP, Zhang W, et al. Prospective comparison of MR imaging and US for the diagnosis of pediatric appendicitis. Radiology 2014;272(1): 233–40.
59. Reddy SB, Kelleher M, Bokhari SAJ, et al. A highly sensitive and specific combined clinical and sonographic score to diagnose appendicitis. J Trauma Acute Care Surg 2017;83(4):643–9.
60. Street D, Bodai BI, Owens LJ, et al. Simple ligation vs stump inversion in appendectomy. Arch Surg 1988;123(6):689–90.
61. Jacobs PP, Koeyers GF, Bruyninckx CM. Simple ligation superior to inversion of the appendiceal stump; a prospective randomized study. Ned Tijdschr Geneeskd 1992;136(21):1020–3 [in Dutch].
62. Litynski GS. Kurt Semm and the fight against skepticism: endoscopic hemostasis, laparoscopic appendectomy, and Semm's impact on the "laparoscopic revolution". JSLS 1998;2(3):309–13.
63. Dai L, Shuai J. Laparoscopic versus open appendectomy in adults and children: a meta-analysis of randomized controlled trials. United European Gastroenterol J 2017;5(4):542–53.
64. Navarra G, Pozza E, Occhionorelli S, et al. One-wound laparoscopic cholecystectomy. Br J Surg 1997;84(5):695.
65. Carter JT, Kaplan JA, Nguyen JN, et al. A prospective, randomized controlled trial of single-incision laparoscopic vs conventional 3-port laparoscopic appendectomy for treatment of acute appendicitis. J Am Coll Surg 2014;218(5):950–9.

66. Wakasugi M, Tei M, Omori T, et al. Single-incision laparoscopic surgery as a teaching procedure: a single-center experience of more than 2100 procedures. Surg Today 2016;46(11):1318–24.
67. Antoniou SA, Koch OO, Antoniou GA, et al. Meta-analysis of randomized trials on single-incision laparoscopic versus conventional laparoscopic appendectomy. Am J Surg 2014;207(4):613–22.
68. Buckley FP, Vassaur H, Monsivais S, et al. Single-incision laparoscopic appendectomy versus traditional three-port laparoscopic appendectomy: an analysis of outcomes at a single institution. Surg Endosc 2014;28(2):626–30.
69. Kumar A, Sinha AN, Deepak D, et al. Single incision laparoscopic assisted appendectomy: experience of 82 cases. J Clin Diagn Res 2016;10(5). Pc01–03.
70. Vettoretto N, Cirocchi R, Randolph J, et al. Acute appendicitis can be treated with single-incision laparoscopy: a systematic review of randomized controlled trials. Colorectal Dis 2015;17(4):281–9.
71. Bulian DR, Kaehler G, Magdeburg R, et al. Analysis of the first 217 appendectomies of the German NOTES registry. Ann Surg 2017;265(3):534–8.
72. Knuth J, Heiss MM, Bulian DR. Transvaginal hybrid-NOTES appendectomy in routine clinical use: prospective analysis of 13 cases and description of the procedure. Surg Endosc 2014;28(9):2661–5.
73. Artifon ELA, Uemura RS, Furuya Junior CK, et al. Endoluminal appendectomy: the first description in humans for acute appendicitis. Endoscopy 2017;49(6):609–10.
74. Ochsner AJ. A handbook of appendicitis. Chicago: G.P. Engelhard & Co; 1902.
75. Stengel A. Appendicitis. In: Osler W, McCrae T, editors. Modern medicine. Vol V. Diseases of the alimentary tract. Philadelphia: Lea & Febinger; 1908.
76. Coldrey E. Treatment of acute appendicitis. Br Med J 1956;2(5007):1458–61.
77. Coldrey E. Five years of conservative treatment of acute appendicitis. J Int Coll Surg 1959;32(3):255–61.
78. Paajanen H, Grönroos JM, Rautio T, et al. A prospective randomized controlled multicenter trial comparing antibiotic therapy with appendectomy in the treatment of uncomplicated acute appendicitis (APPAC trial). BMC Surg 2013;13(1):3.
79. Salminen P, Paajanen H, Rautio T, et al. Antibiotic therapy vs appendectomy for treatment of uncomplicated acute appendicitis: the APPAC randomized clinical trial. JAMA 2015;313(23):2340–8.
80. Sippola S, Gronroos J, Tuominen R, et al. Economic evaluation of antibiotic therapy versus appendicectomy for the treatment of uncomplicated acute appendicitis from the APPAC randomized clinical trial. Br J Surg 2017;104(10):1355–61.
81. DiSaverio S, Sibilio A, Giorgini E, et al. The NOTA Study (Non Operative Treatment for Acute Appendicitis): prospective study on the efficacy and safety of antibiotics (amoxicillin and clavulanic acid) for treating patients with right lower quadrant abdominal pain and long-term follow-up of conservatively treated suspected appendicitis. Ann Surg 2014;260(1):109–17.
82. Findlay JM, Kafsi JE, Hammer C, et al. Nonoperative management of appendicitis in adults: a systematic review and meta-analysis of randomized controlled trials. J Am Coll Surg 2016;223(6):814–24.e2.
83. Georgiou R, Eaton S, Stanton MP, et al. Efficacy and safety of nonoperative treatment for acute appendicitis: a meta-analysis. Pediatrics 2017;139(3) [pii: e20163003].
84. Helling TS, Soltys DF, Seals S. Operative versus non-operative management in the care of patients with complicated appendicitis. Am J Surg 2017;214(6): 1195–200.

85. Hanson AL, Crosby RD, Basson MD. Patient preferences for surgery or antibiotics for the treatment of acute appendicitis. JAMA Surg 2018;153(5):471–8.
86. Davidson GH, Flum DR, Talan DA, et al. Comparison of Outcomes of antibiotic Drugs and Appendectomy (CODA) trial: a protocol for the pragmatic randomised study of appendicitis treatment. BMJ Open 2017;7(11):e016117.
87. Rogers MB, Brower-Sinning R, Firek B, et al. Acute appendicitis in children is associated with a local expansion of fusobacteria. Clin Infect Dis 2016;63(1):71–8.
88. Roberts JP. Quantitative bacterial flora of acute appendicitis. Arch Dis Child 1988;63(5):536–40.
89. Thadepalli H, Mandal AK, Chuah SK, et al. Bacteriology of the appendix and the ileum in health and in appendicitis. Am Surg 1991;57(5):317–22.
90. Jackson HT, Mongodin EF, Davenport KP, et al. Culture-independent evaluation of the appendix and rectum microbiomes in children with and without appendicitis. PLoS One 2014;9(4):e95414.
91. Zhong D, Brower-Sinning R, Firek B, et al. Acute appendicitis in children is associated with an abundance of bacteria from the phylum Fusobacteria. J Pediatr Surg 2014;49(3):441–6.
92. Salö M, Marungruang N, Roth B, et al. Evaluation of the microbiome in children's appendicitis. Int J Colorectal Dis 2017;32(1):19–28.
93. Swidsinski A, Dorffel Y, Loening-Baucke V, et al. Mucosal invasion by fusobacteria is a common feature of acute appendicitis in Germany, Russia, and China. Saudi J Gastroenterol 2012;18(1):55–8.
94. Andersson RE, Petzold MG. Nonsurgical treatment of appendiceal abscess or phlegmon: a systematic review and meta-analysis. Ann Surg 2007;246(5):741–8.
95. St. Peter SD, Aguayo P, Fraser JD, et al. Initial laparoscopic appendectomy versus initial nonoperative management and interval appendectomy for perforated appendicitis with abscess: a prospective, randomized trial. J Pediatr Surg 2010;45(1):236–40.
96. Schurman JV, Cushing CC, Garey CL, et al. Quality of life assessment between laparoscopic appendectomy at presentation and interval appendectomy for perforated appendicitis with abscess: analysis of a prospective randomized trial. J Pediatr Surg 2011;46(6):1121–5.
97. Darwazeh G, Cunningham SC, Kowdley GC. A systematic review of perforated appendicitis and phlegmon: interval appendectomy or wait-and-see? Am Surg 2016;82(1):11–5.
98. Hall NJ, Jones CE, Eaton S, et al. Is interval appendicectomy justified after successful nonoperative treatment of an appendix mass in children? A systematic review. J Pediatr Surg 2011;46(4):767–71.
99. Iqbal CW, Knott EM, Mortellaro VE, et al. Interval appendectomy after perforated appendicitis: what are the operative risks and luminal patency rates? The J Surg Res 2012;177(1):127–30.
100. Kaminski A, Liu IL, Applebaum H, et al. Routine interval appendectomy is not justified after initial nonoperative treatment of acute appendicitis. Arch Surg 2005;140(9):897–901.
101. Ditkofsky NG, Singh A. Challenges in magnetic resonance imaging for suspected acute appendicitis in pregnant patients. Curr Probl Diagn Radiol 2015;44(4):297–302.
102. Smith MP, Katz DS, Lalani T, et al. ACR Appropriateness Criteria(R) right lower quadrant pain–suspected appendicitis. Ultrasound Q 2015;31(2):85–91.

103. Bass JA, Goldman J, Jackson MA, et al. Pediatric Crohn disease presenting as appendicitis: differentiating features from typical appendicitis. Eur J Pediatr Surg 2012;22(4):274–8.
104. AbdullGaffar B. Granulomatous diseases and granulomas of the appendix. Int J Surg Pathol 2010;18(1):14–20.
105. Dorfman S, Cardozo J, Dorfman D, et al. The role of parasites in acute appendicitis of pediatric patients. Invest Clin 2003;44(4):337–40.
106. Dorfman S, Talbot I, Torres R, et al. Parasitic infestation in acute appendicitis. Ann Trop Med Parasitol 1995;89(1):99–101.
107. Singh M, Kapoor V. Tuberculosis of the appendix: a report of 17 cases and a suggested aetiopathological classification. Postgrad Med J 1987;63(744): 855–7.

Emergency Presentations of Diverticulitis

Michael P. Meara, MD*, Colleen M. Alexander, MD

KEYWORDS

• Diverticulitis • Emergency • Surgery • Peritonitis • Lavage

KEY POINTS

- Acute diverticulitis varies in disease severity ranging from mild uncomplicated diverticulitis, which may be treated in the outpatient setting, to perforated complicated diverticulitis, requiring emergent surgical intervention.
- The pathophysiology of acute diverticulitis is still being elucidated but is now believed to have a significant contribution from inflammatory processes rather than being a strictly infectious process. Because of this, the routine use of antibiotics in the treatment of acute diverticulitis has been challenged.
- As nonoperative management of acute diverticulitis has improved, the need for routine colonic resection has been questioned. Multiple options for surgical management of acute diverticulitis exist and at this juncture the selection of what operation is best should be made on a case-by-case basis.
- Further research is needed to be able to recommend strategies for preventing the recurrence of acute diverticulitis. Dietary restrictions have not been proved beneficial.

INTRODUCTION

Acute diverticulitis is a common condition that has been increasing in incidence in the United States.[1–4] It is associated with increasing age, but other factors are believed to contribute to the pathophysiology of diverticular disease as well. As the population of the United States ages, diverticular disease is expected to require significant hospital resources. In 1988, diverticulitis was responsible for 2.2 million hospitalizations in the United States with health care costs of approximately $2.5 billion, and these figures have continued to increase.[4–6] There are still many questions to be answered regarding the optimal management of acute diverticulitis because recent studies have challenged traditional practices, such as the routine use of antibiotics, surgical technique, and dietary restrictions, for prevention of recurrence. Diverticulitis can be

Disclosure Statement: The authors have nothing to disclose.
Division of General and Gastrointestinal Surgery, The Ohio State University, 410 West 10th Avenue, 7th Floor Doan Hall, Columbus, OH 43210, USA
* Corresponding author.
E-mail address: Michael.Meara@osumc.edu

Surg Clin N Am 98 (2018) 1025–1046
https://doi.org/10.1016/j.suc.2018.06.006 surgical.theclinics.com
0039-6109/18/

seen in the right colon and small bowel (such as Meckel or duodenal diverticulitis) but left-sided colonic diverticulitis is the most common form of diverticulitis in the United States and is the focus of this article.[5,7]

EPIDEMIOLOGY

Diverticulitis is the most common nontraumatic cause of colonic perforation and the most common indication for elective colonic resection.[8,9] Although diverticular disease is common—approximately 60% of persons older than age 60 have diverticular disease. Acute diverticulitis develops in 4% to 25% of individuals with diverticular disease, and of these 15% to 40% have recurrent episodes of diverticulitis.[1,9–12] Multiple studies evaluating the Nationwide Inpatient Sample data in the United States have shown an increase in the admission rate for acute diverticulitis after adjustment for age.[1–4] Studies in England have shown an analogous increase in the incidence of acute diverticulitis.[1,13] Multiple explanations for the increasing incidence of diverticulitis have been postulated, including dietary factors, obesity, and bacterial colonization but the pathophysiology of this process still has aspects that are not well understood.[1,10] Up to 95% of patients who present with a diagnosis of acute uncomplicated diverticulitis are able to be managed in an outpatient setting.[1,14–16] After an initial episode of diverticulitis, the risk of recurrence is 15% to 40%, with the risk of developing a third or fourth episode similar to the risk of the first recurrence in some studies or increased in others.[9,11,17,18] A majority of the cases of complicated diverticulitis—characterized by perforation, abscess, fistula, or stricture—are in patients without a previous history of diverticulitis.[11,19]

PATHOPHYSIOLOGY OF DIVERTICULOSIS AND DIVERTICULITIS

The pathophysiology of diverticular disease is an area of continued research. It seems that the development of diverticulitis is triggered by interaction between individual predispositions and environmental factors. Factors suspected to be involved in the etiology of acute diverticulitis include obstruction of diverticula, colonic stasis, composition of the gut flora, and localized ischemia, among others.[11] The processes associated with the development of diverticulitis can be divided into approximately 3 categories: processes relating to weakness in the bowel wall, those relating to increased intraluminal pressure, and other processes (**Box 1**). As understanding of the disease process leading to diverticulitis has continued to develop, there have

Box 1
Factors believed to contribute to the development of colonic diverticulae

Weakness of the Bowel Wall	High Intraluminal Pressure	Other Associated Factors
• Noncircumferential muscular layers • Insertion of the vasa recta • Localized ischemia • Connective tissue disorders • Ehlers-Danlos syndrome	• Increased collagen crosslinking with age → less distensible, more contractile bowel → segmentation • Obstruction of diverticulae • Colonic stasis, chronic constipation • Low fiber intake	• Seasonal variation (summer months) • Smoking • Age • Obesity • Alcohol use • Immunocompromised state • Composition of intestinal flora

Data from Refs.[1,5,11,20–23]

been changes to treatment algorithms and recommendations for the prevention of recurrence.

An enteric diverticulum is classically defined as a true diverticulum, which is an outpouching that contains all layers of the bowel wall, or a false diverticulum, in which the inner mucosal and submucosal layers herniate through the muscular layers.[24] The presence of multiple diverticula commonly seen in the colon is described as diverticulosis. These are false diverticula and are most common in the sigmoid colon. Multiple theories exist for why this area of the colon is more susceptible to formation of diverticula. It may relate to anatomic considerations, such as the noncircumferential nature of the muscle layers or the insertion of the vasa recta.[1,11] Processes that affect collagen composition and distensibility of the bowel area also implicated in the diverticular disease process. It has been noted that collagen cross-linking increases with age resulting in a less distensible bowel wall, which is more contractile.[1,11] This can lead to a disordered motility process known as segmentation—where a segment of bowel contracts all at once instead of sequentially and creates a zone of high pressure—which may contribute to the formation of diverticula.[11] The ratio of type I to type III collagen in the colon has been compared across age groups as a possible etiology for diverticulitis and is known to decrease with age but was not found to be altered in younger patients with diverticulitis.[25]

A genetic predisposition toward diverticulosis may be present in some cases, as it has been observed that individuals with Ehlers-Danlos syndrome have a higher prevalence of diverticular disease.[11,20] The higher prevalence of right-sided colonic diverticulitis among Asian populations suggests a combination of genetic and environmental factors may be at play.[11,26,27] Two Scandinavian twin studies estimated the genetic contribution to diverticulitis to be 40% to 50%, and, although no particular genetic defect could be identified, the risk was noted to be highest in monozygotic twins.[1,28,29]

The pathophysiology of the progression from diverticulosis to acute inflammation and diverticulitis is still being investigated. More recent literature implicates an inflammatory process early in the course of the disease, which has led to questioning of the use of routine antibiotics for uncomplicated acute diverticulitis.[11] Comparison of RNA expression in diverticulitis patients at the time of elective sigmoid resection to normal controls revealed up-regulation of genes associated with immune response (gene ontology pathways).[10] There is also seasonal variation in the incidence of acute diverticulitis, with a peak during summer months noted universally in a study, including the United States, United Kingdom, and Australia.[21] The etiology of this seasonal variation is not well understood.

Patients with diverticulitis have been observed to have more variation in their gut microflora, primarily in the Proteobacteria phylum.[1,30] Some sources hypothesize a link between the chronic inflammatory state seen in obesity with a change in gut microflora, which may help explain the increased prevalence of diverticulitis in obese patients.[1,30–32] The idea of diverticulitis as an inflammatory condition rather than having a purely infectious etiology is also supported by a comparison of biopsies from chronic diverticulitis patients to those with chronic idiopathic inflammatory bowel disease.[31]

The relative risk (RR) of developing acute diverticulitis has been noted to be higher in certain populations. Current or past tobacco use is associated with a moderately increased risk, as is alcohol use, with the highest increase seen in cirrhotic patients (RR 2.9).[1,23,33,34] Multiple studies have shown an increased RR of diverticulitis in obese patients (RR 1.33–1.78), who are also at increased risk of complicated diverticulitis.[1,23,35,36] This is postulated to be due to a state of chronic low-grade inflammation, which is observed in obese patients.[1]

As discussed previously, the prevalence of diverticular disease is known to increase with age and has increased disproportionally more than expected when corrections are made for the aging population of the United States and increased life expectancy.[1–5] Although there is not a clear gender association, it has been observed that hospitalized patients with diverticulitis less than age 45 tend to be male, whereas those older than 54 tend to be female.[2,11]

An immunocompromised state is associated with an increased risk of acute diverticulitis and an increased risk of morbidity and mortality among patients with diverticulitis.[22] Because of this, some sources recommend evaluation for elective sigmoid colon resection in patients with a history of diverticulitis who are currently wait-listed for organ transplantation.[22]

Although the mechanism is unclear, physical activity is associated with a decreased risk of developing acute diverticulitis.[1,36–39] Historically, a high-fiber diet has been postulated to decrease the risk of acute diverticulitis, but many studies have failed to show a significant benefit. Low dietary fiber intake has been suspected of playing a role in the development of diverticulosis, perhaps by having lower stool bulk, which contributes to the process of segmentation.[11]

EVALUATION

The evaluation and treatment of patients who present with suspected acute diverticulitis hinge on the ability to accurately stratify patients along a spectrum of escalating treatment options. Although a majority of patients can be managed without hospital admission and are not likely to be seen by a surgeon, it should not be forgotten that up to 72% of patients who present with complicated diverticulitis do not have had a prior episode.[1,14–16,19] Priority should be given to patient resuscitation if needed and to evaluation for signs and symptoms of sepsis or organ dysfunction. Patients who are critically ill on presentation may benefit from a brief period of resuscitation preoperatively but ultimately require surgical intervention.[11] History and physical examination can help determine if the episode of diverticulitis is recurrent or not and whether there are any findings to suggest complicated diverticulitis, but currently there is no classification system that perfectly predicts which patients will benefit from particular treatment regimens.[1]

CLASSIFICATION

Acute diverticulitis can be classified in multiple ways to aid in treatment decisions. Uncomplicated cases typically have a less acute presentation and lack the features indicative of a complicated diverticulitis (**Table 1**). Abscess is the most common complication of acute diverticulitis.[11] If perforation is suspected, the Hinchey classification system is traditionally used to stratify the stages of abdominal contamination (**Box 2**). Other classification systems have been evaluated, such as endoscopic scoring, imaging-based scoring with CT scan or ultrasound, and combined clinical and radiographic scoring systems.[1,5] The American Association for the Surgery of Trauma (AAST) has proposed a grading scale for 16 emergency general surgery conditions, including acute diverticulitis. This has been based on consensus and although it has been validated retrospectively in a multicenter study, prospective data are not yet available.[40] The AAST system has similarities to the Hinchey classification system but includes nonperforated disease as grade I (**Table 2**).

Table 1
Etiologies of complicated diverticulitis—findings on presentation

Complication	History and Physical Examination Findings	Findings on Imaging
Abscess	• Fever, leukocytosis • Palpable mass	• Spectrum from contained abscess to generalized feculent peritonitis (see Hinchey classification)
Bowel obstruction	• Nausea, vomiting • Abdominal distention	• Dilated bowel proximal to site of inflammation or abscess
Fistula	• Colovesical fistula: pneumaturia, fecaluria, recurrent urinary tract infections • Colovaginal fistula: air or feculent drainage from the vagina • Enterocutaneous or perirectal fistula: external drainage	• Possible visualization of a fistula tract; can be aided by injection of contrast into the fistulous opening (fistulogram) or enteric contrast
Perforation	• May be asymptomatic • Fever, leukocytosis, sepsis • Peritonitis, rebound tenderness	• Free air or free fluid within the abdomen • Gross perforation may be present with a large amount of free air or feculent contamination • Microperforation may be evident with small bubbles of air surrounding the colon
Stricture	• Obstructive symptoms, nausea, vomiting • Previous episodes of diverticulitis	• Narrowing of the affected bowel, often with proximal dilation • May have chronic appearance with scarring

Data from Shah SD, Cifu AS. Management of acute diverticulitis. JAMA 2017;318(3):291–2; and Fagenholz PJ, de Moya MA. Acute inflammatory surgical disease. Surg Clin North Am 2014;94(1):1–30.

Box 2
Hinchey classification for perforated diverticulitis

- Stage I: pericolic or mesenteric abscess
- Stage II: walled off pelvic abscess
- Stage III: generalized purulent peritonitis
- Stage IV: generalized fecal peritonitis

Adapted from Hinchey EJ, Schaal PG, Richards GK. Treatment of perforated diverticular disease of the colon. Adv Surg 1978;12:85; with permission.

PRESENTATION

Acute diverticulitis can present differently depending on the location of the affected colon. Right-sided diverticulitis is more common in Asian populations and can be difficult to differentiate from acute appendicitis.[7] Diverticulitis of the left colon is more common in Western countries and presents with left lower quadrant pain in approximately 70% of cases.[5] The presentation of acute diverticulitis can be anywhere on a spectrum from mild abdominal discomfort in an afebrile patient with a normal white blood cell count to a patient with peritonitis, rebound tenderness, and septic shock. Approximately 85% of patients present with uncomplicated diverticulitis.[9] Many patients have had abdominal pain for more than 24 hours with low-grade fever and either a mild leukocytosis or normal white blood cell count.[5,41] Associated symptoms may include nausea and vomiting, changes in bowel habits, or urinary symptoms.[5] Physical examination and vital signs may reveal fever, left lower quadrant tenderness, abdominal distention, or palpable mass if an abscess is present.[5]

Differential Diagnosis

Lower abdominal pain is often the presenting symptom for acute diverticulitis but has a broad differential, which can lead to misdiagnosis in 34% to 68% of patients (**Box 3**).[5,42–44] A thorough history and physical examination as well as diagnostic imaging may help narrow the possibilities. The differential for female patients must include disorders of the reproductive tract or pregnancy in the appropriate context.

Work-up for a Patient with Suspected Acute Diverticulitis

After initial stabilization and evaluation for sepsis, the evaluation of suspected acute diverticulitis focuses on collection of information from the history, physical

Table 2
American Association for the Surgery of Trauma grading scale for acute colonic diverticulits

Grade	Description
I	Colonic inflammation
II	Colonic microperforation or pericolic phlegmon without abscess
III	Localized pericolonic abscess
IV	Distant abscess
V	Free colonic perforation with generalized peritonitis

Data from Shafi S, Priest EL, Crandall ML, et al. Multicenter validation of American Association for the Surgery of Trauma grading system for acute colonic diverticulitis and its use for emergency general surgery quality improvement program. J Trauma Acute Care Surg 2016;80(3):405–10.

Box 3
Differential diagnosis for common causes of acute lower abdominal pain

- Acute diverticulitis
- Appendicitis
- Infectious or ischemic colitis
- Inflammatory bowel disease
- Bowel obstruction
- Hernia of the abdominal wall (inguinal, ventral)
- Internal hernia
- Nephrolithiasis
- Female patients: gynecologic pathology or pregnancy

Data from Refs.[5,11,42–44]

examination, laboratory studies, and imaging modalities that can guide therapy decisions. What information is gathered may depend in part on what classification system is used (discussed previously). Clinically mild cases may be diagnosed without laboratory studies or imaging if a history of diverticulitis is known, but initial or more acute presentations usually require further evaluation.[11]

History

Attention should be paid to determination of whether an episode is new or recurrent and complicated versus uncomplicated. Review of systems may aid in identification of symptoms suggestive of complicated disease, such as pneumaturia, fecaluria, and vomiting. Associated factors, such as age, obesity, immunocompromised state, or connective tissue disorders, should be noted. It should be determined if a patient is up to date on colonoscopy screenings and if the patient has a personal or family history suggestive of colonic malignancy.

Physical examination

Vital signs may be normal or indicative of sepsis. Examination likely evaluates hemodynamic status and then focuses on the abdomen, assessing for signs of peritonitis, abscess, mass, or fistula. A rectal examination may reveal fluctuance or pain consistent with an abscess.

Laboratory studies

Basic laboratory studies, such as a complete blood cell count and metabolic panel, are useful to determine if a leukocytosis is present as well as renal function or electrolyte abnormalities, which may require correction. Leukocytosis alone has not been useful for differentiating acute diverticulitis from other forms of abdominal pain or for stratification of disease severity but may be used in conjunction with other measures in some scoring systems.[45,46] A urinalysis should be obtained to assist in ruling out complicated diverticular disease with a colovesical fistula.[11]

C-reactive protein (CRP) has been studied as an indicator of acute diverticulitis or its severity but has not been standardized.[45] CRP greater than 20 mg/dL was associated with an increased risk of death in immunocompromised patients with acute diverticulitis but did not remain statistically significant after multivariate analysis.[22] CRP greater than 109 mg/mL has been evaluated to predict complicated diverticulitis, but the area under the curve was 0.64, which indicates poor predictive value.[46]

Diagnostic imaging

Multiple imaging modalities have been used in the evaluation of possible acute diverticulitis. Due to its availability, sensitivity, and specificity, CT scan is the most commonly used.[11] Oral and intravenous contrast are recommended because they improve the sensitivity and specificity of the study.[5] CT scan can be used to help differentiate possible etiologies of abdominal pain and to stratify the severity of diverticulitis but cannot always differentiate acute diverticulitis from a colonic malignancy.[11,47,48]

Preoperative evaluation of psoas muscle mass on CT scan has been studied as a predictor of postoperative complications in patients with diverticulitis. Low psoas muscle mass was associated with postoperative major complications and surgical site infection.[49] Ultrasound has been proposed as an imaging modality to evaluate acute diverticulitis but is not currently a standard of care.[50–52]

For acutely ill patients, abdominal series radiographs may be helpful in establishing if large-volume free air is present, but the amount of free air has been called into question as an indicator for surgery in stable patients (discussed later).[11]

MEDICAL MANAGEMENT

The optimal management of acute diverticulitis continues to be an area of research and controversy. Multiple sets of guidelines have been published, which vary in their recommendations.[1,53–58]

Antibiotic Therapy

Acute diverticulitis has traditionally been considered an infectious process and has been treated with antibiotic therapy, such as a 7-day to 14-day course of antibiotics with concurrent bowel rest until symptoms resolve with gradual reintroduction of the diet.[5,11] Further understanding of the pathophysiology of diverticulitis as well as multiple studies evaluating the safety of treating uncomplicated diverticulitis without antibiotics have called this into question.[9,11,59,60] In 2015 the American Gastroenterological Association published guidelines for the management of acute diverticulitis that included a conditional recommendation to use antibiotics selectively rather than routinely.[9] This recommendation was based on 2 multicenter randomized controlled trials that did not show superiority of antibiotic treatment, but the recommendation was conditional due to low-quality evidence and risk of bias.[9] A cohort study of 244 patients with uncomplicated acute diverticulitis also concluded that treatment without antibiotics is safe and feasible. This study had a 4% ($n = 5$) conversion to antibiotic therapy due to worsening clinical picture and 2 readmissions within 30 days, with complications reported as 1 fistula and a recurrence rate of 5% ($n = 8$).[60]

Antibiotic therapy is still a mainstay of treatment of patients with complicated disease. Empiric coverage should include gram-negative bacteria and anaerobes.[11] Combination treatment with a fluoroquinolone, such as ciprofloxacin or metronidazole, is common, although there are numerous alternative regimens, including use of a β-lactam/β-lactamase, use of clindamycin instead of metronidazole, or monotherapy with a carbapenem or moxifloxacin.[11]

Inpatient Versus Outpatient Treatment

For a majority of patients who present with uncomplicated acute diverticulitis, management in the outpatient setting (with or without antibiotics) can be considered.[5] Studies comparing inpatient versus outpatient therapy with a course of oral antibiotics showed no differences in effectiveness but significantly reduced health care costs.[5,61–63] There is theoretic support for outpatient monitoring of patients with uncomplicated acute diverticulitis without the use of antibiotics, but studies directly evaluating this are lacking. Patient selection is also of importance, because these studies excluded patients with comorbidities or preset criteria from the no-antibiotics or outpatient care groups.[5,63,64] Currently the best approach seems to be to determine admission status and antibiotic use on a case-by-case basis, taking into account a patient's clinical status and comorbidities.

Dietary Changes and Probiotics

Currently there is not sufficient evidence to recommend probiotics or manipulation of the colonic flora in the treatment or prevention of recurrence of diverticulitis.[1,65] The observation that colonic flora differ in patients with diverticulitis suggests that altering the colonic flora may be beneficial in the treatment or prevention of diverticulitis, but studies supporting this are currently lacking.

Many patients with a history of diverticulitis have been cautioned regarding the dietary intake of certain foods, such as seeds or nuts, but there have been multiple studies that showed no difference in outcomes between groups on a restricted diet versus an unrestricted diet.[1,5]

ADJUNCTIVE THERAPY FOR COMPLICATED DIVERTICULITIS

Percutaneous Drainage of Abscess

Because minimally invasive and image-guided approaches to abscess drainage have improved, they have largely replaced the operative management of intra-abdominal abscesses. Percutaneous drainage is successful in resolving intra-abdominal abscesses associated with diverticulitis in 60% to 85% of patients.[11] The size at which an abscess should be drained versus managed with antibiotics alone varies among studies, but generally an abscess of 2 cm or 3 cm or less can be effectively managed with antibiotics alone whereas larger abscesses likely require percutaneous drainage.[11,66,67] The American Society of Colon and Rectal Surgeons (ASCRS) recommends treatment with antibiotics alone for abscesses 2 cm and smaller. Treatment of intermediate-sized abscesses (3–5 cm) with antibiotics alone can be considered for patients with contraindications to percutaneous drainage or anatomically inaccessible abscesses, but they should be clinically stable and monitored for failure to improve or deterioration, which would trigger operative intervention.[11] Percutaneous drains can be removed after a patient has clinically improved, imaging shows resolution of the abscess cavity, and the drain output is low (less than 10–20 mL/d).[11]

OPERATIVE MANAGEMENT

Surgical treatment of acute diverticulitis continues to be an area of controversy among surgeons. Multiple studies have been published comparing laparoscopic lavage to alternatives, such as laparoscopic sigmoid resection with primary anastomosis, or the gold standard of a Hartmann pouch. Variations in study methodology and definitions of treatment failure or recurrence have made meta-analyses difficult and interpretation of results inconsistent.[68] Due to the success of percutaneous drainage in a majority of patients with diverticular abscess, operative intervention is generally reserved for cases of treatment failure or contraindications to percutaneous drainage.[11] Approximately 15% to 25% of patients with acute diverticulitis have complicated disease, which requires surgery.[69] Selection of an appropriate surgical option may be influenced by patient considerations or surgeon preference (**Box 4**).

Box 4
Indications for surgical management of acute diverticulitis

- Failure of medical or percutaneous therapy
- Patient instability or persistent sepsis
- Complicated disease with peritonitis
- Recurrent uncomplicated diverticulitis (number of episodes is controversial)
- Inability to rule out malignancy

Large-volume pneumoperitoneum has historically been viewed as an indication for surgery but more recently has been called into question as an absolute indication for operative intervention and instead is used in combination with other signs or symptoms to identify ongoing contamination of the peritoneum.[11,70]

Hartmann Pouch—Historical Gold Standard

In 2000, the ASCRS recommended the Hartmann procedure as the gold standard for acute perforated diverticulitis with peritonitis.[5,71] Historically, a 3-stage process was used, consisting of a proximal diverting colostomy, later resection of the affected segment of colon, and eventual colostomy closure.[72] A 2-stage process has since been widely adopted, consisting of concurrent diverting colostomy with resection of the affected segment, then a staged colostomy takedown.[5]

Primary Resection with Anastomosis

There is a reasonable body of evidence to support primary resection of the affected colon as an alternative to colostomy alone as the initial treatment of complicated acute diverticulitis.[5,11,73,74] Multiple studies have indicated that primary anastomosis of the colon at the initial operation has comparable morbidity and mortality to the Hartmann procedure as well as higher rates of stoma closure and lower cost.[75] The safety of a single-stage operation without a diverting loop ileostomy is controversial and needs to be in stable, carefully selected patients.[11] Although some patients who present with a partial bowel obstruction respond to medical management, resection or ostomy creation may be necessary for patients who fail medical management or for those who present with a high-grade obstruction.[11] For patients who are not obstructed on presentation, a laparoscopic approach with primary colonic resection and primary anastomosis is feasible, with a conversion rate of 6.8% in a prospective trial.[5]

Laparoscopic Lavage Versus Primary Resection

Laparoscopic lavage without colonic resection has garnered attention as an alternative to the gold standard Hartmann procedure and other variants of colonic resection for the treatment of acute complicated diverticulitis. Multiple trials, reviews, and meta-analyses have been published, some with conflicting conclusions.[76–89] These studies highlight the importance of continued research and careful patient selection (**Table 3**).

Some of the larger trials have been included in meta-analyses and have been the focus of much debate.[90–92] Data derived from these studies and published case series show that laparoscopic lavage has shorter operative times and less cost than surgical resection.[85,88] Whether laparoscopic lavage should be adopted as a new standard of care in the treatment of acute perforated diverticulitis is less clear. Although comparisons are difficult due to differences in definitions and measured outcomes, there seems to be a higher rate of reoperation and percutaneous intervention during the

Table 3
Summary of recent studies on laparoscopic treatment of acute diverticulitis

Study	Description	Major Findings	Comments
LapLAND trial (NCT01019239)	• Comparison of laparoscopic lavage to Hartmann procedure or resection with stoma	• Pending	Hospitals in Ireland
DILALA trial[84]	• Multicenter RCT comparing laparoscopic lavage (n = 39) to colon resection with stoma (n = 36) • Used diagnostic laparoscopy to determine Hinchey stage III, then randomized and followed for 12 wk postoperatively	• No difference in morbidity or mortality • Lavage was associated with shorter times in OR and recovery unit, and shorter hospital stay. • Conclusion: laparoscopic lavage for patients with Hinchey III perforated diverticulitis is feasible and safe in the short term.	Cost analysis published, showed reduced cost in laparoscopic lavage group.[85]
Ref.[86]	• RCT comparing laparoscopic lavage (n = 43) to Hartmann procedure (n = 40) • Primary outcome: number of operations within 12 mo • Secondary outcomes: number of reoperations, readmissions, total length of stay, and adverse events	• Risk of reoperation was lower in the laparoscopic lavage group (n = 12, 28%) vs Hartmann group (n = 25, 62.5%). • There was no difference in mortality or adverse events. • Risk of stoma at 12 mo was lower in lavage group (n = 3 and 11, respectively). • Total length of stay was shorter in the lavage group.	

(*continued on next page*)

Table 3
(continued)

Study	Description	Major Findings	Comments
LOLA arm of LADIES trial (NCT01317485)[87]	• Multicenter RCT, open label • 2 arms: LOLA and DIVA • LOLA—comparing laparoscopic lavage with sigmoidectomy • DIVA—comparing Hartmann to sigmoidecotmy with primary anastomosis (results pending). • LOLA arm: patients with perforated purulent peritonitis were randomized to laparoscopic lavage, Hartmann procedure, or primary anastomosis in a 2:1:1 ratio. Endpoint was morbidity or mortality in 12 mo.	• 90 patients were enrolled in the LOLA arm when it was terminated early for an increased event rate in the laparoscopic lavage group (4 mortalities, 18 reoperations) and in the sigmoidectomy group (6 mortalities, 2 reoperations).	34 teaching hospitals, 8 academic hospitals in Belgium and the Netherlands Cost analysis favored laparoscopic lavage.[88]
SCANDIV trial[89]	• RCT. Laparoscopic lavage (n = 101) compared with primary resection (n = 98). • Perforated diverticulitis was verified in 89 and 83 patients, respectively.	• 1-y rates of complications and mortality were significantly different. • Laparoscopic lavage had more unplanned reoperations than primary resection (27% vs 10%), but secondary operation rates were 28% vs 29% respectively if stoma reversals were included.	

Abbreviation: RCT, randomized controlled trial.

initial hospitalization in the laparoscopic lavage groups. Reoperation rates are reported to be 20% to 53% for laparoscopic lavage, with the majority of studies indicating a lower rate for reoperation after primary resection (Thornell and colleagues[80] cited a 62% reoperation rate in the primary resection group, which is much higher than other studies).[80,86,90–93] The overall rate of ostomy creation and reoperation for ostomy reversal has typically been higher in the primary resection group than in the laparoscopic lavage group. The cited rates for overall morbidity and mortality have been variable with multiple studies showing no difference between surgical resection and laparoscopic lavage, but the LOLA arm of the Ladies trial was stopped early due to an increased event rate.[84,86,87,90,91]

At this point in time, it is difficult to make a generalized recommendation whether it is better to proceed with surgical resection and accept a higher rate of ostomy creation or whether to proceed with laparoscopic lavage and risk an approximately 30% reoperation rate. Based on the current data, this decision is best left to surgeons to be decided on a case-by-case basis given that overall morbidity and mortality seem equal.

As medical management strategies have improved, the trend has been toward operative intervention only in the sickest patients, who are more likely to have associated comorbidities.[93,94] Careful patient selection may help improve the reintervention rate of laparoscopic lavage. Some sources have advocated laparoscopic lavage for Hinchey III disease but not for Hinchey IV disease, whereas others have postulated that many Hinchey III diverticulitis patients would improve without surgical intervention.[11] In particular, immunosuppression, such as with steroids or chemotherapy, has been associated with failure of laparoscopic lavage therapy and merit attention when determining the surgical plan for patients with acute complicated diverticulitis.[93]

Interval Sigmoid Colectomy

Patients who are diagnosed with complicated acute diverticulitis and are treated medically have typically been offered interval sigmoid colectomy, although that practice has recently been challenged.[5,11,95] Exceptions may be made based on patient factors, such as the severity of comorbidities, operative risk, and life expectancy.[96,97] Patients who have persistent sequelae of complicated diverticulitis, such as a fistula, are also typically offered surgery, whereas surgical resection may not be needed in patients whose symptoms completely resolve with medical management.[5] The need for interval surgical resection after laparoscopic lavage for complicated acute diverticulitis has also been called into question.[96–99]

At what point surgical resection should be offered to patients with repeated episodes of uncomplicated diverticulitis is less standardized. Approximately 1 in 3 patients develop a second episode of uncomplicated diverticulitis, with the risk of a third episode being the same or increasing after each episode.[1,18] Patients who are immunosuppressed or have chronic renal failure, collagen vascular disease, or persistent symptoms between episodes have been considered for earlier primary resection due to a higher risk of complicated diverticulitis, but this also has been debated in recent years.[1,5] For patients without these risk factors, guidelines from the American Gastroenterological Association released in 2015 recommend that elective colonic resection is not offered after a first attack of uncomplicated diverticulitis.[9] At least 1 study showed lower mortality and colostomy rates when patients had surgical resection after their fourth episode compared with their second episode of acute diverticulitis.[100] Even when acute diverticulitis recurs (approximately 20% in 5 years), the risk of complications or emergency surgery with the recurrence is less than 5%.[9]

Laparoscopic sigmoid colectomy has become the standard of care due to lower morbidity than open resection and is feasible even in the setting of complications, such as colovesical fistula.[11,101,102]

Other Surgical Considerations

Timing of surgery

In 1 study, retrospective analysis showed a higher rate of morbidity and longer hospital stays in patients whose surgery was delayed more than 24 hours after admission, but there was no difference in 30-day mortality.[103] This highlights the importance of trying to risk stratify patients for nonoperative versus operative therapy.

Loop transverse colostomy

For patients who present with high-grade obstruction and are critically ill or with concurrent dilation of the cecum, a transverse loop colostomy can be a good option. It typically takes less time to perform than a Hartmann procedure and can be done under local anesthesia if necessary—temporizing the patient to allow for later colonic resection with possible anastomosis.[11]

Minimally invasive techniques

Alternative surgical techniques for colonic resection in the treatment of diverticulitis have been published, but remain topics for future research. These include robotic-assisted sigmoid colectomy, single-incision laparoscopic surgery, and natural orifice transluminal endoscopic surgery.[104–106]

Ureteral stents

Use of ureteral stents varies widely. They can be placed prior to surgery in patients where there is concern for risk of ureteral injury during the process of dissection. Ureteral stent placement may not prevent ureteral injury, but some investigators believe it allows for intraoperative recognition and correction of the problem should it occur.[107]

Adjunctive use of indocyanine green dye

Use of indocyanine green (ICG) dye for visualization of the colonic blood supply can be a useful adjunctive measure to determine the viability of colon for creation of an anastomosis.[108] It also has been used for visualization of the ureters intraoperatively via cystoscopic injection (**Fig. 1**).[109]

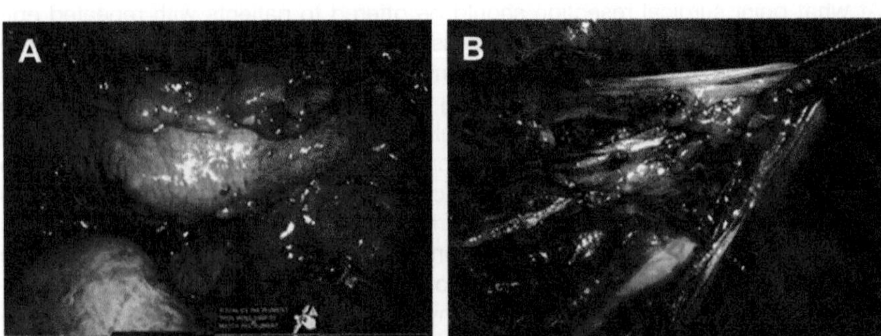

Fig. 1. ICG dye for visualization of the colon vascular supply (*A*) and ureter (*B*). (*Courtesy of* Michael P. Meara, MD, FACS, Columbus, OH.)

FOLLOW-UP

Role of Colonoscopy After Acute Diverticulitis

Whether or not colonoscopy should be performed prior to elective colon resection for diverticular disease has been a topic of debate. The rationale for proceeding with colonoscopy prior to resection is that the presence of malignancy may influence operative planning, and up to 5% of patients initially diagnosed with diverticulitis may be found to have adenocarcinoma on further work-up.[11] Preoperative work-up may not be necessary if a patient has had a recent screening for colon cancer, or a patient can have a screening evaluation, such as colonoscopy approximately 6 weeks after resolution of the episode of acute diverticulitis.[11] Colonoscopy can be used to confirm the presence of diverticular disease, diagnose and treat colonic polyps (up to 26% of patients), or diagnose colorectal malignancy.[11,110] Some institutions have cited lower rates of pathology in patients who had uncomplicated diverticulitis and only recommend colonoscopy after complicated diverticulitis, if CT findings were atypical for acute diverticulitis, or if the patient was otherwise due for screening.[111,112] In contrast, the incidence of colon cancer in a Danish population study was higher (4.3%) in the diverticulitis group than in the group without diverticulitis (2.3%).[113]

Prevention of Recurrence

Multiple approaches to reduce the risk of recurrence of acute diverticulitis have been evaluated, but most lack sufficient evidence to be routinely recommended.

Probiotics

Probiotics, such as lactobacillus or bifidobacteria, have been proposed as a means of altering the microflora of the colon and influencing the pathophysiology contributing to the development of acute diverticulitis, but this requires further studies to demonstrate benefit.[1,114]

Luminal antibiotics and 5-aminosalicylic acid compounds

Treatment with mesalazine derivatives, rifaximin, or other agents to modify gut microflora is appealing for use in the prevention of recurrent diverticulitis, but trials have been contradictory to each other and currently they are not standard practice.[115–119]

Dietary restrictions

Avoidance of seeds and nuts have historically been recommended to patients with a history of diverticulitis, but guidelines from the American Gastroenterological Association have lifted these restrictions due to lack of evidence.[1,9] The guidelines give a conditional recommendation for a fiber-rich diet because there is some evidence that it is helpful, but the quality of the available data is poor.[9,120] A prospective cohort study showed an association between a Western diet (high in red meat and low in fiber) and diverticulitis, but other studies have shown no association with an unrestricted diet.[121,122]

SUMMARY

Acute diverticulitis is a disease process that requires further research to continue elucidating the pathophysiology, ideal treatment algorithms, and strategies to prevent recurrence. Understanding of the inflammatory nature of acute diverticulitis has led to decreased use of antibiotics in uncomplicated cases. Laparoscopic lavage may be considered in carefully selected patients, but the standard of care for treatment of perforated acute diverticulitis continues to be surgical resection. The ideal approach for each patient should be determined on an individual basis. Measures to help prevent the recurrence of acute diverticulitis have been proposed, but further research is needed to demonstrate any benefit from these measures.

REFERENCES

1. Søreide K, Boermeester MA, Humes DJ, et al. Acute colonic diverticulitis: modern understanding of pathomechanisms, risk factors, disease burden and severity. Scand J Gastroenterol 2016;51(12):1416–22.
2. Nguyen GC, Sam J, Anand N. Epidemiological trends and geographic variation in hospital admissions for diverticulitis in the United States. World J Gastroenterol 2011;17:1600–5.
3. Masoomi H, Buchberg BS, Magno C, et al. Trends in diverticulitis management in the United States from 2002 to 2007. Arch Surg 2011;146:400–6.
4. Etzioni DA, Mack TM, Beart RW Jr, et al. Diverticulitis in the United States: 1998-2005: changing patterns of disease and treatment. Ann Surg 2009;249:210–7.
5. Horesh N, Wasserberg N, Zbar AP, et al. Changing paradigms in the management of diverticulitis. Int J Surg 2016;33 Pt A(9):146–50.
6. Sandler RS, Everhart JE, Donowitz M, et al. The burden of selected digestive diseases in the United States. Gastroenterology 2002;122(5):1500–11.
7. Hall JF, Stein SL. Unexpected intra-operative findings. Surg Clin North Am 2013;93(1):45–59.
8. Brown CV. Small bowel and colon perforation. Surg Clin North Am 2014;94(2):471–5.
9. Shah SD, Cifu AS. Management of acute diverticulitis. JAMA 2017;318(3):291–2.
10. Schieffer KM, Choi CS, Emrich S, et al. RNA-seq implicates deregulation of the immune system in the pathogenesis of diverticulitis. Am J Physiol Gastrointest Liver Physiol 2017;313(3):G277–84.
11. Fagenholz PJ, de Moya MA. Acute inflammatory surgical disease. Surg Clin North Am 2014;94(1):1–30.
12. Shahedi K, Fuller G, Bolus R, et al. Long-term risk of acute diverticulitis among patients with incidental diverticulosis found during colonoscopy. Clin Gastroenterol Hepatol 2013;11(12):1609–13.
13. Kang JY, Hoare J, Tinto A, et al. Diverticular disease of the colon on the rise: a study of hospital admissions in England between 1989/1990 and 1999/2000. Aliment Pharmacol Ther 2003;17:1189–95.
14. Chabok A, Pahlman L, Hjern F, et al. Randomized clinical trial of antibiotics in acute uncomplicated diverticulitis. Br J Surg 2012;99:532–9.
15. De Korte N, Unlu C, Boermeester MA, et al. Use of antibiotics in uncomplicated diverticulitis. Br J Surg 2011;98:761–7.
16. Moya P, Arroyo A, Perez-Legaz J, et al. Applicability, safety and efficiency of outpatient treatment in uncomplicated diverticulitis. Tech Coloproctol 2012;16:301–7.
17. Rafferty J, Shellito P, Hyman NH, et al, Standards Committee of American Society of Colon and Rectal Surgeons. Practice parameters for sigmoid diverticulitis. Dis Colon Rectum 2006;49:939–44.
18. Hupfeld L, Burcharth J, Pommergaard HC, et al. Risk factors for recurrence after acute colonic diverticulitis: a systematic review. Int J Colorectal Dis 2017;32(5):611–22.

19. Humes DJ, West J. Role of acute diverticulitis in the development of complicated colonic diverticular disease and 1-year mortality after diagnosis in the UK: population-based cohort study. Gut 2012;61:95–100.
20. Leganger J, Søborg MK, Mortensen LQ, et al. Association between diverticular disease and Ehlers-Danlos syndrome: a 13-year nationwide population-based cohort study. Int J Colorectal Dis 2016;31(12):1863–7.
21. Adler JT, Chang DC, Chan AT, et al. Seasonal variation in diverticulitis: evidence from both hemispheres. Dis Colon Rectum 2016;59(9):870–7.
22. Brandl A, Kratzer T, Kafka-Ritsch R, et al. Diverticulitis in immunosuppressed patients: a fatal outcome requiring a new approach? Can J Surg 2016;59(4): 254–61.
23. Jamal Talabani A, Lydersen S, Ness-Jensen E, et al. Risk factors of admission for acute colonic diverticulitis in a population-based cohort study: the North Trondelag Health Study, Norway. World J Gastroenterol 2016;22(48):10663–72.
24. Mahmoud NN, Bleier JIS, Aarons CB, et al. Colon and rectum. In: Courtney M, Townsend Jr, et al, editors. Sabiston textbook of surgery: the biological basis of modern surgical practice. 19th edition. Philadelphia: Elsevier, Inc; 2012. p. 1294–380.
25. Brown SR, Cleveland EM, Deeken CR, et al. Type I/type III collagen ratio associated with diverticulitis of the colon in young patients. J Surg Res 2017;207: 229–34.
26. Touzios JG, Dozois EJ. Diverticulosis and acute diverticulitis. Gastroenterol Clin North Am 2009;38:513–25.
27. Commane DM, Arasaradnam RP, Mills S, et al. Diet, ageing and genetic factors in the pathogenesis of diverticular disease. World J Gastroenterol 2009;15: 2479–88.
28. Granlund J, Svensson T, Olen O, et al. The genetic influence on diverticular disease - a twin study. Aliment Pharmacol Ther 2012;35:1103–7.
29. Strate LL, Erichsen R, Baron JA, et al. Heritability and familial aggregation of diverticular disease: a population-based study of twins and siblings. Gastroenterology 2013;144:736–42.
30. Daniels L, Budding AE, de Korte N, et al. Fecal microbiome analysis as a diagnostic test for diverticulitis. Eur J Clin Microbiol Infect Dis 2014;33:1927–36.
31. Daniels L, Philipszoon LE, Boermeester MA. A hypothesis: important role for gut microbiota in the etiopathogenesis of diverticular disease. Dis Colon Rectum 2014;57:539–43.
32. Spiller RC. Changing views on diverticular disease: impact of aging, obesity, diet, and microbiota. Neurogastroenterol Motil 2015;27:305–12.
33. Aldoori WH, Giovannucci EL, Rimm EB, et al. A prospective study of alcohol, smoking, caffeine, and the risk of symptomatic diverticular disease in men. Ann Epidemiol 1995;5:221–8.
34. Hjern F, Wolk A, Hakansson N. Smoking and the risk of diverticular disease in women. Br J Surg 2011;98:997–1002.
35. Strate LL, Liu YL, Aldoori WH, et al. Obesity increases the risk of diverticulitis and diverticular bleeding. Gastroenterology 2009;136:115–22.
36. Hjern F, Wolk A, Hakansson N. Obesity, physical activity, and colonic diverticular disease requiring hospitalization in women: a prospective cohort study. Am J Gastroenterol 2012;107:296–302.
37. Strate LL, Liu YL, Aldoori WH, et al. Physical activity decreases diverticular complications. Am J Gastroenterol 2009;104:1221–30.

38. Tursi A, Brandimarte G, Di Mario F, et al. Predictive value of the Diverticular Inflammation and Complication Assessment (DICA) endoscopic classification on the outcome of diverticular disease of the colon: an international study. United European Gastroenterol J 2016;4:604–13.
39. Tursi A, Brandimarte G, Di Mario F, et al. Development and validation of and endoscopic classification of diverticular disease of the colon: the DICA classification. Dig Dis 2015;33:68–76.
40. Shafi S, Priest EL, Crandall ML, et al. Multicenter Validation of American Association for the Surgery of Trauma grading system for acute colonic diverticulitis and its use for emergency general surgery quality improvement program. J Trauma Acute Care Surg 2016;80(3):405–10.
41. Rodkey GV, Welch CE. Changing patterns in the surgical treatment of diverticular disease. Ann Surg 1984;200(4):466–78.
42. Wexner SD, Dailey TH. The initial management of left lower quadrant peritonitis. Dis Colon Rectum 1986;29(10):635–8.
43. Cho KC, Morehouse HT, Alteman DD, et al. Sigmoid diverticulitis: diagnostic role of CT–comparison with barium enema studies. Radiology 1990;176(1):111–5.
44. Farag Soliman M, Wüstner M, Sturm J, et al. Primary diagnostics of acute diverticulitis of the sigmoid. Ultraschall Med 2004;25(5):342–7.
45. Jamal Talabani A, Endreseth BH, Lydersen S, et al. Clinical diagnostic accuracy of acute colonic diverticulitis in patients admitted with acute abdominal pain, a receiver operating characteristic curve analysis. Int J Colorectal Dis 2017;32(1): 41–7.
46. Hogan J, Sehgal R, Murphy D, et al. Do inflammatory indices play a role in distinguishing between uncomplicated and complicated diverticulitis? Dig Surg 2017;34(1):7–11.
47. Sartelli M, Moore FA, Ansaloni L, et al. A proposal for a CT driven classification of left colon acute diverticulitis. World J Emerg Surg 2015;10:3.
48. Flor N, Maconi G, Sardanelli F, et al. Prognostic value of the diverticular disease severity score based on CT colonography: follow up in patients recovering from acute diverticulitis. Acad Radiol 2015;22:1503–9.
49. Matsushima K, Inaba K, Jhaveri V, et al. Loss of muscle mass: a significant predictor of postoperative complications in acute diverticulitis. J Surg Res 2017; 211:39–44.
50. Lembcke BJ. Ultrasonography in acute diverticulitis - credit where credit is due. Z Gastroenterol 2016;54:47–57.
51. Lembcke BJ, Strobel D, Dirks K, et al. Statement of the section internal medicine of the DEGUM - ultrasound obtains pole position for clinical imaging in acute diverticulitis. Ultraschall Med 2015;36:191–5.
52. Thorisson A, Smedh K, Torkzad MR, et al. CT imaging for prediction of complications and recurrence in acute uncomplicated diverticulitis. Int J Colorectal Dis 2015;31:451–7.
53. Jacobs DO. Clinical practice. Diverticulitis. N Engl J Med 2007;357:2057–66.
54. SSAT. SSAT patient care guidelines: surgical treatment of diverticulitis. 2007. Available at: http://www.ssat.com/cgi-bin/divert.cgi. Accessed December 31, 2014.
55. Andersen JC, Bundgaard L, Elbrond H, et al. Danish national guidelines for treatment of diverticular disease. Dan Med J 2012;59:C4453.
56. Fujita T. Feasibility of the practice guidelines for colonic diverticulitis. Surgery 2012;151:491–2.

57. Kruis W, Germer CT, Leifeld L. Diverticular disease: guidelines of the German society for gastroenterology, digestive and metabolic diseases and the German society for general and visceral surgery. Digestion 2014;90:190–207.
58. Vennix S, Morton DG, Hahnloser D, et al. Systematic review of evidence and consensus on diverticulitis: an analysis of national and international guidelines. Colorectal Dis 2014;11:866–78.
59. Daniels L, Ünlü Ç, de Korte N, et al. Randomized clinical trial of observational versus antibiotic treatment for a first episode of CT-proven uncomplicated acute diverticulitis. Br J Surg 2017;104(1):52–61.
60. Brochmann ND, Schultz JK, Jakobsen GS, et al. Management of acute uncomplicated diverticulitis without antibiotics: a single-centre cohort study. Colorectal Dis 2016;18(11):1101–7.
61. Biondo S, Golda T, Kreisler E, et al. Outpatient versus hospitalization management for uncomplicated diverticulitis: a prospective, multicenter randomized clinical trial (DIVER Trial). Ann Surg 2014;259(1):38–44.
62. Jackson JD, Hammond T. Systematic review: outpatient management of acute uncomplicated diverticulitis. Int J Colorectal Dis 2014;29(7):775–81.
63. Balasubramanian I, Fleming C, Mohan HM, et al. Out-patient management of mild or uncomplicated diverticulitis: a systematic review. Dig Surg 2017;34(2): 151–60.
64. Sirany AE, Gaertner WB, Madoff RD, et al. Diverticulitis diagnosed in the emergency room: is it safe to discharge home? J Am Coll Surg 2017;225(1):21–5.
65. Lahner E, Bellisario C, Hassan C, et al. Probiotics in the treatment of diverticular disease. A systematic review. J Gastrointestin Liver Dis 2016;25:79–86.
66. Gregersen R, Mortensen LQ, Burcharth J, et al. Treatment of patients with acute colonic diverticulitis complicated by abscess formation: a systematic review. Int J Surg 2016;35:201–8.
67. Forshaw MJ, Sankararajah D, Stewart M, et al. Self-expanding metallic stents in the treatment of benign colorectal disease: indications and outcomes. Colorectal Dis 2006;8:102–11.
68. Garfinkle R, Boutros M. Recurrent versus persistent diverticulitis: an important distinction. Dis Colon Rectum 2016;59(10):e437.
69. Elagili F, Stocchi L, Ozuner G, et al. Outcomes of percutaneous drainage without surgery for patients with diverticular abscess. Dis Colon Rectum 2014;57(3): 331–6.
70. Costi R, Cauchy F, Le Bian A, et al. Challenging a classic myth: pneumoperitoneum associated with acute diverticulitis is not an indication for open or laparoscopic emergency surgery in hemodynamically stable patients. A 10-year experience with a nonoperative treatment. Surg Endosc 2012;26:2061–71.
71. Wong WD, Wexner SD, Lowry A, et al. Practice parameters for the treatment of sigmoid diverticulitis–supporting documentation. The Standards Task Force. The American Society of Colon and Rectal Surgeons. Dis Colon Rectum 2000; 43(3):290–7.
72. Large JM. Treatment of perforated diverticulitis. Lancet 1964;1(7330):413–4.
73. Eng K, Ranson JH, Localio SA. Resection of the perforated segment. A significant advance in treatment of diverticulitis with free perforation or abscess. Am J Surg 1977;133(1):67–72.
74. Miller DW, Wichern WA. Perforated sigmoid diverticulitis. Appraisal of primary versus delayed resection. Am J Surg 1971;121(5):536–40.
75. Oberkofler CE, Rickenbacher A, Raptis DA, et al. A multicenter randomized clinical trial of primary anastomosis or Hartmann's procedure for perforated left

colonic diverticulitis with purulent or fecal peritonitis. Ann Surg 2012;256(5): 819–26.
76. Afshar S, Kurer MA. Laparoscopic peritoneal lavage for perforated sigmoid diverticulitis. Colorectal Dis 2012;14(2):135–42.
77. Alamili M, Gogenur I, Rosenberg J. Acute complicated diverticulitis managed by laparoscopic lavage. Dis Colon Rectum 2009;52(7):1345–9.
78. Liang S, Russek K, Franklin ME. Damage control strategy for the management of perforated diverticulitis with generalized peritonitis: laparoscopic lavage and drainage vs. laparoscopic Hartmann's procedure. Surg Endosc 2012;26(10): 2835–42.
79. Rogers AC, Collins D, O'Sullivan GC, et al. Laparoscopic lavage for perforated diverticulitis: a population analysis. Dis Colon Rectum 2012;55(9):932–8.
80. Thornell A, Angenete E, Gonzales E. Treatment of acute diverticulitis laparoscopic lavage vs. resection (DILALA): study protocol for a randomised controlled trial. Trials 2011;12:186.
81. Toorenvliet BR, Swank H, Schoones JW, et al. Laparoscopic peritoneal lavage for perforated colonic diverticulitis: a systematic review. Colorectal Dis 2010; 12(9):862–7.
82. White SI, Frenkiel B, Martin PJ. A ten-year audit of perforated sigmoid diverticulitis: highlighting the outcomes of laparoscopic lavage. Dis Colon Rectum 2010;53(11):1537–41.
83. Gralista P, Moris D, Vailas M, et al. Laparoscopic approach in colonic diverticulitis: dispelling myths and misperceptions. Surg Laparosc Endosc Percutan Tech 2017;27(2):73–82.
84. Angenete E, Thornell A, Burcharth J, et al. Laparoscopic lavage is feasible and safe for the treatment of perforated diverticulitis with purulent peritonitis: the first results from the randomized controlled trial DILALA. Ann Surg 2016;263:117–22.
85. Gehrman J, Angenete E, Björholt I, et al. Health economic analysis of laparoscopic lavage versus Hartmann's procedure for diverticulitis in the randomized DILALA trial. Br J Surg 2016;103(11):1539–47.
86. Thornell A, Angenete E, Bisgaard T, et al. Laparoscopic lavage for perforated diverticulitis with purulent peritonitis: a randomized, controlled trial. Ann Intern Med 2016;164:137–45.
87. Vennix S, Musters GD, Mulder IM, et al, Ladies Trial Collaborators. Laparoscopic peritoneal lavage or sigmoidectomy for perforated diverticulitis with purulent peritonitis: a multicentre, parallel-group, randomised, open-label trial. Lancet 2015;386:1269–77.
88. Vennix S, van Dieren S, Opmeer BC, et al. Cost analysis of laparoscopic lavage compared with sigmoid resection for perforated diverticulitis in the Ladies trial. Br J Surg 2017;104(1):62–8.
89. Schultz JK, Yaqub S, Wallon C, et al. Laparoscopic lavage vs primary resection for acute perforated diverticulitis: the SCANDIV randomized clinical trial. JAMA 2015;314:1364–75.
90. Shaikh FM, Stewart PM, Walsh SR, et al. Laparoscopic peritoneal lavage or surgical resection for acute perforated sigmoid diverticulitis: a systematic review and meta-analysis. Int J Surg 2017;38:130–7.
91. Angenete E, Bock D, Rosenberg J, et al. Laparoscopic lavage is superior to colon resection for perforated purulent diverticulitis-a meta-analysis. Int J Colorectal Dis 2017;32(2):163–9.

92. Ceresoli M, Coccolini F, Montori G, et al. Laparoscopic lavage in perforated purulent diverticulitis-is it time for definitive conclusions? Int J Colorectal Dis 2017; 32(1):159.
93. Greilsamer T, Abet E, Meurette G, et al. Is the failure of laparoscopic peritoneal lavage predictable in Hinchey III diverticulitis management? Dis Colon Rectum 2017;60(9):965–70.
94. Rosen DR, Hwang GS, Ault GT, et al. Operative management of diverticulitis in a tertiary care center. Am J Surg 2017;214(1):37–41.
95. Bridoux V, Antor M, Schwarz L, et al. Elective operation after acute complicated diverticulitis: is it still mandatory? World J Gastroenterol 2014;20(25):8166–72.
96. Constantinides VA, Tekkis PP, Senapati A. Prospective multicentre evaluation of adverse outcomes following treatment for complicated diverticular disease. Br J Surg 2006;93(12):1503–13.
97. Alves A, Panis Y, Slim K, et al. French multicentre prospective observational study of laparoscopic versus open colectomy for sigmoid diverticular disease. Br J Surg 2005;92(12):1520–5.
98. Sarin S, Boulos PB. Long-term outcome of patients presenting with acute complications of diverticular disease. Ann R Coll Surg Engl 1994;76(2):117–20.
99. Myers E, Hurley M, O'Sullivan GC, et al. Laparoscopic peritoneal lavage for generalized peritonitis due to perforated diverticulitis. Br J Surg 2008;95(1): 97–101.
100. Salem L, Veenstra DL, Sullivan SD, et al. The timing of elective colectomy in diverticulitis: a decision analysis. J Am Coll Surg 2004;199(6):904–12.
101. Klarenbeek BR, Veenhof AA, Bergamaschi R, et al. Laparoscopic sigmoid resection for diverticulitis decreases major morbidity rates: a randomized control trial: short-term results of the Sigma Trial. Ann Surg 2009;249:39–44.
102. Badic B, Leroux G, Thereaux J, et al. Colovesical fistula complicating diverticular disease: a 14-Year experience. Surg Laparosc Endosc Percutan Tech 2017;27(2):94–7.
103. Mozer AB, Spaniolas K, Sippey ME, et al. Post-operative morbidity, but not mortality, is worsened by operative delay in septic diverticulitis. Int J Colorectal Dis 2017;32(2):193–9.
104. Elliott PA, McLemore EC, Abbass MA, et al. Robotic versus laparoscopic resection for sigmoid diverticulitis with fistula. J Robot Surg 2015;9(2):137–42.
105. D'Hondt M, Pottel H, Devriendt D, et al. SILS sigmoidectomy versus multiport laparoscopic sigmoidectomy for diverticulitis. JSLS 2014;18(3) [pii:e2014.00319].
106. Steinemann DC, Zerz A, Germann S, et al. Anorectal function and quality of life after transrectal rigid-hybrid natural orifice translumenal endoscopic sigmoidectomy. J Am Coll Surg 2016;223(2):299–307.
107. Chiu AS, Jean RA, Gorecka J, et al. Trends of ureteral stent usage in surgery for diverticulitis. J Surg Res 2018;222:203–11.e3.
108. Boni L, David G, Dionigi G, et al. Indocyanine green-enhanced fluorescence to assess bowel perfusion during laparoscopic colorectal resection. Surg Endosc 2016;30(7):2736–42.
109. Autorino R, Zargar H, White WM, et al. Current applications of near-infrared fluorescence imaging in robotic urologic surgery: a systematic review and critical analysis of the literature. Urology 2014;84(4):751–9.
110. Lau KC, Spilsbury K, Farooque Y, et al. Is colonoscopy still mandatory after a CT diagnosis of left-sided diverticulitis: can colorectal cancer be confidently excluded? Dis Colon Rectum 2011;54:1265–70.

111. Suhardja TS, Norhadi S, Seah EZ, et al. Is early colonoscopy after CT-diagnosed diverticulitis still necessary? Int J Colorectal Dis 2017;32(4):485–9.
112. Walker AS, Bingham JR, Janssen KM, et al. Colonoscopy after Hinchey I and II left-sided diverticulitis: utility or futility? Am J Surg 2016;212(5):837–43.
113. Mortensen LQ, Burcharth J, Andresen K, et al. An 18-year nationwide cohort study on the association between diverticulitis and colon cancer. Ann Surg 2017;265(5):954–9.
114. Unlu C, Daniels L, Vrouenraets BC, et al. Systematic review of medical therapy to prevent recurrent diverticulitis. Int J Colorectal Dis 2012;27:1131–6.
115. Tursi A, Brandimarte G, Daffinà R. Long-term treatment with mesalazine and rifaximin versus rifaximin alone for patients with recurrent attacks of acute diverticulitis of colon. Dig Liver Dis 2002;34:510–5.
116. Raskin JB, Kamm MA, Jamal MM, et al. Mesalamine did not prevent recurrent diverticulitis in phase 3 controlled trials. Gastroenterology 2014;147:793–802.
117. Stollman N, Magowan S, Shanahan F, et al. A randomized controlled study of mesalamine after acute diverticulitis: results of the DIVA trial. J Clin Gastroenterol 2013;47:621–9.
118. Parente F, Bargiggia S, Prada A, et al. Intermittent treatment with mesalazine in the prevention of diverticulitis recurrence: a randomized multicentre pilot double-blind placebo-controlled study of 24-month duration. Int J Colorectal Dis 2013;28:1423–31.
119. Tursi A, Brandimarte G, Elisei W, et al. Randomised clinical trial: mesalazine and/or probiotics in maintaining remission of symptomatic uncomplicated diverticular disease – a double-blind, randomised, placebo-controlled study. Aliment Pharmacol Ther 2013;38:741–51.
120. Carabotti M, Annibale B, Severi C, et al. Role of fiber in symptomatic uncomplicated diverticular disease: a systematic review. Nutrients 2017;9(2) [pii:E161].
121. Strate LL, Keeley BR, Cao Y, et al. Western dietary pattern increases, and prudent dietary pattern decreases, risk of incident diverticulitis in a prospective cohort study. Gastroenterology 2017;152(5):1023–30.
122. Stam MA, Draaisma WA, van de Wall BJ, et al. An unrestricted diet for uncomplicated diverticulitis is safe: results of a prospective diverticulitis diet study. Colorectal Dis 2017;19(4):372–7.

The Acute Upper Gastrointestinal Bleed

David W. Nelms, MD[a], Carlos A. Pelaez, MD[a,b,c,*]

KEYWORDS

- Upper gastrointestinal bleed • Peptic ulcer disease • Variceal bleeding • Endoscopy
- Operative management

KEY POINTS

- Although only 2% to 8% of upper gastrointestinal (GI) bleeds require operative intervention, early surgeon involvement remains imperative.
- Initial evaluation and treatment of upper GI bleeding requires a systematic approach starting with airway, breathing, and circulation.
- Peptic ulcer disease remains the most common cause of upper GI bleeds despite the increased use of proton pump inhibitors and understanding of *Helicobacter pylori*.
- Endoscopy is the main diagnostic and therapeutic tool for most upper GI bleeds.
- Bleeding varices due to portal hypertension can fail medical and endoscopic treatment in 10% to 15% of cases in which transjugular intrahepatic portosystemic shunt may be required. Consideration of facility capabilities and need for transfer should be considered early.

INTRODUCTION

Upper gastrointestinal bleeding (UGIB), defined as intraluminal hemorrhage proximal to the ligament of Treitz, can range from mild and asymptomatic to massive life-threatening hemorrhage.[1–3] For the purposes of this article, the authors define an acute UGIB to be one that results in new acute symptoms and is, therefore, potentially life-threatening. The incidence of UGIB is approximately 100 cases per 100,000 population per year.[4] Although the incidence of hospitalization for acute UGIB is decreasing (4% decrease from 1998–2006),[5] it remains a common problem encountered by the acute-care and general surgeon.

Disclosure: The authors have nothing to disclose.
[a] General Surgery Residency Program, UnityPoint Health, 1415 Woodland Avenue, Suite 130, Des Moines, IA 50309, USA; [b] General Surgery, Trauma and Critical Care, The Iowa Clinic, 1212 Pleasant Street, Suite 211, Des Moines, IA 50309, USA; [c] Trauma Services, UnityPoint Health, Iowa Methodist Medical Center, 1200 Pleasant Street, Des Moines, IA 50309, USA
* Corresponding author. Trauma Services, UnityPoint Health, Iowa Methodist Medical Center, 1200 Pleasant Street, Des Moines, IA 50309.
E-mail address: cpelaezgil@iowaclinic.com

Surg Clin N Am 98 (2018) 1047–1057
https://doi.org/10.1016/j.suc.2018.05.004
0039-6109/18/

The surgeon continues to play a key role in the outcome of patients with UGIBs. Even though only approximately 2.5% to 5% of UGIBs ultimately require operative intervention,[1,2] early surgeon consultation remains critical for a variety of reasons. In many practice settings, the surgeon represents the primary endoscopist, but even when this role is assumed by gastroenterology, early surgeon involvement allows for aid in appropriate resuscitation of unstable patients, streamlining of preoperative assessment, early establishment of the goals of the patient and family, and judgment regarding the limits of nonoperative management.

PRESENTATION

UGIB typically presents with hematemesis or melena, but brisk UGIB can present with hematochezia. The redder the blood, the more rapid the bleed. Approximately 80% of all GI bleeds and 11% to 15% of cases of hematochezia are due to an upper source[6,7]; therefore, it is important to include upper sources in the differential diagnosis for all GI bleeds. Conversely, melena can occur from lower GI bleed that originate in the small bowel or right colon especially when there is slow transit time. Hematemesis almost always represents an upper source of bleeding, although nasal and oropharyngeal sources must also be kept in mind.

TRIAGE

Effective initial evaluation and treatment of an UGIB requires a systematic approach. One organized approach is to divide priorities into a primary survey (airway, breathing, and circulation) and a secondary survey (completion of history and physical examination). The purpose of this division is to emphasize that lack of definitive diagnosis or detailed history and physical examination (H&P) should never impede initiation of airway protection and treatment of shock. Baradarian and colleagues[8] demonstrated that early intensive resuscitation with correction of hemodynamics, hemoglobin, and coagulopathy can reduce mortality in patients with UGIB. In the massively bleeding patient, it may not be possible to move beyond the primary survey until definitive source control of bleeding has been obtained. However, in most cases, the bleeding stops spontaneously[9] or the patient is stable enough to allow further details of the H&P to be obtained. Consideration must be given during the primary survey as to whether the health care facility is capable of providing definitive bleeding source control, and arrangements for transfer should be initiated if the facility is unable to care for the patient.

On the opposite extreme, if the patient is found to be stable on the primary survey and the secondary survey does not reveal comorbidities that increase the risk for complications, the patient can potentially be managed as an outpatient. Several clinical decision tools have been created to assist with risk stratification and triage. One is the Glascow-Blatchford Score (GBS) (**Table 1**). This scale is based on clinical parameters that are available before endoscopy. The GBS has been validated and can be used to safely manage patients with a GBS of either 0 or 1 as an outpatient.[10]

INITIAL MANAGEMENT (THE PRIMARY SURVEY)

The primary survey is outlined in **Box 1**. The following key points are emphasized:

1. *Airway and breathing are always the initial priority.*[11] Assessment should be performed quickly, and if the airway is compromised a definitive airway is required. Ongoing reassessment of the airway must be performed. Mental status changes due to shock may lead to patient inability to protect their own airway. Pragmatic

Table 1
Glasgow-Blatchford score

Admission Risk Marker	Score Component Value
Blood urea (mmol/L)	
≥6.5 <8.0	2
≥8.0 <10.0	3
≥10.0 <25	4
≥25	6
Hemoglobin (g/dL) for men	
≥12 <13	1
≥10 <12	3
<10	6
Hemoglobin (g/dL) for women	
≥10 <12	1
<10	6
Systolic blood pressure (mm Hg)	
100–109	1
90–99	2
<90	3
Other markers	
Pulse ≥100 (per min)	1
Presentation with melena	1
Presentation with syncope	2
Hepatic disease	2
Cardiac failure	2

From Blatchford O, Murray WR, Blatchford M. A risk score to predict need for treatment for upper gastrointestinal haemorrhage. Lancet 2000;356:1319; with permission.

Box 1
The primary survey priorities

1. Airway
2. Breathing
3. Circulation
   a. Access
   b. Blood volume restoration
   c. CBC, CMP, cross-match, and coagulation laboratory studies
   d. Drug history of anticoagulants/antiplatelets
   e. Source control and localization
      i. Preendoscopy initiation of PPI has a low risk to benefit ratio
      ii. Evaluate for portal hypertension/varices; consider need for transfer
      iii. Develop plan for endoscopy and treatment

Abbreviations: CBC, complete blood count; CMP, comprehensive metabolic panel; PPI, proton pump inhibitor.

consideration must be given to whether airway protection is required before the initiation of procedures such as endoscopy, but there is a lack of evidence that prophylactic intubation before endoscopy decreases complications.[12]

2. *Circulation is an issue in all acute GI bleeds. The degree of the problem must be quickly assessed.* Key data for this rapid assessment include presence of tachycardia, hypotension, anxiety/mental status changes, cool/clammy extremities, and recent syncope. Checking for orthopnea is a simple way to rapidly assess for hypovolemia when other clinical signs of shock are not present. However, it must be remembered that a patient can lose a significant blood volume without any clinical signs of shock.
    a. *Access—Establishing vascular access is the initial priority for treating the circulation problem.* Placement of at least 2 large-bore (18 or smaller gauge) peripheral intravenous devices is preferred because wide and short catheters offer the lowest resistance to flow for large volume resuscitation (flow is proportional to the radius to the fourth power and inversely proportional to length).
    b. *Blood volume restoration.* Hypotensive patients with active bleeding should be resuscitated with a 1:1:1 (packed red blood cell:fresh frozen plasma:platelet) transfusion strategy as translated from recent guidelines for treatment of traumatic bleeding.[13] Crystalloid may be used while blood products are being obtained, but the massively bleeding, hemodynamically unstable patient requires blood regardless of hemoglobin level. Uncross-matched blood may be used while waiting for completion of the cross-match. Foley catheter placement may be considered for hourly monitoring and guidance of resuscitation in an unstable patient. Finally, the principle of permissive hypotension should be followed with avoidance of overresuscitation beyond what is required to maintain perfusion and consciousness. Vasopressors should be avoided, other than for variceal bleeding. When the patient is hemodynamically stable, a restrictive transfusion strategy with a transfusion trigger of less than 7 g/dL is recommended.[14] In addition, recent evidence has not been able to demonstrate superiority of tranexamic acid in the treatment of UGIB when compared with current standard using proton pump inhibitors (PPIs) and endoscopic therapy.[15]
    c. Complete blood count, comprehensive metabolic panel, cross-match, and coagulation laboratory studies should be obtained. It should be emphasized that hemoglobin can remain normal in the setting of massive acute bleeding; therefore a normal value does not rule out massive hemorrhage. Assessment of total bilirubin and international normalized ratio are essential to screen for liver disease. In addition, coagulation studies provide information regarding potential coagulopathy associated with massive hemorrhage or due to medications. When available, thromboelastography can be useful for guiding product resuscitation in massive hemorrhage. All laboratory values should be trended based on the acuity of bleeding. Cross-match should be sent and units ordered to stay ahead of transfusion.
    d. *Drug history of any anticoagulant or antiplatelet medications is essential in the primary survey.* Depending on the severity of the bleeding and the indication for taking these medications, the patient may require emergent reversal. There are a growing number of anticoagulant and antiplatelet agents on the market, and specific reversal strategy is beyond the scope of this article. It should be remembered that GI bleeding in patients taking anticoagulant medications is still most commonly due to GI disease and should not be ascribed to the anticoagulant alone.[16] All nonsteroidal antiinflammatory drugs (NSAIDs) and selective

serotonin reuptake inhibitors (SSRIs) should be held due to their known association with increased risk of GI bleeding.[17]

e. *Source control. A plan for localization and source control should be developed during the primary survey.* The best way to help any bleeding patient is to stop the bleed. External soft-tissue hemorrhage bleeding can usually be stopped by applying pressure, but with bleeding in the GI tract, it is necessary to both localize the bleed and determine a method to stop it. Because this takes time (such as setting up endoscopy), the prior steps of initial management are listed earlier, but it must always be remembered that the primary goal is to stop the bleed. Therefore, a plan for localization and source control must be part of the primary survey.
   i. Because of the low risk to benefit ratio, the authors recommend starting a PPI during the early stage of workup because peptic ulcer disease represents the most common cause of UGIB.[18] Lau and colleagues[19] demonstrated that high-dose intravenous PPI in patients admitted for UGIB reduced the stigmata of recent hemorrhage and the need for intervention with endoscopy performed the following day. However, preendoscopy initiation did not change patient outcomes of rebleeding, need for surgery, or death.[19] Recommended intravenous dosing is an 80 mg bolus followed by an 8 mg/h infusion.
   ii. Nasogastric tube placement can be considered but is not required for diagnosis, prognosis, visualization, or therapeutic effect.[14] Intuitively, ongoing aspiration of bright red blood portends a more severe bleed, but there is no proven benefit for it. A Canadian study demonstrated that in retrospective review of the aspirate character did stratify risk, but there was low diagnostic accuracy. In addition, 13% of patients with known UGIB could have a clear or bile-stained aspirate.[20]
   iii. If portal hypertension/varices is known or suspected, the patient should be treated at a facility with an endoscopist experienced in banding. If this is not available or banding is not successful, the patient may require transjugular intrahepatic portosystemic shunt (TIPS) and should be transferred to a capable center. A Sengstaken–Blakemore tube or Minnesota tube can be a lifesaving temporizing device in unstable patients with bleeding varices requiring transfer. The patient should also have octreotide and antibiotics initiated before transfer.
   iv. The primary method for definitively localizing and treating most UGIB is endoscopy. Most of the UGIBs can be controlled with endoscopy alone. Urgent endoscopy is required for hemodynamically unstable patients, but studies have confirmed that for patients with stabilized acute bleeds there is no benefit from endoscopy at 6 to 12 hours compared with endoscopy within 24 hours.[21,22] Endoscopy may be performed in the intensive care unit or operating room setting (see specific causes of GI bleeds in the later discussion for further details of endoscopic treatment). If endoscopy is not available at the surgeon's institution within the necessary timeframe, the patient requires transfer to a capable facility. Plans for angiography or surgical intervention should be considered based on the cause of the bleed, patient comorbidities, and patient status.

COMPLETION OF THE HISTORY AND PHYSICAL EXAMINATION (SECONDARY SURVEY)

Once the priorities of the primary survey are initiated or completed, there is then time to gather more information. The H&P can provide information to narrow the differential diagnosis, tailor appropriate management, and conduct risk stratification of the patient based on probable cause and medical comorbidities.

Specific causes of UGIB may be suggested by the patient's symptoms:[23]

- Peptic ulcer: epigastric or right upper quadrant pain
- Esophageal ulcer: odynophagia, gastroesophageal reflux, dysphagia
- Mallory-Weiss tear: emesis, retching, or coughing before hematemesis
- Variceal hemorrhage or portal hypertensive gastropathy: jaundice, weakness, fatigue, anorexia, abdominal distention
- Malignancy: dysphagia, early satiety, involuntary weight loss, cachexia

History of recent trauma should be ruled out. A complete list of the medical comorbidities should be obtained. Knowledge of previous surgeries can help narrow the differential diagnosis and is important before any operative intervention. For example, history of aortic aneurysm repair provides a clue to possible aortoenteric fistula, and a history of GI anastomosis raises the possibility of a marginal ulcer. A complete medication list should again be verified for use of any anticoagulants, NSAIDs, salicylates, or SSRIs that are common in the elderly.[24]

DEFINITIVE TREATMENT OF SPECIFIC CAUSES

Nonvariceal Bleeding

Nonvariceal bleeding accounts for approximately 80% of all UGIBs.[25]

Peptic Ulcer Disease

Peptic ulcer disease is the most common cause of UGIB, representing nearly 40% of all cases.[26] The vast majority are related to *Helicobacter pylori* and NSAID use. The incidence has declined in the era of PPI use and the understanding of *H pylori*.[27]

Upper endoscopy is the diagnostic and therapeutic study of choice. Although most of the bleeds stop on their own, approximately 25% require an intervention at the time of endoscopy.[27] Endoscopic findings can be classified according to the Forrest classification[28] for guidance regarding need for intervention and risk of rebleeding (**Table 2**). Endoscopic treatment modalities include injection of epinephrine or sclerosants, bipolar electrocoagulation, band ligation, heater probe coagulation, constant probe pressure tamponade, argon plasma coagulator, laser photocoagulation, and hemoclips. Evidence has revealed improved rates of control when treatment modalities are used in combination than in isolation (eg, epinephrine injection followed by clipping). Injection of epinephrine is performed in 4 quadrants around the lesion, starting most distally in order to prevent obscuring the view for subsequent injections. Biopsies of all gastric ulcers should be performed due to their relatively high rate of

Table 2
The Forrest classification

Class	Description	Endoscopic Intervention[14]	Rebleeding Rate[42]
1A	Active spurting	Yes	55%
1B	Active oozing	Yes	55%
2A	Nonbleeding visible vessel	Yes	43%
2B	Adherent clot	Consider	22%
2C	Flat pigmented spot	No	10%
3	Clean ulcer base	No	5%

malignancy (6%).[29] When duodenal ulcers are encountered, control of the bleeding should be performed, followed by biopsy not of the ulcer but of the antrum obtained for evidence of *H pylori*. *H pylori* testing may be falsely negative in the setting of an acute bleed, so repeat testing should be obtained later if the test is negative for *H pylori* followed by confirmation of eradication.

Risk of recurrent bleeding after endoscopic control is approximately 15% to 20%.[30] The risk of rebleeding can be predicted based on the initial endoscopic appearance of the ulcer (Forrest classification, see **Table 2**) When rebleeding does recur, repeat endoscopy should be attempted because long-term bleeding control can be obtained in approximately 75% of cases without increased risk of death and with fewer complications than those treated with surgery for first recurrent bleed.[30]

Operative intervention should be considered based on initial or recurrent magnitude of bleeding, ability of patient to withstand continued bleeding, and probability of recurrent bleeding. A Canadian review from 2004 to 2010 revealed a need for surgical intervention in 4.3% of cases of hospitalized UGIB caused by peptic ulcer disease.[31–33] In general, older patients with less physiologic reserve to withstand ongoing bleeding should undergo earlier operative intervention. Ulcers that are high-risk based on the Forrest classification, are larger than 2 cm, or are located in the stomach or posterior duodenum should all be considered for early surgical intervention.[34,35] The choice of operation depends on the location of the ulcer. Duodenal ulcers most commonly occur in the first portion (bulb) and erode posteriorly into the gastroduodenal artery. Approach for these ulcers consists of a longitudinal duodenotomy, oversewing of ulcer with triple stitch including the medially located transverse pancreatic artery, and closure transversely with Heineke-Mikulicz pyloroplasty. Historically, vagotomy ± antrectomy was also performed, but in the era of PPIs and understanding of H pylori, the utility of this acid-reducing procedure has greatly diminished. Gastric ulcers in favorable locations should be resected with primary closure of the gastrotomy site. Unfavorably located ulcers may have hemorrhage controlled with oversewing followed by biopsy to rule out malignancy.

The role of angiographic embolization for peptic ulcer disease is less well defined. Many patients now undergo an attempt at angiography and embolization before surgery, particularly in patients at high risk for surgery. Angiography is minimally invasive, it often allows precise localization of bleeding, and it enables the use of therapeutic options, which include embolization or vasopressin infusion. A hemorrhage rate of 0.5 to 1.0 mL/min is required before it can be visualized with angiography. Initial success rates for patients with acute peptic ulcer bleeding are between 52% and 98%, with recurrent bleeding rates of 10% to 20%.[36]

Mallory-Weiss Tears

Mallory-Weiss tear is a laceration in the cardia caused by forceful emesis. These are commonly seen in alcoholic patients who retch after belching. Tears are usually single and longitudinal. The lesions have a high rate of spontaneous cessation of bleeding, and intervention is only required in only 10% of cases. It spontaneously resolves in 50% to 80% of the patients by the time endoscopy is performed. Rebleeding is rare (7%) and tears that are not actively bleeding can be managed with acid suppression and antiemetics alone. Endoscopic therapy is indicated for treatment of actively bleeding tears and should be treated with a combination of thermal coagulation, hemoclips, and/or endoscopic band ligation, with or without epinephrine injection. Patients who have failed endoscopic therapy should undergo angiography with transarterial embolization. Surgery with oversewing of the bleeding vessel is reserved for those who fail angiographic therapy.

Dieulafoy Lesions

Dieulafoy vascular malformations consist of an unusually dilated submucosal vessel with erosion of a small portion of the overlying mucosa. The lesions typically occur along the lesser curve of the stomach within 6 cm of the gastroesophageal junction.[37] Because of the small size of the mucosal defect (2–5 mm) they can be difficult to identify.[38] Given the large size of the underlying artery, the bleeding can be massive. Usually they can be controlled endoscopically. If this fails, angiography and embolization is an excellent option. If both options are unsuccessful, which is rare, surgical intervention is required. An anterior gastrotomy should be performed with oversewing of the lesion. If the lesion cannot be identified, sometimes partial gastrectomy is required.

Aortoenteric Fistula

Although primary aortoenteric fistulas can occur, primarily these are the result of prosthetic graft to duodenum fistula. Patients often present with an initial herald bleed before massive hemorrhage. Upper endoscopy to the ligament of Treitz is the diagnostic modality of choice. Treatment options for this challenging problem includes extra-anatomic bypass with resection of the infected graft and closure of the duodenal defect. Perioperative mortality rates are high.

Hemobilia and Hemosuccus Pancreaticus

Hemobilia is bleeding into the biliary tract. Hemosuccus pancreaticus is bleeding in to the pancreatic ducts. These are rare causes of UGIB and are usually related to recent instrumentation or trauma. The treatment of choice for both entities is angiographic embolization.[39]

VARICEAL BLEEDING

Gastroesophageal Varices

For esophageal variceal bleeding, treatment consists of controlling the acute hemorrhage and reducing the risk of rebleeding. The 6-week mortality rate following the first episode of variceal bleeding is almost 20%.[40] Acute treatment consists of judicious fluid resuscitation, octreotide or vasopressin along with attempted endoscopic banding. When banding fails, TIPS can be lifesaving. This is required in approximately 10% of cases of variceal bleeding.[3] TIPS is associated with 50% rate of hepatic encephalopathy within 1 year.[41] Antibiotics are recommended for all acutely bleeding varices due to a high rate of underlying aggravating infection that led to the bleeding; there is evidence that a 7-day course of a broad spectrum antibiotic will lower the rebleeding rate.[40] A nonselective beta blocker such as propranolol should also be initiated for long-term prevention of rebleeding. Endoscopic banding should also be repeated every 10 to 14 days until all varices have been eradicated.

Portal Hypertensive Gastropathy

Bleeding from portal hypertensive gastropathy is not amenable to endoscopic therapy due to its diffuse nature. It requires pharmacologic therapy to reduce portal venous pressure and if this fails, then TIPS.

Gastric Varices

Gastric varices are isolated to the stomach and are caused by left-sided (sinistral) hypertension that usually results from splenic vein thrombosis in the setting of pancreatitis. The treatment of choice is splenectomy.

SUMMARY

UGIB requires a systematic approach to evaluation and treatment, similar to the management of a trauma patient. Surgeon involvement in UGIBs remains integral despite the rare need for operative management. Endoscopy is the primary tool for diagnosis and treatment.

REFERENCES

1. Clarke MG, Bunting D, Smart NJ, et al. The surgical management of acute upper gastrointestinal bleeding: a 12-year experience. Int J Surg 2010;8(5):377–80.
2. Botianu A, Matei D, Tantau M, et al. Mortality and need of surgical treatment in acute upper gastrointestinal bleeding: a one year study in a tertiary center with a 24 hours/day-7 days/week endoscopy call. Has anything changed? Chirurgia (Bucur) 2013;108(3):312–8.
3. Garcia-Pagan JC, Caca K, Bureau C, et al. Early use of TIPS in patients with cirrhosis and variceal bleeding. N Engl J Med 2010;362(25):2370–9.
4. Fallah MA, Prakash C, Edmundowicz S. Acute gastrointestinal bleeding. Med Clin North Am 2000;84(5):1183–208.
5. Zhao Y, Encinosa W. Hospitalizations for gastrointestinal bleeding in 1998 and 2006: statistical brief #65. Healthcare Cost and Utilization Project (HCUP) Statistical Briefs [Internet]. Rockville (MD): Agency for Healthcare Research and Quality (US); 2006.
6. Barnert J, Messmann H. Management of lower gastrointestinal tract bleeding. Best Pract Res Clin Gastroenterol 2008;22(2):295–312.
7. Laine L, Shah A. Randomized trial of urgent vs. elective colonoscopy in patients hospitalized with lower GI bleeding. Am J Gastroenterol 2010;105(12):2636–41 [quiz: 42].
8. Baradarian R, Ramdhaney S, Chapalamadugu R, et al. Early intensive resuscitation of patients with upper gastrointestinal bleeding decreases mortality. Am J Gastroenterol 2004;99(4):619–22.
9. Wee E. Management of nonvariceal upper gastrointestinal bleeding. J Postgrad Med 2011;57(2):161–7.
10. Stanley AJ, Ashley D, Dalton HR, et al. Outpatient management of patients with low-risk upper-gastrointestinal haemorrhage: multicentre validation and prospective evaluation. Lancet 2009;373(9657):42–7.
11. Meltzer AC, Klein JC. Upper gastrointestinal bleeding: patient presentation, risk stratification, and early management. Gastroenterol Clin North Am 2014;43(4): 665–75.
12. Rehman A, Iscimen R, Yilmaz M, et al. Prophylactic endotracheal intubation in critically ill patients undergoing endoscopy for upper GI hemorrhage. Gastrointest Endosc 2009;69(7):e55–9.
13. Baraniuk S, Tilley BC, del Junco DJ, et al. Pragmatic randomized optimal platelet and plasma ratios (PROPPR) Trial: design, rationale and implementation. Injury 2014;45(9):1287–95.
14. Laine L, Jensen DM. Management of patients with ulcer bleeding. Am J Gastroenterol 2012;107(3):345–60 [quiz: 61].
15. Bennett C, Klingenberg SL, Langholz E, et al. Tranexamic acid for upper gastrointestinal bleeding. Cochrane Database Syst Rev 2014;(11):CD006640.
16. Rubin TA, Murdoch M, Nelson DB. Acute GI bleeding in the setting of supratherapeutic international normalized ratio in patients taking warfarin: endoscopic diagnosis, clinical management, and outcomes. Gastrointest Endosc 2003;58(3):369–73.

17. Paton C, Ferrier IN. SSRIs and gastrointestinal bleeding. BMJ 2005;331(7516): 529–30.
18. Barkun AN, Bardou M, Kuipers EJ, et al. International consensus recommendations on the management of patients with nonvariceal upper gastrointestinal bleeding. Ann Intern Med 2010;152(2):101–13.
19. Lau JY, Leung WK, Wu JC, et al. Omeprazole before endoscopy in patients with gastrointestinal bleeding. N Engl J Med 2007;356(16):1631–40.
20. Aljebreen AM, Fallone CA, Barkun AN. Nasogastric aspirate predicts high-risk endoscopic lesions in patients with acute upper-GI bleeding. Gastrointest Endosc 2004;59(2):172–8.
21. Tsoi KK, Ma TK, Sung JJ. Endoscopy for upper gastrointestinal bleeding: how urgent is it? Nat Rev Gastroenterol Hepatol 2009;6(8):463–9.
22. Sarin N, Monga N, Adams PC. Time to endoscopy and outcomes in upper gastrointestinal bleeding. Can J Gastroenterol 2009;23(7):489–93.
23. Cappell MS, Friedel D. Initial management of acute upper gastrointestinal bleeding: from initial evaluation up to gastrointestinal endoscopy. Med Clin North Am 2008;92(3):491–509, xi.
24. Tata LJ, Fortun PJ, Hubbard RB, et al. Does concurrent prescription of selective serotonin reuptake inhibitors and non-steroidal anti-inflammatory drugs substantially increase the risk of upper gastrointestinal bleeding? Aliment Pharmacol Ther 2005;22(3):175–81.
25. Enestvedt BK, Gralnek IM, Mattek N, et al. An evaluation of endoscopic indications and findings related to nonvariceal upper-GI hemorrhage in a large multicenter consortium. Gastrointest Endosc 2008;67(3):422–9.
26. Rockey DC. Gastrointestinal bleeding. Gastroenterol Clin North Am 2005;34(4): 581–8.
27. Wang YR, Richter JE, Dempsey DT. Trends and outcomes of hospitalizations for peptic ulcer disease in the United States, 1993 to 2006. Ann Surg 2010;251(1):51–8.
28. Forrest JA, Finlayson ND, Shearman DJ. Endoscopy in gastrointestinal bleeding. Lancet 1974;2(7877):394–7.
29. Selinger CP, Cochrane R, Thanaraj S, et al. Gastric ulcers: malignancy yield and risk stratification for follow-up endoscopy. Endosc Int Open 2016;4(6):E709–14.
30. Lau JY, Sung JJ, Lam YH, et al. Endoscopic retreatment compared with surgery in patients with recurrent bleeding after initial endoscopic control of bleeding ulcers. N Engl J Med 1999;340(10):751–6.
31. Quan S, Frolkis A, Milne K, et al. Upper-gastrointestinal bleeding secondary to peptic ulcer disease: incidence and outcomes. World J Gastroenterol 2014; 20(46):17568–77.
32. Sung JJ, Tsoi KK, Ma TK, et al. Causes of mortality in patients with peptic ulcer bleeding: a prospective cohort study of 10,428 cases. Am J Gastroenterol 2010;105(1):84–9.
33. Straube S, Tramer MR, Moore RA, et al. Mortality with upper gastrointestinal bleeding and perforation: effects of time and NSAID use. BMC Gastroenterol 2009;9:41.
34. Guglielmi A, Ruzzenente A, Sandri M, et al. Risk assessment and prediction of rebleeding in bleeding gastroduodenal ulcer. Endoscopy 2002;34(10):778–86.
35. Chung IK, Kim EJ, Lee MS, et al. Endoscopic factors predisposing to rebleeding following endoscopic hemostasis in bleeding peptic ulcers. Endoscopy 2001; 33(11):969–75.
36. Gralnek IM. Will surgery be a thing of the past in peptic ulcer bleeding? Gastrointest Endosc 2011;73(5):909–10.

37. Lara LF, Sreenarasimhaiah J, Tang SJ, et al. Dieulafoy lesions of the GI tract: localization and therapeutic outcomes. Dig Dis Sci 2010;55(12):3436–41.
38. Nguyen DC, Jackson CS. The dieulafoy's lesion: an update on evaluation, diagnosis, and management. J Clin Gastroenterol 2015;49(7):541–9.
39. Millward SF. ACR Appropriateness Criteria on treatment of acute nonvariceal gastrointestinal tract bleeding. J Am Coll Radiol 2008;5(4):550–4.
40. Herrera JL. Management of acute variceal bleeding. Clin Liver Dis 2014;18(2): 347–57.
41. Riggio O, Angeloni S, Salvatori FM, et al. Incidence, natural history, and risk factors of hepatic encephalopathy after transjugular intrahepatic portosystemic shunt with polytetrafluoroethylene-covered stent grafts. Am J Gastroenterol 2008;103(11):2738–46.
42. Laine L, Peterson WL. Bleeding peptic ulcer. N Engl J Med 1994;331(11):717–27.

Lower Gastrointestinal Bleeding

Brandt D. Whitehurst, MD, MS

KEYWORDS

- Lower gastrointestinal bleeding • Emergency • Surgery

KEY POINTS

- Most episodes of lower gastrointestinal bleeding stop spontaneously and can be effectively managed with common clinical tools.
- Computed tomography angiography is widely available and expeditious for localization of gastrointestinal bleeding.
- Resuscitative endovascular balloon occlusion of the aorta (REBOA) may temporize the unstable patient with gastrointestinal bleed, allowing definitive therapy.
- Standard upper and lower endoscopy allows diagnosis and therapeutic management for most presentations of gastrointestinal bleeding.

INTRODUCTION

Gastrointestinal bleeding, responsible for 612,000 hospital days and $1.2 billion in aggregate health care expenditures in 2009,[1] is a common clinical problem encountered by general surgeons. Hospitalization for gastrointestinal bleeding increased 22% between 2000 to 2009,[1] likely a consequence of an increasing elderly population and proliferating anticoagulant usage.

Hematochezia or melena are frequent clinical impetus for patients to seek evaluation. Although not definitive for localization, their presence in the absence of hematemesis raises the suspicion of lower gastrointestinal bleeding (LGIB), defined as gastrointestinal bleeding with a source distal to the ligament of Treitz. LGIB is associated with colonic sources, such as diverticulosis or angiodysplasia, but can include small bowel sources. LGIB outcomes are more favorable than upper gastrointestinal bleeding (UGIB) and 80% resolve spontaneously.[2] Less invasive efficacious interventions likely contributed to the decline in mortality and morbidity over the preceding 20 years.[3]

Because general surgeons have clinical expertise in hemorrhagic shock, critical care, vascular access, endoscopy, and definitive surgical interventions, they are

Disclosure Statement: The author has nothing to disclose.

Department of Surgery, Southern Illinois University School of Medicine, PO Box 19663, Springfield, IL 62794-9663, USA
E-mail address: bwhitehurst81@siumed.edu

Surg Clin N Am 98 (2018) 1059–1072
https://doi.org/10.1016/j.suc.2018.06.007 surgical.theclinics.com

well-equipped to manage LGIBs, particularly in resource-limited settings. Evaluation and management goals for LGIB are constant: resuscitate the patient, localize the source, control the bleeding, and prevent recurrence. We review diagnostic and management modalities the general surgeon should be prepared to execute when managing LGIB.

INITIAL EVALUATION

Bleeding acuteness, duration, number of episodes, pain, melena, heartburn, hematemesis, recent endoscopic, colorectal or aortic procedures, nonsteroidal anti-inflammatory drug (NSAID) use, smoking, and caffeine consumption may direct suspicions to an upper or lower etiology. Comorbid conditions such as heart disease, heart failure, chronic kidney disease, or cirrhosis may also suggest etiologies and affect management decisions.

Physical examination findings, such as irregularly irregular heart rhythm, spider angiomas, palmar erythema, scleral icterus, jaundice, caput medusa, or abdominal guarding may suggest etiologies and exacerbating factors. Because hemorrhoids were the most common etiology for hematochezia in one series of emergency department patients, rectal examination or anoscopy should be considered.[4]

Impaired mentation, confusion, stupor, agitation, obtundation, pallor, cyanosis, diaphoresis, tachypnea, accessory muscle use, extensive hematemesis, gross hematochezia, or objective findings, such as tachycardia, hypoxemia, or hypotension, suggest an unstable patient in need of urgent resuscitation.

Complete blood count, complete metabolic panel, ionized calcium, prothrombin time, international normalized ratio, partial thromboplastin time, fibrinogen, lactate, and arterial blood gas are considered based on severity of presentation. Thromboelastography allows rapid characterization of coagulation deficits or anticoagulant effect and may aid in targeting component blood therapy.

After initial workup, the patient may be categorized as stable or unstable to clarify the subsequent algorithm for localization and control. Patients not anticoagulated, with hemoglobin greater than 13 g/dL, and systolic blood pressure greater than 115 mm Hg, may be managed with interval endoscopy as an outpatient.[5] Other patients may be admitted to a level of care appropriate to the severity of presentation.

RESUSCITATION OF THE UNSTABLE PATIENT

Patients in extremis or pulseless may require initiation of cardiopulmonary resuscitation and consideration of dramatic salvage options. Like penetrating injuries, gastrointestinal bleeding is frequently a point source, and trauma management principles can be applied to catastrophic LGIB. Resuscitative thoracotomy allows rapid control of infra-diaphragmatic bleeding, though outcomes in LGIB are not reported and likely poor.

Resuscitative endovascular balloon occlusion of the aorta (REBOA), with relatively low cost and growing availability, is increasingly used for nontraumatic hemorrhage. REBOA for nontraumatic hemorrhage had a lower 24-hour mortality (19% vs 51%, P = .001) but prolonged critical care course and similar overall mortality (68% vs 64%) to traumatic hemorrhage.[6] Another report found a mortality rate of 36% (n = 11) despite 64% of patients presenting in arrest.[7] REBOA for salvage in life-threatening LGIB is feasible, and future data may elucidate the optimal application.

Unstable patients with a pulse may be initially managed following principles of trauma resuscitation. Supplementary oxygen will pre-oxygenate for possible airway control and optimize oxygen delivery. Pulse oximetry, cardiac rhythm, and blood pressure monitoring should be continuous. Should the airway require control, ketamine or etomidate have favorable hemodynamic profiles for sedation.[8] Dual intravenous access (18 g or larger) is critical for therapeutic interventions. Intraosseous access, even in multiple extremities, is a rapid alternative, preventing delays in therapeutic intervention when peripheral access is difficult. If adequate access remains difficult, large-bore infusion catheters or introducer sheaths are preferred over standard size central venous catheters. Femoral placement in the urgent setting can be performed using landmarks, is easily compressible if hematoma occurs, and reserves alternative locations for clean placement in the nonurgent setting.

Prolonged attempts to measure blood pressure or place invasive lines should not delay empiric treatment with blood products. Transfusion of packed red blood cells, fresh frozen plasma (FFP), and platelets in at least 1:2:2 ratio is a standard of care in traumatic hemorrhagic shock. As applied to nontraumatic hemorrhage, several reports found no benefit of higher ratio (1:1:1) transfusion.[9,10] Massive transfusion, with a rapid hemodynamic response to fewer than 10 units, is associated with increased morbidity.[11] Should access to blood products be exhausted, isotonic crystalloid or albumin solution are alternatives. Volume can be infused concurrently through multiple sites with rate titrated to hemodynamic response. Pressure bags, manual compression, or rapid transfusion devices allow faster infusion than standard pumps set to maximum rate. If available, in-line warming should be used, as insufficient evidence of harm to blood products exists.[12]

Hypocalcemia, acidosis, and hypothermia contribute to coagulopathy and empiric administration of calcium and bicarbonate, as well as active patient rewarming are warranted. Tranexamic acid, a low-cost antifibrinolytic agent with a mild risk profile, reduces mortality in traumatic hemorrhagic shock. Despite a possible benefit in UGIB, a recent randomized controlled trial did not corroborate any benefit in LGIB.[13]

Reversal of anticoagulant agents should be considered. Clinical status and underlying indication can be considered in determining the duration and degree of reversal. Warfarin can be reversed in approximately 10 minutes with prothrombin-complex concentrates (PCC). PCC has durable effect at 48 hours and may be useful in comorbid conditions in which large-volume transfusion is less desirable.[14] FFP reversal of warfarin is slower and less durable than PCC but more cost-effective. If prolonged reversal is acceptable, vitamin K provides reversal within 12 to 24 hours and may minimize the risk of rebleeding, as effect of acute reversal wanes. Platelet transfusion occurs empirically with massive transfusion, but is commonly practiced in patients taking antiplatelet agents. Platelet transfusion in gastrointestinal bleeding with platelet counts greater than 100×10^9/L has limited benefit and may increase mortality.[15]

Proliferating novel oral anticoagulants (NOACs) and absence of reversal agents has created difficulty managing severe hemorrhage. For doses taken less than 2 hours prior, activated charcoal may limit absorption but can obscure endoscopic visualization. PCC may partially reverse NOAC agents, but thromboembolic risk, cost, and lack of evidence may limit use to unstable patients. Dabigatran can be reversed with the monoclonal antibody agent idarucizumab. Oral factor Xa inhibitors (rivaroxaban, apixaban, edoxaban, and betrixaban) currently have no reversal agents approved by the Food and Drug Administration and cannot be dialyzed, thus rendering care supportive. Depending on renal function and agent half-life, the anticoagulant effect may subside after 24 hours. When approved, investigational agents andexanet alfa (universal factor Xa antidote) and ciraparantag (direct thrombin inhibitors, factor Xa inhibitors, and heparins) should alleviate this dilemma.[16]

URGENT LOCALIZATION AND CONTROL IN THE UNSTABLE PATIENT

With resuscitation initiated, gross localization of bleeding source to upper or lower gastrointestinal tract aids in determining the appropriate treatment algorithm. Although melena or hematochezia without hematemesis suggests LGIB, the prevalence of UGIB in this scenario is between 32% and 74%.[17] Known liver disease or presence of stigmata suggests variceal UGIB better suited to nonsurgical interventions, such as endoscopic banding or transjugular intrahepatic portosystemic shunting. Nasogastric tube aspiration is described to differentiate UGIB and LGIB, but numerous reports suggest both poor sensitivity and negative predictive value.[17,18] Of patients with melena but not hematemesis, 93% with a confirmed UGIB source had at least 2 of the following: presence of melena, age younger than 50, or blood urea nitrogen:creatinine ratio less than 30.[19]

Detailed later, several options for rapid localization and control of bleeding exist. Computed tomography angiography (CTA) for localization is rapid, widely available, and has excellent sensitivity in identifying bleeding sources. In the unstable patient, angioembolization is frequently recommended as the initial diagnostic and therapeutic modality due to its favorable risk profile and hemostasis efficacy. Upper endoscopy is the gold standard for localization and control if UGIB suspicion is high, but aspiration risk and airway protection must be considered. If the above resources are unavailable, empiric operative intervention may be appropriate. A suggested algorithm for diagnosis and management of LGIB is presented in **Fig. 1**.

CONSIDERATION OF TRANSFER

Patient transfer is associated with increased in-hospital mortality for diverticular bleeds.[20] Spontaneous resolution occurs in 80% of LGIB, only 18% require

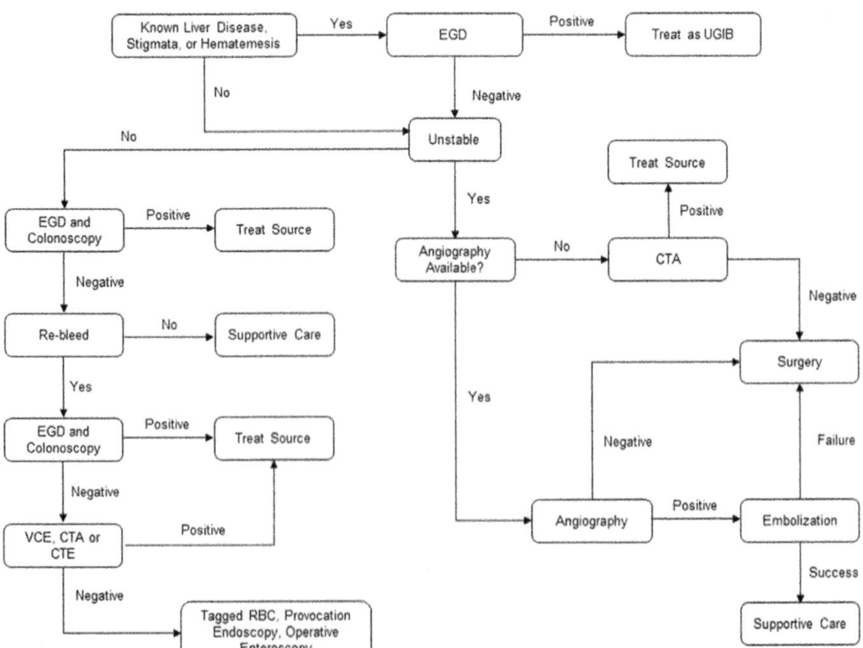

Fig. 1. Suggested algorithm for LGIB management. EGD, esophagogastroduodenoscopy.

transfusion, and only 8.5% require more than 2 units.[4,21] Of patients meeting traditional indications for operative intervention, 60% were managed nonoperatively without mortality.[22] Multiple prediction tools are described to identify high-risk patients with LGIB, but none has achieved universal acceptance. Commonly described characteristics include hypotension, tachycardia, gross blood on rectal examination, recurrent hematochezia within 4 hours, and increasing number of comorbidities (chronic obstructive pulmonary disease, chronic kidney disease, diabetes mellitus).[23]

For stable patients, these reports highlight most patients can be safely managed with limited resources and avoid costly transfer. For unstable patients, however, the need and availability of significant resources is an important determinant of whether transfer to high care should be considered. Emergent surgical intervention to control LGIB bleeding may be appropriate even in the patient requiring subsequent transfer for additional resources. Dao and colleagues[20] suggest deference of urgent surgical intervention for diverticular bleeding may be a source of increased mortality noted in transfer patients. The decision to transfer is a complex assessment of variables the surgeon must make based on clinical experience and available resources.

ENDOSCOPIC TECHNIQUES FOR LOCALIZATION AND CONTROL

Flexible endoscopy is the standard of care for localization and control of gastrointestinal bleeding in the stable patient. In evaluation of LGIB, upper endoscopy should be considered to exclude UGIB sources. Urgent (<24 hours) colonoscopy is recommended in some LGIB management guidelines suggesting benefits of increased localization, reduced rebleeding, and reduced need for surgery.[24] Meta-analyses report similar findings of improved localization, but no difference in bleeding recurrence, transfusion requirement, or surgical intervention was evident.[25] Improved source localization favors urgent colonoscopy in patients with recurrent LGIB following prior unsuccessful localization attempts. Regardless of timing, adequate bowel preparation increases diagnostic yield, success of cecal intubation, and reduces perforation risk. Suspected postpolypectomy bleeding is a notable exception in which enema alone may be adequate for successful localization and intervention.[26] High-volume (4 to 6 L) polyethylene glycol preparations have been associated with better visualization.[27] Nasogastric tube placement and prokinetic agent administration may facilitate completion of bowel preparation in the patient intolerant of oral intake. The benefit of aggressive bowel preparation must be weighed against risks of aspiration and airway compromise in the unstable or debilitated patient.

The potential of therapeutic intervention, in addition to diagnostic ability, makes colonoscopy the standard of care in stable patients with LGIB patients. Powered irrigation systems are beneficial for clearing residual intraluminal blood and breaking up clots. Visualized active bleeding, a nonbleeding visible vessel, or adherent clot may herald a hemorrhagic source and prompt intervention, but the possibility of additional proximal sources should not be excluded. Initial epinephrine injection may temporize active bleeding and improve visualization for additional interventions. Mucosal lift with saline injection may improve access to technically difficult locations enabling interventions. Diverticular and postpolypectomy bleeding are frequently amenable to epinephrine injection and hemostatic clip placement, although band ligation has been described. Emerging topical hemostatic agents offer a technically easy and rapid approach to achieving high rates of immediate endoscopic hemostasis (96.5%, n = 108), but may be associated with higher bleeding recurrence.[28] Argon beam coagulation is frequently described for colonic angiodysplasia with a reported success rate of 85% and may achieve hemostasis in radiation colitis or gastrointestinal tumors as well.[29] Equipment availability and local experience will determine the precise techniques used. The ACG Guideline for Management of Patients with Acute LGIB (2016) is available for free on the Internet[30] and is a rich source of technical details for performing endoscopic hemostatic therapies.[24]

RADIOGRAPHIC TECHNIQUES FOR LOCALIZATION AND CONTROL

CTA, with a reported sensitivity of 84.8% and specificity of 96.9%, is a useful resource to localize gastrointestinal bleeding, particularly when localization may aid urgent transfer or surgical decision-making.[31] CTA more frequently identified an active bleeding source (31.3% vs 14.8%, $P = .031$) with a similar rate of inconclusive examinations when compared with endoscopy.[32] The shorter time to performance of CTA versus endoscopy underscores the utility of CTA for rapid diagnosis. Compared with tagged-red blood cell (RBC) scintigraphy, CTA was found to have a superior localization rate (38% vs 53%, $P = .008$).[33] CTA before traditional angiography reduced the number studies performed and, despite an increase in contrast administration, did not adversely affect renal function.[34]

Tagged-RBC scintigraphy is a well-described diagnostic modality in gastrointestinal bleeding with a reported accuracy of 75% in localization.[35] Advantages may include high sensitivity for slow bleeding and ability to perform repeat examinations to identify intermittent bleeding up to 48 hours after tagged-RBC infusion. Despite advances in imaging acquisition technology, the true positive rate was only 39% in one recent retrospective series.[36] The investigators noted a false-positive rate of 10%, which resulted in 5 surgeries that they labeled as “incorrect surgeries.” Positivity within 2 hours was associated with higher accuracy (86%) in localization.[35] Positivity $\leq$9 minutes from injection has a sensitivity of 92% and a 6.1-fold increase ($P = .020$) in likelihood of a positive finding on subsequent angiography. This relationship was inversely correlated with increasing time between positive scan and angiography, underscoring the need to expeditiously obtain CTA or angiographic confirmation of a positive tagged-RBC scan.[37] Delayed positivity (3–24 hours after injection) was associated with greater frequencies of transfusion, surgery, and bleeding source located in the stomach or small bowel.[38] Additional weakness of scintigraphy, beyond lacking therapeutic value, include imprecise localization, time requirement for the examination, and false positives or incorrect localization due to radiotracer migration and pooling. The current role of scintigraphy is less clear than historically, but likely most applicable in stable patients with unrevealing endoscopic and/or angiographic examinations.

Catheter angiography is the only radiologic modality imparting both diagnostic and therapeutic capability, making it critical in the unstable patient where time required for bowel preparation and endoscopy is prohibitive. In LGIB, angiography following a positive CTA has a localization success rate between 48% and 67% with less than 90 minutes to angiography enhancing the detection rate.[39] Among identified active bleeding, selective angiography and embolization achieved a 100% rate of immediate hemostasis, but was associated with recurrent bleeding in as frequently as 35% of cases within 30 days.[40] Ischemic events were reported in only 0% to 5% of embolizations performed in several recent retrospective series.[39,41] Success of embolization for active tumor-associated hemorrhage was reported in 91% ($n = 11$) of cases without an incident of intestinal ischemia.[41] Considering resource utilization, invasiveness, and potential morbidity (eg, hematoma, infection, pseudoaneurysm, arteriovenous-fistula), angiography seems best used when therapeutic interventions are likely, such as in unstable patients.

Impaction of diverticula via high-dose barium enema is reported as an effective therapy for hemostasis in patients with acute diverticular bleeding with a source not identifiable by urgent colonoscopy.[42] A small randomized controlled trial of barium enema after resolution of diverticular bleeding demonstrated a reduction of recurrent bleeding at 1 year. Although these reports have limitations, given its safety, the utility of barium impaction therapy as a salvage therapy for multiply-comorbid patients to avoid surgery is intriguing.

RECURRENT AND OBSCURE LOWER GASTROINTESTINAL BLEEDING

Recurrence of LGIB is common. Reported readmission rate for recurrent LGIB is 13.7% at 14 days, and 19.0% at 1 year.[43,44] Risk factors identified include malignancy, nonsteroidal anti-inflammatory use, nonaspirin antiplatelet agents, dual antiplatelet therapy, and age older than 65.[43,44]

Early rebleeding in the unstable patient can be evaluated and treated with angiography and embolization or, if previously localized, surgical intervention. Previously localized sources in the stable patient can be addressed based on management of the underlying etiology. The most challenging scenarios occur with recurrent bleeding after inconclusive attempts at localization. Repeat (ie, "second-look") upper and lower endoscopy has diagnostic yield of 40% to 65% and should be considered.[45] Continued failure to localize bleeding should prompt evaluation for suspected small bowel source.

Obscure gastrointestinal bleeding was defined as unlocalized recurrent bleeding despite standard upper and lower endoscopy as well as radiographic evaluations. Because small bowel pathology in identified in most cases, this scenario is alternatively referred to as "suspected small bowel bleeding." Angiodysplasia, inflammatory bowel disease, Dieulafoy lesions, neoplasms, and NSAID ulcers are frequently cited etiologies.[46] Evaluation of small bowel bleeding sources may include a combination of CTA, computed tomography enterorrhaphy (CTE), or video capsule endoscopy (VCE). VCE has become the primary endoscopic modality for initial evaluation of suspected small bowel bleeding with a diagnostic yield of 38% to 83%.[47] Abdominal pain, signs of bowel obstruction, history of inflammatory bowel disease, or suspected adhesive disease should prompt abdominal imaging with CTE before performing VCE. In the stable patient with suspected active bleeding, CTA is preferred over CTE. A negative CTE can be subsequently evaluated with VCE. Dissolvable patency capsules can evaluate passage if capsule entrapment is a concern. Identified lesions, most commonly angiodysplasia, can be managed with deep enteroscopy (eg, push, single-balloon, double-balloon) and endoscopic hemostatic methods (ie, argon beam coagulation) although some question the long-term efficacy of this technique.[48] Regardless, deep enteroscopy is an uncommon surgeon skill and may require collaboration with experienced gastroenterologists.

Rarely, a bleeding source remains elusive despite extensive attempts at localization. Repeat VCE within 2 weeks, particularly with overt rebleeding or a >4 g/dL drop in hemoglobin, has a 50% to 75% diagnostic yield.[49] Pharmacologic provocation using fibrinolytics, anticoagulants, and vasodilators during angiography is another approach to identify occult bleeding sources, with a success rate of 29% to 80%.[50] Endoscopy with heparin and clopidogrel provocation had a diagnostic yield of 71% for occult bleeding sources, frequently angiodysplasia or Dieulafoy lesions, without any adverse events.[51] Intraoperative small bowel enteroscopy is an effective but morbid diagnostic option when surgical therapy is undertaken or all other modalities are exhausted. Recurrent obscure gastrointestinal bleeding is a challenging scenario that requires a methodical and persistent approach to successfully manage.

SURGICAL INTERVENTIONS FOR LOCALIZATION AND CONTROL

Indications for surgical intervention may include unavailable or unsuccessful angiography in the unstable patient, recurrent bleeding despite repeated endoscopic or angiographic interventions in the stable patient, or etiology best managed by definitive resection, such as neoplasm. Although 60% of patients meeting them can be managed nonoperatively without mortality, traditional indications for surgery include more than 6 units of blood, hemodynamic instability, continued bleeding longer than 72 hours, or rebleeding more than 24 hours after presentation.[22] A suggestive algorithm for surgical decision-making is presented in **Fig. 2**.

Most literature on LGIB surgical interventions are retrospective and published before damage control surgery was widely adopted. Without adequate evidence to guide decisions, a variety of approaches are reasonable and ultimately a judgment of the surgeon. We present an approach using patient stability and localization as major determinants for surgical decision-making.

If a bleeding source has been localized, in the stable patient, anatomic resection and anastomosis is an ideal approach, although patient factors may exclude primary anastomosis. In the unstable patient with localized LGIB, anatomic resection for bleeding control with temporary abdominal closure may be considered. Anastomosis or ostomy creation can be subsequently considered depending on comorbidities and resuscitation response.

If a bleeding source has not been localized, upper endoscopy to exclude UGIB sources may prevent morbid empiric resections. If an UGIB source is identified and endoscopic hemostasis is unsuccessful, operative intervention can be immediately performed to achieve control of nonvariceal sources. Variceal bleeding can be addressed endoscopically by an appropriately skilled endoscopist or temporized with tamponade catheters, such as the Blakemore or Minnesota tube, allowing

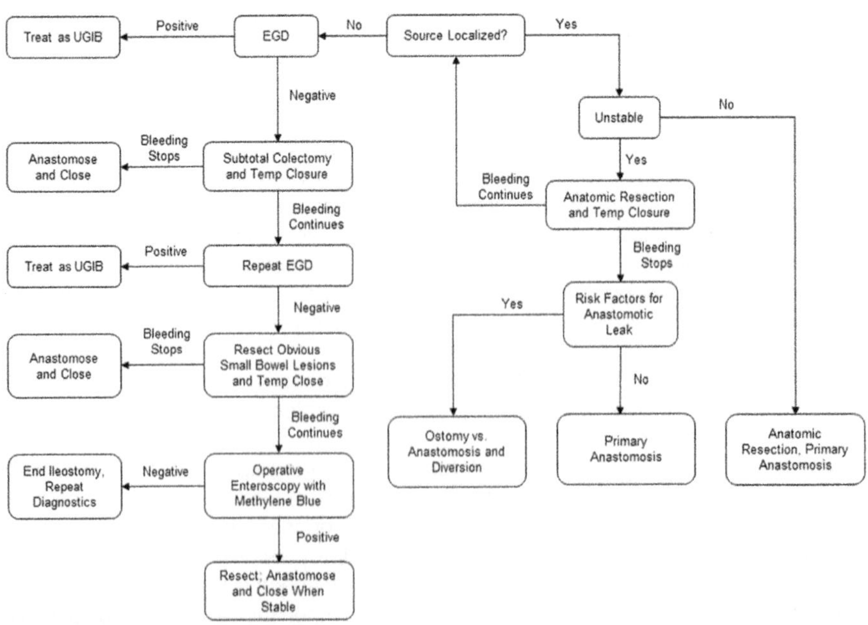

Fig. 2. Suggested algorithm for surgical management of LGIB. EGD, esophagogastroduodenoscopy; Temp, temporary.

transfer to a facility with appropriate resources. Depending on patient stability, colonoscopy may be attempted for suspected postpolypectomy bleeding, but is less successful for other etiologies in the unprepped patient. If a bleeding source remains elusive, abdominal exploration is indicated.

In the unstable patient with unlocalized LGIB, subtotal colectomy is the traditional empiric surgical intervention. Rebleeding risk with segmental colon resection is greater than with subtotal colectomy, although the limited evidence does not agree whether this confers increased mortality.[52–55] Ileorectal anastomosis was described in most of these series, a practice avoided today in unstable patients. Unsurprisingly, anastomotic leak was the primary source of mortality in one series.[54] Resection with temporary closure and delayed anastomosis is a reasonable approach. Oncologic mesenteric resection should be performed for suspicions of a neoplastic process if feasible. Before colonic mobilization, if an intact ileocecal valve is present, an enterotomy in the distal ileum may allow identification of proximal blood, suggesting a small bowel etiology. Exploration for a Meckel diverticulum or mass can be performed before empiric colon resection.

In stable patients with unlocalized LGIB, all endoscopic and radiographic modalities for localization of small bowel bleeding should be exhausted before any surgical intervention. Intraoperative enteroscopy may exclude small bowel etiology before performing an empiric resection. Intraoperative methylene blue injection may aid in the identification of bleeding source.[56] Voron and colleagues[57] provide a detailed technical review on the performance of this infrequently used technique. If intraoperative enteroscopy is unsuccessful, options include empiric resection of any bowel lesions (ie, Meckel diverticulum or mass), anatomic segmental resection based on suspicions (ie, sigmoidectomy for extensive diverticulosis), or an empiric subtotal colectomy with anastomosis. Surgical intervention for unlocalized bleeding in the stable patient is a vexing challenge.

OTHER MANAGEMENT ISSUES IN LOWER GASTROINTESTINAL BLEEDING

High-risk patients not requiring immediate intervention should be closely monitored. Invasive hemodynamic monitoring may be beneficial and adequate vascular access is critical. Urgently placed semi-sterile access should be replaced when prudent. Hemoglobin, lactate, electrolyte, creatinine, and coagulation parameters can be followed at a frequency appropriate to patient stability. Dynamic measures of volume responsiveness (pulse-pressure variability) have superior predictive value than traditional static measurements (central venous pressure) and may guide volume resuscitation.[58] Point-of-care transthoracic ultrasonography may aid assessment of cardiac function and volume status. Persistent hypotension despite adequate volume resuscitation suggests concurrent cardiac pathology, which electrocardiogram, serial troponins, and transthoracic echocardiography may elucidate.

Resuscitation goals may include mean arterial pressure greater than 65 mm Hg, systolic blood pressure higher than 90 mm Hg, central venous saturation of greater than 60%, urine output of greater than 0.5 mL/kg/h, and normalization of lactic acid or base deficit. Goals of 0.9 mmol/L for ionized calcium, pH >7.1, and temperature higher than 34°C may correct and prevent coagulopathy. Maintenance of hemoglobin greater than 7.0 g/dL is standard of care for critically ill patients with a goal of greater than 8.0 g/dL in the setting of acute coronary syndrome or chronic cardiovascular disease.[59] Several studies examined liberal (<9 g/dL) and restrictive (<7 g/dL) transfusion triggers in UGIB and found no difference in mortality, morbidity, and myocardial infarction, but advantages including reduced blood product usage and shorter length of stay.[60,61]

Evidence to guide resumption of anticoagulants after LGIB is limited. Deep venous thrombosis prophylaxis may be safe 24 hours after LGIB.[62] Review of medications and indications may identify anticoagulants for discontinuation to reduce rebleeding risk, although risk-benefit discussion with the prescribing physician may be required. Resumption of non-NOAC anticoagulation 7 days after LGIB does not increase risk of recurrent bleeding, but does reduce risk of thromboembolic events.[63] NSAID use may increase risk of recurrent LGIB and should be avoided.[64] Proton pump inhibitor prophylaxis is recommended by some guidelines to mitigate this risk. Future evidence will clarify the best approach to managing anticoagulation post-LGIB.

SUMMARY

LGIB is a common entity in general surgery practice. Familiarity with the various diagnostic and therapeutic modalities is necessary for optimal patient care. Evolving resuscitation strategies, pharmaceuticals, diagnostic technology, and management devices are altering traditional management algorithms. As less invasive interventions become more efficient, surgical interventions are becoming less frequent. With experience in managing hemorrhagic shock, endoscopy, and definitive surgical interventions, the surgeon knowledgeable of the evolving practice landscape is well-positioned to provide efficient and complete care to most patients with LGIB.

REFERENCES

1. Peery AF, Dellon ES, Lund J, et al. Burden of gastrointestinal disease in the United States: 2012 update. Gastroenterology 2012;143(5):1179–87.e3.
2. Qayed E, Dagar G, Nanchal RS. Lower gastrointestinal hemorrhage. Crit Care Clin 2016;32(2):241–54.
3. Laine L, Yang H, Chang S-C, et al. Trends for incidence of hospitalization and death due to GI complications in the United States from 2001 to 2009. Am J Gastroenterol 2012;107(8):1190–5.
4. Chong V, Hill AG, MacCormick AD. Accurate triage of lower gastrointestinal bleed (LGIB)–a cohort study. Int J Surg 2016;25:19–23.
5. Patel R, Clancy R, Crowther E, et al. A rectal bleeding algorithm can successfully reduce emergency admissions. Colorectal Dis 2014;16(5):377–81.
6. Matsumura Y, Matsumoto J, Idoguchi K, et al. Non-traumatic hemorrhage is controlled with REBOA in acute phase then mortality increases gradually by non-hemorrhagic causes: DIRECT-IABO registry in Japan. Eur J Trauma Emerg Surg 2017. https://doi.org/10.1007/s00068-017-0829-z.
7. Brenner M, Teeter W, Hoehn M, et al. Use of resuscitative endovascular balloon occlusion of the aorta for proximal aortic control in patients with severe hemorrhage and arrest. JAMA Surg 2017. https://doi.org/10.1001/jamasurg.2017.3549.
8. Heffner AC, Swords DS, Nussbaum ML, et al. Predictors of the complication of postintubation hypotension during emergency airway management. J Crit Care 2012;27(6):587–93.
9. Etchill EW, Myers SP, McDaniel LM, et al. Should all massively transfused patients be treated equally? An analysis of massive transfusion ratios in the nontrauma setting. Crit Care Med 2017;45(8):1311–6.
10. Mesar T, Larentzakis A, Dzik W, et al. Association between ratio of fresh frozen plasma to red blood cells during massive transfusion and survival among patients without traumatic injury. JAMA Surg 2017;152(6):574.

11. Sambasivan CN, Kunio NR, Nair PV, et al. High ratios of plasma and platelets to packed red blood cells do not affect mortality in nonmassively transfused patients. J Trauma 2011;71(2 Suppl 3):S329–36.
12. Thomas D, Wee M, Clyburn P, et al. Blood transfusion and the anaesthetist: management of massive haemorrhage. Anaesthesia 2010;65(11):1153–61.
13. Smith SR, Murray D, Pockney PG, et al. Tranexamic acid for lower GI hemorrhage. Dis Colon Rectum 2017;61(1):1.
14. Pabinger I, Brenner B, Kalina U, et al. Prothrombin complex concentrate (Beriplex P/N) for emergency anticoagulation reversal: a prospective multinational clinical trial. J Thromb Haemost 2008;6(4):622–31.
15. Zakko L, Rustagi T, Douglas M, et al. No benefit from platelet transfusion for gastrointestinal bleeding in patients taking antiplatelet agents. Clin Gastroenterol Hepatol 2017;15(1):46–52.
16. Samuelson BT, Cuker A. Measurement and reversal of the direct oral anticoagulants. Blood Rev 2017;31(1):77–84.
17. Palamidessi N, Sinert R, Falzon L, et al. Nasogastric aspiration and lavage in emergency department patients with hematochezia or melena without hematemesis. Acad Emerg Med 2010;17(2):126–32.
18. Rockey DC, Ahn C, de Melo SW. Randomized pragmatic trial of nasogastric tube placement in patients with upper gastrointestinal tract bleeding. J Investig Med 2017;65(4):759–64.
19. Witting MD, Magder L, Heins AE, et al. ED predictors of upper gastrointestinal tract bleeding in patients without hematemesis. Am J Emerg Med 2006;24(3):280–5.
20. Dao HE, Miller PE, Lee JH, et al. Transfer status is a risk factor for increased inhospital mortality in patients with diverticular hemorrhage. Int J Colorectal Dis 2013;28(2):273–6.
21. Das A, Wong RCK. Prediction of outcome of acute GI hemorrhage: a review of risk scores and predictive models. Gastrointest Endosc 2004;60(1):85–93. Available at: http://www.ncbi.nlm.nih.gov/pubmed/15229431. Accessed October 25, 2017.
22. Yi WS, Vegeler R, Hoang K, et al. Watch and wait: conservative management of lower gastrointestinal bleeding. J Surg Res 2012;177(2):315–9.
23. Newman J, Fitzgerald JEF, Gupta S, et al. Outcome predictors in acute surgical admissions for lower gastrointestinal bleeding. Colorectal Dis 2012;14(8):1020–6.
24. Strate LL, Gralnek IM. ACG clinical guideline: management of patients with acute lower gastrointestinal bleeding. Am J Gastroenterol 2016;111(4):459–74.
25. Kouanda AM, Somsouk M, Sewell JL, et al. Urgent colonoscopy in patients with lower GI bleeding: a systematic review and meta-analysis. Gastrointest Endosc 2017;86(1):107–17.e1.
26. Lim DS, Kim HG, Jeon SR, et al. Comparison of clinical effectiveness of the emergent colonoscopy in patients with hematochezia according to the type of bowel preparation. J Gastroenterol Hepatol 2013;28(11):1733–7.
27. Saito K, Inamori M, Sekino Y, et al. Management of acute lower intestinal bleeding: what bowel preparation should be required for urgent colonoscopy? Hepatogastroenterology 2009;56(94–95):1331–4. Available at: http://www.ncbi.nlm.nih.gov/pubmed/19950786. Accessed December 28, 2017.
28. Haddara S, Jacques J, Lecleire S, et al. A novel hemostatic powder for upper gastrointestinal bleeding: a multicenter study (the "GRAPHE" registry). Endoscopy 2016;48(12):1084–95.

29. Olmos JA, Marcolongo M, Pogorelsky V, et al. Long-term outcome of argon plasma ablation therapy for bleeding in 100 consecutive patients with colonic angiodysplasia. Dis Colon Rectum 2006;49(10):1507–16.
30. Available at: http://gi.org/wp-content/uploads/2016/03/ACGGuideline-Acute-Lower-GI-Bleeding-03012016.pdf. Accessed July 10, 2018.
31. Kim J, Kim YH, Lee KH, et al. Diagnostic performance of CT angiography in patients visiting emergency department with overt gastrointestinal bleeding. Korean J Radiol 2015;16(3):541.
32. Clerc D, Grass F, Schäfer M, et al. Lower gastrointestinal bleeding—computed tomographic angiography, colonoscopy or both? World J Emerg Surg 2017; 12(1):1.
33. Feuerstein JD, Ketwaroo G, Tewani SK, et al. Localizing acute lower gastrointestinal hemorrhage: CT angiography versus tagged RBC scintigraphy. Am J Roentgenol 2016;207(3):578–84.
34. Jacovides CL, Nadolski G, Allen SR, et al. Arteriography for lower gastrointestinal hemorrhage. JAMA Surg 2015;150(7):650.
35. Dusold R, Burke K, Carpentier W, et al. The accuracy of technetium-99m-labeled red cell scintigraphy in localizing gastrointestinal bleeding. Am J Gastroenterol 1994;89(3):345–8. Available at: http://www.ncbi.nlm.nih.gov/pubmed/8122642. Accessed December 28, 2017.
36. Tabibian JH, Wong Kee Song LM, Enders FB, et al. Technetium-labeled erythrocyte scintigraphy in acute gastrointestinal bleeding. Int J Colorectal Dis 2013; 28(8):1099–105.
37. Chung M, Dubel GJ, Noto RB, et al. Acute lower gastrointestinal bleeding: temporal factors associated with positive findings on catheter angiography after (99m) Tc-labeled RBC scanning. AJR Am J Roentgenol 2016;207(1):170–6.
38. Jacobson AF, Cerqueira MD. Prognostic significance of late imaging results in technetium-99m-labeled red blood cell gastrointestinal bleeding studies with early negative images. J Nucl Med 1992;33(2):202–7. Available at: http://www.ncbi.nlm.nih.gov/pubmed/1732441. Accessed December 28, 2017.
39. Pham T, Tran BA, Ooi K, et al. Super-selective mesenteric embolization provides effective control of lower GI bleeding. Radiol Res Pract 2017;2017:1–5.
40. Chan DKH, Soong J, Koh F, et al. Predictors for outcomes after super-selective mesenteric embolization for lower gastrointestinal tract bleeding. ANZ J Surg 2016;86(6):459–63.
41. Tandberg DJ, Smith TP, Suhocki PV, et al. Early outcomes of empiric embolization of tumor-related gastrointestinal hemorrhage in patients with advanced malignancy. J Vasc Interv Radiol 2012;23(11):1445–52.
42. Fujimoto A, Sato S, Kurakata H, et al. Effectiveness of high-dose barium enema filling for colonic diverticular bleeding. Colorectal Dis 2011;13(8):896–8.
43. Sengupta N, Tapper EB, Patwardhan VR, et al. Risk factors for adverse outcomes in patients hospitalized with lower gastrointestinal bleeding. Mayo Clin Proc 2015; 90(8):1021–9.
44. Aoki T, Nagata N, Niikura R, et al. Recurrence and mortality among patients hospitalized for acute lower gastrointestinal bleeding. Clin Gastroenterol Hepatol 2015;13(3):488–94.e1.
45. Gerson LB. Small bowel bleeding: updated algorithm and outcomes. Gastrointest Endosc Clin N Am 2017;27(1):171–80.
46. Gerson LB, Fidler JL, Cave DR, et al. ACG clinical guideline: diagnosis and management of small bowel bleeding. Am J Gastroenterol 2015;110(9):1265–87.

47. Rondonotti E, Villa F, Mulder CJJ, et al. Small bowel capsule endoscopy in 2007: indications, risks and limitations. World J Gastroenterol 2007;13(46):6140–9. Available at: http://www.ncbi.nlm.nih.gov/pubmed/18069752. Accessed December 29, 2017.
48. Romagnuolo J, Brock AS, Ranney N. Is endoscopic therapy effective for angioectasia in obscure gastrointestinal bleeding? J Clin Gastroenterol 2015;49(10): 823–30.
49. Viazis N, Papaxoinis K, Vlachogiannakos J, et al. Is there a role for second-look capsule endoscopy in patients with obscure GI bleeding after a nondiagnostic first test? Gastrointest Endosc 2009;69(4):850–6.
50. Johnston C, Tuite D, Pritchard R, et al. Use of provocative angiography to localize site in recurrent gastrointestinal bleeding. Cardiovasc Intervent Radiol 2007; 30(5):1042–6.
51. Raines DL, Jex KT, Nicaud MJ, et al. Pharmacologic provocation combined with endoscopy in refractory cases of GI bleeding. Gastrointest Endosc 2017;85(1): 112–20.
52. Farner R, Lichliter W, Kuhn J, et al. Total colectomy versus limited colonic resection for acute lower gastrointestinal bleeding. Am J Surg 1999;178(6):587–91. Available at: http://www.ncbi.nlm.nih.gov/pubmed/10670878. Accessed October 25, 2017.
53. Parkes BM, Obeid FN, Sorensen VJ, et al. The management of massive lower gastrointestinal bleeding. Am Surg 1993;59(10):676–8. Available at: http://www.ncbi.nlm.nih.gov/pubmed/8214970. Accessed October 27, 2017.
54. Plummer JM, Gibson TN, Mitchell DIG, et al. Emergency subtotal colectomy for lower gastrointestinal haemorrhage: over-utilised or under-estimated? Int J Clin Pract 2009;63(6):865–8.
55. Eaton AC. Emergency surgery for acute colonic haemorrhage–a retrospective study. Br J Surg 1981;68(2):109–12. Available at: http://www.ncbi.nlm.nih.gov/pubmed/6970059. Accessed October 27, 2017.
56. Pai M, Frampton AE, Virk JS, et al. Preoperative superselective mesenteric angiography and methylene blue injection for localization of obscure gastrointestinal bleeding. JAMA Surg 2013;148(7):665.
57. Voron T, Rahmi G, Bonnet S, et al. Intraoperative enteroscopy: is there still a role? Gastrointest Endosc Clin N Am 2017;27(1):153–70.
58. Marik PE, Cavallazzi R, Vasu T, et al. Dynamic changes in arterial waveform derived variables and fluid responsiveness in mechanically ventilated patients: a systematic review of the literature. Crit Care Med 2009;37(9):2642–7.
59. Docherty AB, O'Donnell R, Brunskill S, et al. Effect of restrictive versus liberal transfusion strategies on outcomes in patients with cardiovascular disease in a non-cardiac surgery setting: systematic review and meta-analysis. BMJ 2016; 352:i1351.
60. Holst LB, Petersen MW, Haase N, et al. Restrictive versus liberal transfusion strategy for red blood cell transfusion: systematic review of randomised trials with meta-analysis and trial sequential analysis. BMJ 2015;350. https://doi.org/10.1136/bmj.h1354.
61. Wang J, Bao Y-X, Bai M, et al. Restrictive vs liberal transfusion for upper gastrointestinal bleeding: a meta-analysis of randomized controlled trials. World J Gastroenterol 2013;19(40):6919.
62. Deutsch GB, Kandel AR, Knobel D, et al. Bleeding risk secondary to deep vein thrombosis prophylaxis in patients with lower gastrointestinal bleeding. J Intensive Care Med 2012;27(6):379–83.

63. Kido K, Scalese MJ. Management of oral anticoagulation therapy after gastrointestinal bleeding: whether to, when to, and how to restart an anticoagulation therapy. Ann Pharmacother 2017;51(11). https://doi.org/10.1177/1060028017717019.
64. Nagata N, Niikura R, Aoki T, et al. Impact of discontinuing non-steroidal antiinflammatory drugs on long-term recurrence in colonic diverticular bleeding. World J Gastroenterol 2015;21(4):1292.

Rapid Reversal of Novel Anticoagulant and Antiplatelet Medications in General Surgery Emergencies

Lisa L. Schlitzkus, MD*, Jessica I. Summers, MD,
Paul J. Schenarts, MD

KEYWORDS

- Nonvitamin K antagonist oral anticoagulants • Reversal agents
- Perioperative management • Emergent • Urgent

KEY POINTS

- Nonvitamin K antagonist oral anticoagulants (NOACs) are a new class of medications that present challenges in reversal.
- The emergent nature must be determined in every situation, because it will guide the reversal strategy and help determine risk stratification.
- Most NOACs do not have an antidote. Providers must consider other alternatives to mitigating the effect of NOACs.

INTRODUCTION

In the past decade, a new drug class – nonvitamin K antagonist oral anticoagulants (NOACs) – have been rapidly introduced and popularized. For patients, the benefits of these drugs are stable doses without the need for frequent laboratory monitoring. Clinically, these medications are as effective as vitamin K antagonists (VKAs) in preventing stroke and systemic embolic events in nonvalvular atrial fibrillation and preventing and treating venous thromboembolism (VTE).[1–4] Moreover, the risk of bleeding is similar to or less than VKAs with NOACs.[2] Specifically, they are of less risk of intracranial bleeding.[2] Although the phase III trials of each of the drugs were performed without an antidote available, the mortality rates of major bleeding while taking a NOAC were the same or less than those taking VKAs.[5]

Disclosure: The authors have nothing to disclose.
Trauma, Surgical Critical Care and Emergency General Surgery, Department of Surgery, University of Nebraska Medical Center, Nebraska Medical Center, Omaha, NE 68198-3280, USA
* Corresponding author. Department of Surgery, University of Nebraska Medical Center, Nebraska Medical Center, Omaha, NE 68198-3280.
E-mail address: lisa.schlitzkus@unmc.edu

Surg Clin N Am 98 (2018) 1073–1080
https://doi.org/10.1016/j.suc.2018.05.005 surgical.theclinics.com

DABIGATRAN

In October of 2010, dabigatran, the first NOAC was introduced.[6] Its mechanism of action is to directly inhibit thrombin, thus preventing thrombus development.[6] Initially it was only approved for the reduction of stroke and embolic events in nonalvular atrial fibrillation; its scope was expanded to include treatment and reduction in the risk of recurrent VTE and prophylaxis of VTE in patients undergoing hip or knee replacement.[6] It is a prodrug, and estimated bioavailability is 3% to 7%.[6] It has a relatively low protein-binding capability at 35%.[6] Dabigatran is dosed twice a day, 150 mg except for as prophylaxis during hip and knee replacements, where 110 mg is given the first day and 220 mg each day thereafter.[6]

The half-life of dabigatran is 12 to 18 hours (**Table 1**).[6] It peaks after 2 to 4 hours.[6] It is primarily eliminated by the kidneys. When administered intravenously, dabigatran is 80% cleared by the kidneys. When given orally, only 7% is excreted in urine, 86% in the feces.[6] Activated partial thromboplastin time (aPTT) or ecarin clotting time (ECT) can assess for dabigatran's activity. These and thrombin time (TT) may be prolonged while taking dabigatran.

Idarucizumab was developed specifically as a reversal agent for dabigatran. It binds to dabigatran with a 350 times higher affinity than thrombin.[7] It is a humanized monoclonal Fab antibody fragment. The dose is 5 g intravenously.[7] It has a 47-minute half-life and a terminal half-life of 10.3 hours.[7] Furthermore, hemodialysis can remove dabigatran, but the data are limited. Protamine and vitamin K are not expected to affect the drug's activity. Prothrombin complex concentrate (PCC) and recombinant factor VIIa may be used but have not been studied. Dabigatran may be restarted immediately following an operation or invasive procedure. Finally, platelet administration should be undertaken in thrombocytopenia and when long-acting antiplatelet medications are involved.

RIVAROXABAN

Rivaroxaban is a factor Xa inhibitor[8] approved for use by the US Food and Drug Administration (FDA) in November 2011 to reduce the risk of stroke and embolic events in nonvalvular atrial fibrillation, treat VTE and reduce the recurrent risk, and VTE prophylaxis during hip or knee replacements.[8] It does not require antithrombin III or other cofactors, and it is not a prodrug.[8] Its bioavailability is strictly dose dependent; for the 10 mg dose, its estimated bioavailability is 80% to 100%.[8] Rivaroxaban

Table 1
Non-vitamin K antagonist oral anticoagulants

	Dabigatran	Rivaroxaban	Apixaban	Edoxaban	Betrixaban
Half-life	12–18 h	5–9 h	12 h	5.8–10.7 h	19–27 h
Antidote	Idarucizumab	Andexanet[a] Ciraparantag[b]	Andexanet[a] Ciraparantag[b]	Andexanet[a] Ciraparantag[b]	Andexanet[a] Ciraparantag[b]
Adjuncts	PCC, recombinant factor VIIa	PCC	PCC, aPCC (FEIBA), recombinant Factor VIIa, activated charcoal	PCC, aPCC (FEIBA), recombinant factor VIIa	No data
Dialyzable	Yes	No	No	No	No data

[a] In ongoing phase III trial.
[b] In phase II trial.

has extremely high protein-binding capabilities (92%–95%).[8] The recommended dose is 20 mg with the evening meal for atrial fibrillation, 15 mg twice daily for treatment of VTE, 10 mg to reduce recurrent risk after 6 months of full treatment, and 10 mg daily during hip and knee replacements.[8]

Following administration, concentration levels peak at 2 to 4 hours with a half-life of 5 to 9 hours.[8] Effects may be seen up to 24 hours.[8] Rivaroxaban is eliminated by both the kidneys (33%) and liver.[8] The effect of rivaroxaban on PT, aPTT, HepTest, and anti-factor Xa levels are also dose dependent.[8] Once therapeutic, aPTT, ECT, and TT maybe prolonged, but aPTT provides the best approximation of the drug's effect.

Unfortunately, there are currently no FDA-approved reversal agents for rivaroxaban. Andexanet, a recombinant variant of human factor Xa, is in an on-going phase III ANNEXA-4 trial[9] and under review by the FDA. Its reversal of rivaroxaban is short lived and dose dependent.[10] An intravenous bolus must be given followed by a 2-hour infusion, but thrombin generation was normalized by 8 hours and lasted 3 days.[10] Ciraparantag, a cationic molecule that binds to all NOACs, is also being investigated. It is in on-going trials to reverse rivaroxaban. It has demonstrated clot stabilization, but has not begun a phase III trial. Dialysis is not an option in reversing rivaroxaban because of the high protein-binding capability. Protamine and vitamin K are thought to be ineffective in reversal. Although partial reversal demonstrated by a reduced aPTT has been demonstrated with the use of PCC, there are no data to support activated prothrombin complex concentrates (aPCCs), factor VIII inhibitor bypassing activity (FEIBA; Shire), or recombinant factor VIIa. Rivaroxaban can be restarted immediately following an operation or invasive procedure once hemostasis is achieved.[8]

APIXABAN

Apixaban is also a selective factor Xa inhibitor approved by the FDA in December 2012 with the same indications as rivaroxaban. It does not require antithrombin III and inhibits both free and clot-bound factor Xa.[11] It also is not a prodrug, and its bioavailability is about 50% for doses up to 10 mg.[11] At 87%, it has a high protein-binding capability. For many qualities, it is dosing dependent – 5 mg twice daily for atrial fibrillation, 2.5 mg twice daily for hip and knee VTE prophylaxis, 10 mg twice daily for 7 days for VTE treatment followed by 5 mg twice daily for the remaining treatment period, and 2.5 mg twice daily for recurrent VTE.

Apixaban's half-life is about 12 hours,[11] with a peak concentration of 1 to 3 hours.[12–15] The effect may last up to 24 hours.[11] It is eliminated in the urine and feces – kidneys accounting for about 27%. Subtle changes may be appreciated in PT, INR, and aPTT, but are so small that these conventional laboratory tests are not reliable for efficacy testing.[11]

Currently, there are no antidotes for apixaban. Andexanet is a promising treatment given as a bolus followed by an infusion.[9,10] Ciraparantag is earlier in the development stages, and is not being tested yet for apixaban, but again may treat all NOACs. Hemodialysis is not an option in reversing apixaban. Protamine and vitamin K are not expected to alter the efficacy. No literature describes the use of tranexamic acid (TXA) in the reversal of apixaban. Systemic hemostatic agents like desmopressin and aprotinin also are not expected to reverse apixaban. PCC, aPCC (FEIBA), and recombinant factor VIIa have been used but not clinically studied. We do know that clotting studies (prothrombin time [PT], international normalized ratio [INR,], and aPTT) or anti-factor Xa levels are not useful or recommended when assessing if reversal has been successful. Apixaban may be immediately restarted after hemostasis has been achieved.

Lastly, activated charcoal can be given at 2 and 6 hours after a dose, which reduces the body's exposure by reducing absorption of apixaban.[11]

EDOXABAN

In January 2015, edoxaban became an FDA-approved medication to decrease the risk of cerebral vascular events and embolic events in nonvalvular atrial fibrillation, as well as the treatment of VTE.[16] It is a selective inhibitor of factor Xa and does not require antithrombin III.[16] It is not a prodrug and exhibits 62% bioavailablity.[16] Because it has relatively low protein binding capabilities (40%–59%), the concentration is consistent at 2, 6, and 12 hours following administration.[17] The usual dose is a 60 mg tablet daily, with dose adjusted for poor creatinine clearance.[16]

Peak effect occurs within 1 to 2 hours of administration.[16] Its half-life is 5.8 to 10.7 hours,[17] with complete elimination of 10 to 14 hours, but its effects may last up to 24 hours.[17] Although the drug manufacturer states it is excreted in the urine, renal clearance only accounts for 50% of the total clearance. Metabolism and gastrointestinal excretion also play a large role.[16] Elevated PT and aPTT may be seen in edoxaban, as it prolongs the clotting time, but because the changes in PT, INR, and aPTT are so insignificant, these are not reliable tests for efficacy.[16]

Again, there are no approved FDA reversal agents for edoxaban. The ANNEXA-4 phase III trial for andexanet includes edoxaban. Given the daily dosing, the dose to reverse edoxaban is still being determined and more patients are needed in the edoxaban arm. Ciraparantag is not yet being investigated to reverse edoxaban. Hemodialysis does not effectively clear edoxaban. Also, protamine, vitamin K, and TXA are ineffective. PCC, aPCC (FEIBA), and recombinant factor VIIa should be considered, but there are no data to support their use. In fact, when PCC is used, checking traditional coagulation studies (PT, INR, aPTT) are not recommended.[16] It is safe to restart edoxaban 24 hours after hemostasis has been achieved.

BETRIXABAN

The newest NOAC on the market is betrixaban approved in June 2017. It, too is a factor Xa inhibitor that selectively blocks the active site of Factor Xa and does not need a cofactor for activity. Unlike the other NOACs, it is only indicated for "the prophylaxis of VTE in adult patients hospitalized for an acute medical illness who are at risk for thromboembolic complications due to moderate or severe restricted mobility and other risk factors for VTE."[18] As more trials are completed, its indications should expand like the other NOACs.

Betrixaban's bioavailability is 34% when administered orally.[18] It is not a prodrug.[18] It has a 60% protein binding capacity.[18] The first oral daily dose is 160 mg, then 80 mg every day after given at the same time daily.[18]

Peak concentrations can be seen in 3 to 4 hours after oral administration.[18] Several characteristics other than its indication set betrixaban apart from the other NOACs. Its half-life is 19 to 27 hours, and its effect will last at least 72 hours from the last dose.[18] It maximum concentration and body's exposure is reduced by low (20%) and high (60%) fat diets.[18] The primary form of excretion is feces (85%) instead of renal (11%).[18] Traditional standard laboratory testing does not demonstrate the anticoagulant effects of betrixaban.[19]

Like the other NOACs, there is no reversal agent for betrixaban.[18] Interestingly, the pharmaceutical company that owns betrixaban is the developer of andexanet. No data exist to evaluate the effectiveness of hemodialysis removal of betrixaban. Moreover, there is no role for protamine, vitamin K, or TXA.[18] Data do not exist regarding the effect of PCC, recombinant factor VIIa, or FEIBA. There is no information of timing of restarting betrixaban following an operation or other invasive procedure.

TRADITIONAL ANTICOAGULANTS AND ANTIPLATELET MEDICATIONS

The reversal of traditional anticoagulants – heparin, enoxaparin, and warfarin – have all been well documented in the literature.[20–25] For many of the older, well-known medications, not only is a specific antidote available, but there are several other mechanisms for reversal, including fresh-frozen plasma transfusion or PCC or vitamin K administration. Conversely, argatroban and bivalirudin specifically used in the setting of heparin induced-thrombocytopenia do not have any reversal options.

OVERALL APPROACH

First and foremost, when encountering a perioperative situation where the patient is taking one of these medications, hold the medication. The patient can be supported with intravenous fluids and transfusion if needed. Second, the emergent nature of the situation must be assessed. Do the risks of thrombotic events due to reversal outweigh the risks of bleeding caused by one of these medications? Is this an emergent or urgent situation? The Thrombolysis in Myocardial Infarction (TIMI) bleeding criteria, frequently used in cardiovascular trials, defines major life-threatening bleeding (emergent) as an intracranial bleed (excluding microhemorrhages <10 mm seen only on MRI), clinical signs of hemorrhage with a decrease in hemoglobin (Hg) of at least 5 g/dL or at least a 15% absolute decrease in hematocrit (Hct), or fatal bleeding (death within 7 days). Urgent situations according to the TIMI criteria are clinically overt hemorrhage with a Hg drop of 3 - less than 5 g/dL or at least a 10% decrease in Hct, no overt signs of blood loss with a greater than or equal to 4 g/dL drop in Hg or at least a 12% decrease in Hct, or signs of hemorrhage requiring intervention, cause of or prolonging hospitalization, or when the patient seeks medical evaluation.[26–29] The GUSTO, or Global Utilization of Streptokinase and Tpa for Occluded Arteries criteria, used as frequently as TIMI only considers intracerebral hemorrhage or hemorrhage leading to hemodynamic instability requiring intervention as severe or life-threatening. Although a patient may need a transfusion, if he or she does not have hemodynamic instability, the risk is moderate.[26,30]

Certainly in any nonurgent setting, the NOACs can be held, allowing passage of time, before proceeding with any surgical or other invasive intervention. For operations or invasive procedures deemed urgent, requiring intervention in the next several hours, consideration should include the timing of the last dose versus the risk of reversal and the urgency. Although an antidote may be given and reversal agents considered, risk of thrombosis, cost, resource availability, and patient factors must be considered (**Table 2**). Only thrombotic risk can truly be estimated as low with a CHA_2DS_2-VASc score of 1 to 4 and no prior thrombotic event; moderate risk with a CHA_2DS_2-VASc score of 5 or 6 or prior thrombotic event greater than 3 months in the past; or high risk with a CHA_2DS_2-VASc score of at least 7 or a thrombotic event no more than months.[31,32]

Due to daily or twice daily dosing of NOACs, the current recommendation is to hold the medication, allow passage of time and then proceed with surgical or other intervention. During this time the patient may be supported with fluids or transfusion. In an emergent situation, administering 4-factor PCC is indicated, followed by factor VIII inhibitor bypassing activity (FEIBA; Shire) and recombinant factor VIIa (rFVIIa).

Table 2
Thrombosis risk versus bleeding risk

Thrombosis		Bleeding
Anticoagulant (dose, frequency, time of last dose)	versus	Prehospital loss (scene, home, etc.)
Presence of hypercoagulable state/risk factors • Underlying medical etiology • Recent trauma • Cancer • Female gender or pregnancy/ estrogen use (OCP) • Tobacco use • Immobility		Physical examination findings consistent with hemorrhage: • Scalp laceration • Hemothorax • Intraabdominal hemorrhage • Retroperitoneal hemorrhage/pelvic fractures • Long bone fractures
Nonvalvular atrial fibrillation (CHA_2DS_2-Vasc score)		Vital signs, hemodynamic instability
Cardiac valve (mechanical vs tissue, aortic vs mitral)		Diagnosis of internal hemorrhage (+FAST, CT, DPA)
Thrombus on recent echocardiogram		Localization of bleeding, ease of access (OR, IR, compressible vs non-compressible)
Recent history of VTE (past 6–12 months)		Major bleed or intracranial hemorrhage in past 3 months
Medications that potentiate thrombus • Assess indication • Consider another medication class • Risk of withholding medication		Abnormal laboratory findings • Coagulopathy (INR, fibrinogen, TEG) • Platelet dysfunction (qualitative or quantitative) • Physiologic markers of hemorrhage (H/H, Lactate, acidosis, base deficit) • Organ function (LFTs, Cr) • Transfusion considerations (K, Ca)
Implants (mechanical devices, vascular hardware)		Emergent need for intervention
Recent administration of other clotting factors (FFP, PCC, vitamin K, etc.)		Anticoagulant rebound after transient antidote administration
Pre-existing thromboembolic disease		Concern for heparin induced thrombocytopenia Prior allergy to anticoagulants

Data from Refs.[31,32,34]

Tranexamic acid may also be considered. Because of the protein-binding capabilities of edoxaban, dialysis is not an option for reversal.

FINANCIAL CONSIDERATIONS

Finally, providers should consider the cost of these reversal agents when the emergent versus urgent nature is at the provider's discretion. Vitamin K is less than $50 per dose. Fresh-frozen plasma can cost several hundred dollars per unit transfused. PCCs costs $1 to $2 per unit in the United States.[33] For a 70 kg patient, a 25 IU/kg dose costs $1750 to $3500 and a 50 IU/kg dose, about $3500 to $7000. Recombinant factor VIIa costs several thousand dollars for a single dose. Idarucizumab also costs several thousand dollars. The cost of andexanet and ciraparantag is not known, because they have not been FDA approved and are not on the market. However, one could assume as with all new medications, they will be costly.

REFERENCES

1. Yeh CH, Gross PL, Weitz JI. Evolving use of new oral anticoagulants for treatment of venous thromboembolism. Blood 2014;124:1020–8.
2. Ruff CT, Giugliano RP, Braunwald E, et al. Comparison of the efficacy and safety of new oral anticoagulants with warfarin in patients with atrial fibrillation: a meta-analysis of randomised trials. Lancet 2014;383:955–62.
3. Levy JH, Spyropoulos AC, Samama CM, et al. Direct oral anticoagulants: new drugs and new concepts. JACC Cardiovasc Interv 2014;7:1333–51.
4. Chan NC, Eikelboom JW, Weitz JI. Evolving treatments for arterial and venous thrombosis: role of the direct oral anticoagulants. Circ Res 2016;118:1409–24.
5. Weitz JI, Harenberg J. New developments in anticoagulants: past, present and future. Thromb Haemost 2017;117:1283–8.
6. Pradaxa prescribing information. Ridgefield (CT): Boehringer Ingelheim Pharmaceuticals, Inc; 2014.
7. Praxbind prescribing information. Ridgefield (CT): Boehringer Ingelheim Pharmaceuticals, Inc; 2015.
8. Xarelto prescribing information. Titusville (NJ): Janssen Pharmaceuticals, Inc; 2014.
9. Connolly SJ, Milling TJ Jr, Eikelboom JW, et al. Andexanet alfa for acute major bleeding associated with factor Xa inhibitors. N Engl J Med 2016;375:1131–41.
10. Siegal DM, Curnette JT, Connolly SJ, et al. Andexanet alfa for the reversal of factor Xa inhibitor activity. N Engl J Med 2015;373:2413–24.
11. Eliquis prescribing information. Princeton (NJ): Bristol-Myers Squibb Company and Pfizer Inc; 2014.
12. Frost C, Yu Z, Nepal S, et al. Apixaban, a direct factor Xa inhibitor: single-dose pharmacokinetics and pharmacodynamics of an intravenous formulation [abstract 142]. J Clin Pharmacol 2008;48:1132.
13. Frost C, Yu Z, Moore K, et al. Apixaban, an oral direct factor Xa inhibitor: multiple-dose safety, pharmacokinetics, and pharmacodynamics in healthy subjects. XXIst ISTH Congress; August 2007 [abstract]. J Thromb Haemost 2007; 5(Supplement 2):P-M-664.
14. Raghavan N, Frost CE, Yu Z, et al. Apixaban metabolism and pharmacokinetics after oral administration to humans. Drug Metab Dispos 2009;37:74–81.
15. Eriksson BI, Quinlan DJ, Weitz JI. Comparative pharmacodynamics and pharmacokinetics of oral direct thrombin and factor Xa inhibitors in development. Clin Pharmacokinet 2009;48:1–22.
16. Savaysa prescribing information. Basking Ridge (NJ): Daiichi Sankyo, Inc; 2017.
17. Hughes GJ, Hilas O. Edoxaban: an investigational factor Xa inhibitor. P T 2014; 39(10):686–715.
18. Bevyxxa prescribing information. South San Francisco (CA): Portola Pharmaceuticals, Inc; 2017.
19. Betrixaban – drug summary. In: prescribers' digital reference. Available at: http://m.pdr.net/drug-summary/Bevyxxa-betrixaban-24114. Accessed February 19, 2018.
20. Gordon JL, Fabian TC, Lee MD, et al. Anticoagulant and antiplatelet medications encountered in emergency surgery patients: a review of reversal strategies. J Trauma Acute Care Surg 2013;75(3):475–86.
21. Holzmacher JL, Sarani B. Indications and methods of anticoagulation reversal. Surg Clin North Am 2017;97:1291–305.

22. McCoy CC, Lawson JH, Shapiro ML. Management of anticoagulation agents in trauma patients. Clin Lab Med 2014;34:563–74.
23. Nitzki-George D, Wozniak I, Caprini JA. Current state of knowledge on oral anticoagulant reversal using procoagulant factors. Ann Pharmacother 2013;47: 841–55.
24. Frontera JA, Lewin JJ III, Rabinstein AA, et al. Guideline for reversal of antithrombotics in intracranial hemorrhage: a statement for healthcare professionals from the Neurocritical Care Society and Society of Critical Care Medicine. Neurocrit Care 2016;24:6–46.
25. Levi M, Eerenberg E, Kamphuisen PW. Bleeding risk and reversal strategies for old and new anticoagulants and antiplatelet agents. J Thromb Haemost 2011; 9:1705–12.
26. Mehran R, Rao SV, Bhatt DL, et al. Standardized bleeding definitions for cardiovascular clinical trials: a consensus report from the bleeding academic research consortium. Circulation 2011;123:2736–47.
27. Rao SV, O'Grady K, Pieper KS, et al. Impact of bleeding severity on clinical outcomes among patients with acute coronary syndromes. Am J Cardiol 2005;96(9): 1200–6.
28. Bovill EG, Terrin ML, Stump DC, et al. Hemorrhagic events during therapy with recombinant tissue-type plasminogen activator, heparin, and aspirin for acute myocardial infarction. Results of the Thrombolysis in Myocardial Infarction (TIMI), phase II trial. Ann Intern Med 1991;115(4):256–65.
29. Wiviott SD, Braunwald E, McCabe CH, et al. Prasugrel versus clopidogrel in patients with acute coronary syndromes. N Engl J Med 2007;357(20):2001–15.
30. Sabatine MS, Morrow DA, Giugliano RP, et al. Association of hemoglobin levels with clinical outcomes in acute coronary syndromes. Circulation 2005;111(16): 2042–9.
31. Doherty JU, Gluckman TJ, Hucker WJ, et al. 2017 ACC expert consensus decision pathway for periprocedural management of anticoagulation in patients with nonvalvular atrial fibrillation. J Am Coll Cardiol 2017;69(7):871–98.
32. Rechenmacher SJ, Fang JC. Bridging anticoagulation. J Am Coll Cardio 2015; 66(12):1392–403.
33. Shander A, Ozawa S, Hofmann A. Activity-based costs of plasma transfusions in medical and surgical inpatients at a US hospital. Vox Sang 2016;11(1):55–61.
34. Nutescu EA, Dager WE, Kalus JS, et al. Management of bleeding and reversal strategies for oral anticoagulant: clinical practice considerations. Am J Health Syst Pharm 2013;70(1):1914–29.

Acute Limb Ischemia

Michael M. McNally, MD*, Junior Univers, MD

KEYWORDS

• Acute limb ischemia • Limb thrombus • Limb embolus • Phlegmasia
• Myoglobinuria • Compartment syndrome

KEY POINTS

- Acute limb ischemia is classified according to clinical findings and severity. Accurate classification of the limb ischemia is essential in determining the timing and type of intervention.
- Despite the cause, class II ischemia (threatened limb) encompasses most patients presenting with acute limb ischemia and requires intervention. Familiarity with the different types of limb ischemia cause will assist in the further workup and treatment options.
- Upper-extremity ischemia is relatively uncommon with different disease processes compared with lower-extremity ischemia. Differentiation between small vessel and large vessel disease in the upper extremity leads to a significantly different workup. Open surgical therapy remains the mainstay of therapy for large vessel upper-extremity ischemia.
- Postoperative complications attributed to myoglobinuria and compartment syndrome are crucial to monitor and have specific treatments. Operative technique, as discussed in the article, is based on different anatomic locations for compartment syndrome and should be familiar for all surgeons performing revascularization of acutely ischemic extremities.

INTRODUCTION

Acute limb ischemia is defined as any sudden decrease in limb perfusion causing a potential threat to limb viability.[1] Acute limb ischemia is a critical, potentially end-of-life, clinical condition that presents in patients with multiple medical comorbidities. This critical condition threatens the viability of the extremity and the patient's survival due to systemic acid-base, electrolyte, and other abnormalities. The diagnosis and initial assessment are mainly clinical. Diagnostic errors have severe consequences resulting in amputation or possible death. A variety of treatment modalities are available to the clinician, including anticoagulation, catheter-directed thrombolysis, pharmacomechanical thrombectomy, percutaneous mechanical thrombectomy, and operative intervention. Depending on the patient and underlying limb ischemia cause, the most appropriate intervention is essential to the final limb outcome.

Department of Surgery, Division of Vascular Surgery, University of Tennessee, 1940 Alcoa Highway, Building E, Suite 120, Knoxville, TN 37920, USA
* Corresponding author.
E-mail address: mmcnally@utmck.edu

Surg Clin N Am 98 (2018) 1081–1096
https://doi.org/10.1016/j.suc.2018.05.002
surgical.theclinics.com

This article details the classification of limb ischemia, outlines the numerous causes of limb ischemia, highlights the diagnosis with treatment options and describes common postoperative conditions after limb ischemia intervention. The acute limb ischemia causes in the article are divided into sections, including the presentation, diagnosis, and therapy for each cause. The broad limb ischemia causes include the following:

- Embolism
- Thrombosis
- Venous obstruction
- Trauma
- Upper extremity: uncommon causes

Postoperative management is extremely important after revascularization of an acutely ischemic extremity. Reperfusion injury, myoglobinuria, and compartment syndrome are summarized in the postoperative section.

CLASSIFICATION OF ACUTE LIMB ISCHEMIA

The classification system of acute limb ischemia is based on the severity of the ischemia, which determines the therapy and timing of intervention plus implications for outcomes. The Rutherford classification of limb ischemia is accepted as the standard reporting system for limb ischemia (**Table 1**). The three ischemia categories are based on clinical findings and Doppler measurements, which can be performed bedside.[2,3]

Class I: Viable, nonthreatened extremity, no neurologic deficit, audible Doppler signal

Class II: Threatened extremity, manifested by neurologic deficit and sluggish/absent Doppler signals in the affected limb. Class II is divided into 2 subcategories: class IIA has mild sensory deficits, whereas Class IIB is associated with both motor and sensory deficits

Class III: Irreversible ischemic nerve and sensory deficits

Table 1
Rutherford's acute limb ischemia classification

		Findings		Doppler Signals	
Category	Description/ Prognosis	Sensory Loss	Muscle Weakness	Arterial	Venous
I. Viable	Not immediately threatened	None	None	Audible	Audible
II. Threatened					
a. Marginally	Salvageable if promptly treated	Minimal (toes) or none	None	Inaudible	Audible
b. Immediately	Salvageable with immediate revascularization	More than toes, associated with rest pain	Mild, moderate	Inaudible	Audible
III. Irreversible	Major tissue loss or permanent nerve damage inevitable	Profound, anesthetic	Profound, paralysis (rigor)	Inaudible	Inaudible

From Rutherford RB, Baker JD, Ernst C, et al. Recommended standards for reports dealing with lower extremity ischemia: revised version. J Vasc Surg 1997;26:518; with permission.

Class I limb ischemia may only require medical therapy such as anticoagulation. Any revascularization, endovascular or open therapy, can be scheduled electively.

Class II acute limb ischemia encompasses most patients with acute limb ischemia and requires intervention. There is a distinct difference between class IIA (marginally threatened) and IIB (immediately threatened). Class IIA patients should undergo either endovascular or open intervention on an urgent basis depending on the duration of their symptoms. With less than 2 weeks of symptoms, prospective studies comparing thrombolytic and surgical interventions favor percutaneous endovascular options, such as thrombolytic or pharmacomechanical thrombectomy. Ischemic symptoms presenting duration are better treated with open surgical intervention.[4] Class IIB ischemia, manifested by motor and sensory deficits, requires emergency intervention. Surgical therapy has been the preferred therapy; however, advances in catheter-based thrombolytic therapy and pharmacomechanical thrombectomy have shortened the time to reperfusion. In addition, the hybrid operating room has allowed surgeons to perform diagnostic imaging, endovascular intervention, and open surgical therapy in a single setting.

Class III ischemia presents with profound neurologic deficits (insensate, paretic limb), muscle rigidity, and the absence of arterial or venous Doppler signals in the affected limb region. Revascularization is usually futile and potentially harmful if therapy leads to myoglobinuria. Primary amputation should be considered.

CAUSE

Embolism

Presentation

Embolism as a cause of acute limb ischemia is defined by debris in the vascular system that obstructs a distal artery. The most common source for an embolus is the heart, where mural thrombus dislodges and obstructs smaller peripheral arteries leading to acute disruption of blood flood to the extremity.[5] Proximal atherosclerotic debris is another source of emboli, where debris from the proximal aorta dislodges and obstructs peripheral arteries.[6] Whether from the heart or proximal aorta, the emboli travels through the vascular system, and as the caliber of vessels decreases, the likelihood of obstructing a peripheral vessel increases. The embolus tends to obstruct at bifurcations, where the lumen of the arteries is narrowed. In the lower extremity, this occurs most frequently at the common femoral artery and popliteal artery. In the upper extremity, the embolus obstructs most commonly at the origin of the profunda brachialis or brachial artery bifurcation.

Acute embolic ischemia presentation is dramatic in nature because it likely occurred in a healthy artery without established collaterals. The patient usually presents with an acute white extremity and a neurosensory deficit. As time passes, the occlusion also worsens because of secondary thrombus that forms both proximal and distal to the emboli.[7] Early diagnosis and treatment are paramount because secondary clot can propagate into distal vessels making revascularization difficult if not impossible.

Diagnosis

Patients presenting with acute limb ischemia from an embolic source have an acutely white leg or arm secondary to the lack of time for collaterals to form. Neurosensory deficit is one of the early signs of acute limb ischemia because sensory nerves are the first to be affected. Motor nerve deficit then appears, leading to muscle weakness in the extremity. Extremity musculature is the last to show symptoms exhibited with extremity tenderness in the affected compartment followed by muscle rigidity. Neurosensory and motor deficit with muscle rigidity is considered end-stage signs of acute limb ischemia.

Duplex ultrasonography is used to evaluate the level of arterial occlusion in acute limb ischemia due to embolic disease. Computed tomographic arteriography (CTA) is widely available in hospitals and has become the imaging modality most frequently used to evaluate acute limb ischemia. Image quality of computed tomographic scanners using intravenous (IV) contrast is comparable to arteriograms. Arteriogram, which was once the mainstay imagining for acute limb ischemia, has been replaced by CTA. Arteriography is the best choice when the problem could be treated endovascularly because it is both diagnostic and therapeutic.

Management

Systemic therapeutic anticoagulation with unfractionated heparin should be started as soon as the diagnosis of acute limb ischemia is made as long as there are no contraindications. An IV bolus of 80 to 100 units/kg should be given and then titrated to maintain partial thromboplastin time between 2.0 and 3.0 times normal values (60–100 seconds). The patient should receive IV analgesia and hydration because they are volume depleted and in tremendous pain. Volume repletion may mitigate the contrast load they will receive and the potential myoglobinuria from reperfusion.

Treatment of acute limb ischemia is based on the Rutherford's classification, extent of clinical ischemia present, and available expertise with endovascular technology.[2] Class I acute limb ischemia, where the limb is not immediately threatened, can be treated with anticoagulation. If revascularization is deemed necessary, both endovascular and open surgical interventions are available.

Acute subcritical ischemia (class IIA) with stable acute ischemia has both endovascular and open surgical options. All obvious emboli should be treated with open embolectomy. With the clear embolus exception, intra-arterial thrombolysis is the primary treatment option for class IIa ischemia. The patient should be interrogated for contraindications to thrombolysis (**Box 1**), and the surgeon should have a low threshold for embolectomy and possible open bypass if a contraindication is present.

Acute critical limb ischemia (class IIB) needs urgent intervention. If institutions are limited in vascular and endovascular resources, transferring a patient with a full range of vascular and endovascular services should be considered. With time to reperfusion as a key factor, most class IIB patients are best treated in the operating room with embolectomy, surgical bypass, or catheter-directed thrombolysis. Hybrid operating rooms now allow surgeons to perform repeated diagnostic imaging, endovascular intervention with catheter-based thrombolysis, or percutaneous mechanical thrombectomy and open surgical revascularization.

In patients presenting with class III acute limb ischemia wherein major tissue loss has occurred along with permanent nerve damage, revascularization is not indicated and amputation should be considered.[8]

Thrombosis

Presentation

Thrombosis as a cause of acute limb ischemia is caused by a blood clot within an artery; this can be caused by atherosclerotic obstruction or hypercoagulability. When thrombosis is due to progressive atherosclerotic narrowing in peripheral arteries, this leads to a platelet thrombus forming once the stenosis becomes critical and leads to acute arterial occlusion. Unlike embolic disease, thrombosis is progressive, and thus rich collaterals have formed over time. Acute critical limb ischemia occurs when this process occurs at multiple levels. In hypercoagulable states, thrombosis can occur within the arterial systems that do not have atherosclerotic disease.

Box 1
Contraindications to pharmacologic thrombolysis

Absolute contraindications

Active bleeding disorder

Gastrointestinal bleeding within 10 days

Cerebrovascular event within 6 months

Intracranial or spinal surgery within 3 months

Head injury within 3 months

Relative contraindications

Major surgery or trauma within 10 days

Hypertension (systolic >180 mm Hg or diastolic >110 mm Hg)

Cardiopulmonary resuscitation within 10 days

Puncture of noncompressible vessel

Intracranial tumor

Pregnancy

Diabetic hemorrhagic retinopathy

Recent eye surgery

Hepatic failure

Bacterial endocarditis

From Kwolek CJ, Shuja F. Acute ischemia: treatment. In: Cronenwett JL, Johnston KW, editors. Rutherford's vascular surgery. 8th edition. Philadelphia: Elsevier; 2014. p. 2528–43; with permission.

Hypercoagulable thrombosis is usually seen in small arterial vessels and is associated with malignancy, hyperviscosity, and low flow states.[9]

Diagnosis

Patients presenting with acute limb ischemia from thrombosis usually present with worsening claudication symptoms and rest pain. Owing to their rich collaterals that have formed, the leg does not appear acutely white like embolic acute limb ischemia. Similar to embolic disease, neurosensory deficit is one of the early signs of acute limb ischemia because sensory nerves are the first to be affected. Muscle weakness in the extremity from the ischemic motor neurons follows. Finally, extremity tenderness followed by rigidity in the muscle compartment is seen. Unlike embolic disease wherein these changes are seen within hours, thrombosis is more forgiving owing to the collaterals that have formed over time.

Duplex ultrasonography can be used to evaluate the level of arterial occlusion in acute limb ischemia due to thrombosis. CTA has replaced invasive arteriography in the setting of acute ischemia. The exception is when the patient is brought to the hybrid operating room for diagnostic arteriography followed by immediate intervention.

Management

Management of acute limb ischemia from thrombosis is similar to embolic limb ischemia treatment. If no contraindication, therapeutic anticoagulation with unfractionated heparin should be initiated.[10] A bolus of 80 to 100 units/kg should be given and then titrated to maintain partial thromboplastin time between 2.0 and 3.0 times normal values (60–100 seconds). The patient should receive IV analgesia and hydration because they are volume depleted and in tremendous pain. Volume repletion may mitigate the contrast load they will receive and the potential myoglobinuria from reperfusion.

Treatment of acute limb ischemia from thrombosis is based on Rutherford's classification, extent of clinical ischemia, and available expertise with endovascular technology.[8] As previously noted in the embolism section, class I acute limb ischemia is treated with anticoagulation alone. If revascularization is deemed necessary, both endovascular and open surgical interventions are available. Class II acute limb ischemia, where the limb is salvageable with prompt intervention, requires revascularization by either endovascular or open surgical technique or hybrid approach.[11] Because of the thrombosis cause, most class II patients will benefit from an endovascular technique involving either low-dose arterial thrombolysis, high-dose pulse spray thrombolysis, or pharmacomechanical thrombectomy due to the acute thrombus present. Additional open techniques might be warranted especially in the class IIB setting. In patients presenting with class III acute limb ischemia where major tissue loss has occurred along with permanent nerve damage, revascularization is not indicated and amputation should be considered.

Venous Obstruction: Phlegmasia Cerulea Dolens

Presentation

Phlegmasia cerulea dolens is a rare venous condition caused by a severe form of venous thrombosis. The venous thrombosis extends into collateral veins resulting in severe venous congestion with massive fluid sequestration and significant edema. Approximately 40% to 60% of phlegmasia cerulean dolens cases progress to venous gangrene when there is retrograde progression of the venous thrombosis to include the capillary bed.[12,13] Phelgmasia cerulea dolens is identified by sudden pain, swelling, purple ecchymosis, and arterial ischemia with loss of distal pulses in the extremity[14] (**Fig. 1**). Risk factors include malignancy, femoral vein catheterization, heparin-induced thrombocytopenia, antiphospholipid syndrome, recent surgery, heart failure, and pregnancy.[15]

Diagnosis

The diagnosis of phlegmasia cerulea dolens is clinical with a high index of suspicion for the severity of the venous disease process. The 4 key diagnostic signs include edema, violaceous discoloration, pain, and severe venous outflow obstruction. Duplex ultrasonography remains the diagnostic test of choice for the detection of deep vein thrombosis. Duplex ultrasound diagnostic criteria for acute deep vein thrombosis require intraluminal echogenicity, increased venous diameter, noncompressibility of the vein with pressure from the transducer, and absence of flow augmentation with distal compression.[16] Computed tomographic venography and magnetic resonance venography are useful additional diagnostic modalities when imaging larger venous segments, especially the inferior vena cava and iliofemoral veins; however, sensitivities diminish for these expensive modalities when smaller diameter veins are evaluated.[17,18]

Management

Treatment of phlegmasia cerulean dolens with systemic anticoagulation should be initiated as soon as the diagnosis is suspected. Heparin administration is started with IV bolus (80–100 U/kg) followed by continuous infusion rate of 15 to 18 U/kg/h. Activated partial thromboplastin time should be monitored with a goal of 2.0 to 3.0 times normal values (60–100 seconds). Newer oral Factor Xa inhibitors (apixiban, rivaroxban) are approved for DVT treatment, however, after all interventions are completed and the patient is clinically improved.

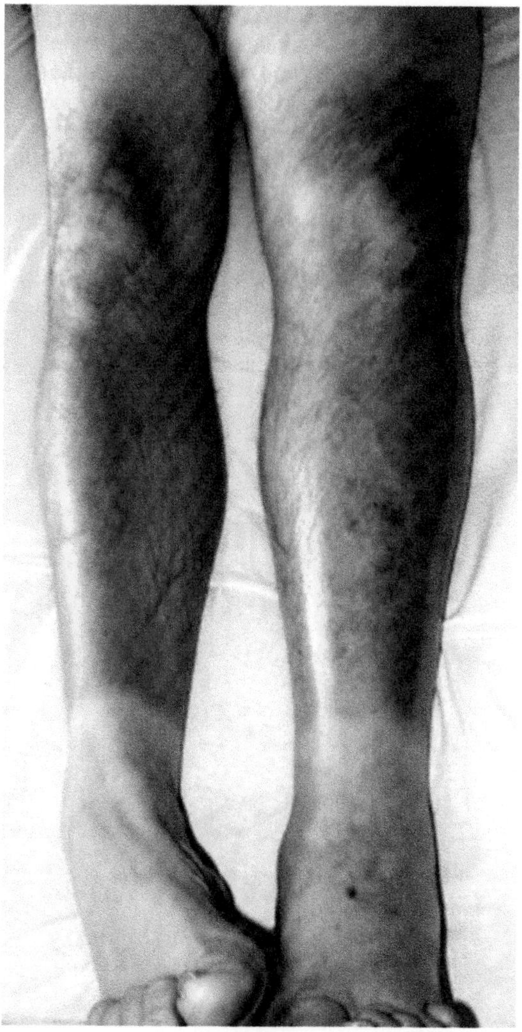

Fig. 1. Phelgmasia cerulea dolens. (*From* Comerota AJ, Aziz F. Acute deep venous thrombosis: surgical and interventional treatment. In: Cronenwett JL, Johnston KW, editors. Rutherford's vascular surgery. 8th edition. Philadelphia: Elsevier; 2014. p. 792–810; with permission.)

Surgical therapy for phlegmasia cerulea dolens centers around relief of proximal large-caliber vein thrombosis to allow for maximal venous outflow. If the patient has no contraindications to thrombolysis, catheter-directed thrombolytic therapy is the primary treatment of extensive DVT associated with phlegmasia. Under ultrasound guidance, the popliteal or tibial vein is accessed. After crossing the segment of thrombus, a multihole infusion catheter is placed across the clot, and thrombolysis infusion is started. For patients with tissue compromise, aggressive maneuvers such as pharmacomechanical thrombolysis, aspiration thrombectomy, or angioplasty can be performed in addition to initiating thrombolysis on the initial venogram.[19,20] With the thrombolysis infusion, patients are monitored in the intensive care unit setting and returned for repeat angiograms every 24 hours for 1 to 3 days. Venous occlusive or stenotic lesions are treated with stenting after the resolution of acute thrombus.

If the patient has a contraindication to thrombolysis, open surgical thrombectomy is indicated (**Fig. 2**). Under general anesthesia in the operating room, the patient is placed in the Trendelenburg position. The femoral vein is exposed from a longitudinal incision. After circumferential vessel control, a longitudinal venotomy in the common femoral vein is performed to allow for a Fogarty balloon (no. 8 or 10 balloon catheter) passage proximally into the iliofemoral veins. For infrainguinal thrombus, the leg is elevated and compressed with an esmarch wrap from the foot toward the groin. If thrombus persists, the posterior tibial vein is exposed in the distal lower extremity. To preserve the lower-extremity vein valves, advanced technique calls for passage of Fogarty catheters from both the femoral and the tibial veins by connecting each with silastic stem from an IV catheter (12–14 gauge). A no. 4 femoral Fogarty catheter is pulled down to the tibial venotomy (by the connected tibial catheter) and then inflated and pulled back from the infrainguinal veins to perform the thrombectomy.

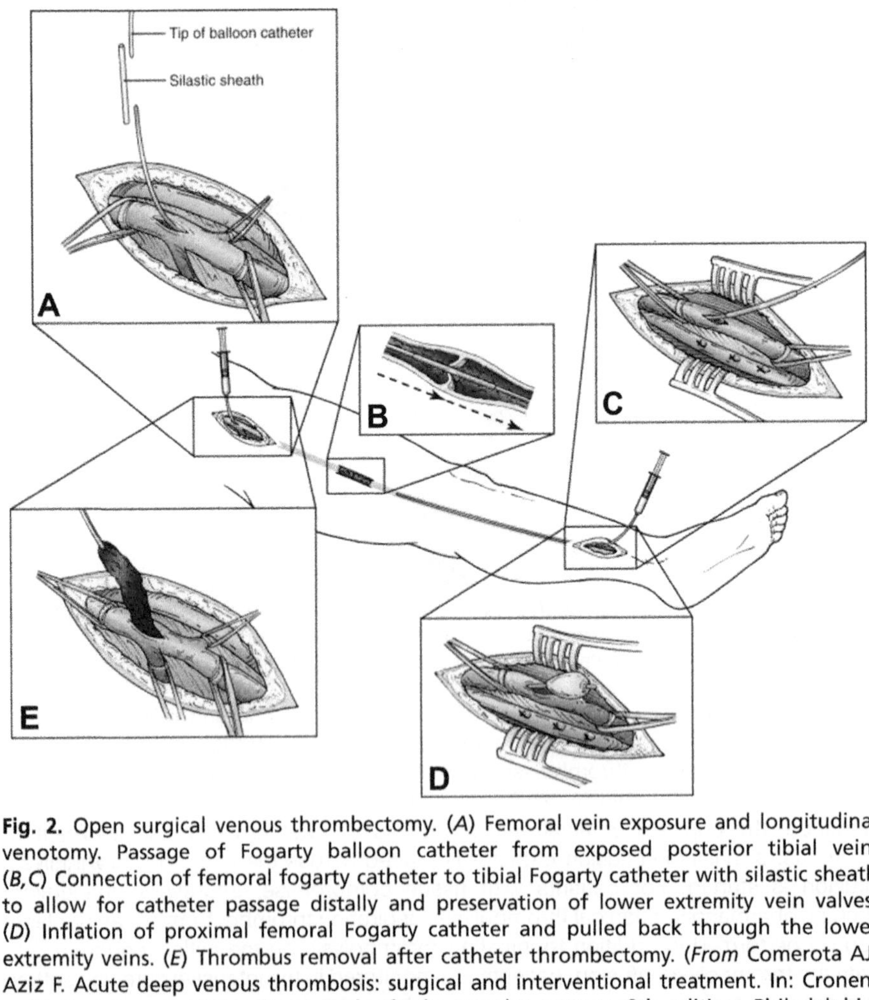

Fig. 2. Open surgical venous thrombectomy. (*A*) Femoral vein exposure and longitudinal venotomy. Passage of Fogarty balloon catheter from exposed posterior tibial vein. (*B,C*) Connection of femoral fogarty catheter to tibial Fogarty catheter with silastic sheath to allow for catheter passage distally and preservation of lower extremity vein valves. (*D*) Inflation of proximal femoral Fogarty catheter and pulled back through the lower extremity veins. (*E*) Thrombus removal after catheter thrombectomy. (*From* Comerota AJ, Aziz F. Acute deep venous thrombosis: surgical and interventional treatment. In: Cronenwett JL, Johnston KW, editors. Rutherford's vascular surgery. 8th edition. Philadelphia: Elsevier; 2014. p. 792–810; with permission.)

After the venous thrombectomy, the venous system is flushed with a red rubber catheter placed in the tibial venotomy. Completion venogram is carried out with any iliac vein stenosis treated with angioplasty or stenting at that time. After femoral venotomy closure, an end-to-side arteriovenous fistula is created between the femoral artery and vein using the proximal saphenous vein to assure patency of the revascularized venous segment.[21] Frequently, 4-compartment fasciotomy will be required for acute compartment syndrome. If venous revascularization is unsuccessful, amputation is sometimes required.

Trauma

Presentation

Acute limb ischemia caused by traumatic disruption of blood flow to a limb presents with either hard or soft signs of vascular injury. Hard signs of vascular injury are pulsatile bleeding, expanding hematoma, absent distal pulses, cold limb, palpable thrill, and audible bruit. Soft signs are significant hemorrhage on history, nerve deficit, reduced palpable pulse, and injury in proximity to major artery.[22] Patients who present with hard signs of vascular injury need to be taken emergently to the operating room for exploration and definitive repair. Traumatic injuries, whether blunt or penetrating, that are in close proximity to vascular structures need to be thoroughly investigated to rule out vascular injury.

Diagnosis

The diagnosis of acute limb ischemia due to trauma is usually identified on initial physical examination because there is usually trauma near to the vasculature of that extremity. Whether it is a gunshot wound to the leg that is actively hemorrhaging or a fracture without distal pulses, knowing the anatomy of the extremity with certain vascular injuries is expected as is the case with posterior knee dislocations and high incidence of popliteal artery injury. Evaluation of the extremity and evidence of hard or soft vascular signs will dictate whether further imagining is necessary versus operative exploration. Patients presenting with soft signs of vascular injury can be further evaluated with Doppler ultrasound, CTA, or angiography.[23]

Management

In acute limb ischemia caused by trauma, the goal is restoration of flow to extremity as soon as possible. If the patient is actively hemorrhaging, a tourniquet is placed proximally for hemostasis and the patient is taken to operating room for surgical exploration. In the operating room, the following basic principles of vascular surgery should be adhered to:

1. Obtain proximal and distal control of the injured vessel
2. Repair: primary repair, venous angioplasty, or bypass with suitable conduit

After perfusion has been restored, it is important to determine whether the extremity requires a fasciotomy. In most instances, if an extremity has gone 6 hours or more with ischemia, a fasciotomy should be performed.[24] Patients who do not receive a fasciotomy during initial revascularization should be watched closely for the development of compartment syndrome and taken promptly back to the operating room for a fasciotomy. Special consideration should be given to blunt trauma in which patient has a posterior knee dislocation because physical examination may not be revealing. A high index of suspicion is required for posterior knee dislocations with CTA or arteriography needed to rule out vascular injury. Undiagnosed popliteal injuries have as high as a 50% amputation rate.[25]

Upper Extremity: Uncommon Causes

Acute ischemia of the upper extremity is relatively uncommon, accounting for only one-fifth of all patients presenting with acute limb ischemia.[26] Women are affected twice as often as men, and patients are significantly older than those with acute lower-extremity ischemia.[27] Numerous different disease processes affect the upper-extremity vasculature versus atherosclerosis, accounting for most of the lower-extremity vascular disease. The cause, pathophysiology, and treatment of upper-extremity ischemia can be differentiated between small vessel and large vessel disease. Small vessel arteriopathies in the upper extremity lead to distal extremity and hand ischemia. These small vessel diseases include autoimmune or connective tissue disease, such as scleroderma, rheumatoid arthritis, systemic lupus, Buerger's disease (thromboangiitis obliterans), and Raynaud phenomenon.[28] Large vessel artery disease in the upper extremity is mainly attributed to atherosclerosis. The most common location of occlusive disease in the upper extremity is the left subclavian artery origin. Other specific large vessel pathologic conditions potentially leading to acute ischemia are arterial thoracic outlet syndrome, thromboembolism from subclavian or axillary artery aneurysms, iatrogenic trauma from cardiac catheterization, steal syndrome after dialysis access placement, aortic dissection with great vessel involvement, trauma, or embolic occlusion from atrial fibrillation.

Presentation

Acute ischemia presents with upper extremity symptoms, such as sudden pain, paresthesias, pallor, and paralysis. Physical examination reveals diminished or absent brachial, radial, or ulnar pulses. Other examination findings reveal arm pallor, dependent hand rubor, and reduced extremity temperature. Because of the diffuse arterial collateral network, acute occlusion in the upper extremity rarely results in tissue loss.[27]

Diagnosis

A detailed history and physical examination can help narrow down the ischemia cause. Important questions in the history regard signs and symptoms for connective tissue disorders (dry eyes, dry mouth, arthritis), remote trauma, recent arterial access for peripheral or coronary catheterization, or occupational history with vibrating tools. In addition to the vascular examination, bilateral blood pressures are assessed with greater than 20 mm Hg difference, suggestive of arterial inflow disease. Auscultation of the supraclavicular and infraclavicular fossa for a bruit can signify subclavian artery stenosis. Splinter hemorrhages in the nail beds are seen with chronic emboli and can give a clue as to the acute pathologic condition, such as cardiac valve vegetation with embolic phenomenon.

The initial diagnostic test is noninvasive segmental pressure measurements of the upper extremity and fingers. Arterial pressures are compared with a wrist to brachial pressure index ratio, where a normal index range is 0.85 to 1.0 and an index less than 0.85 is abnormal. CTA and magnetic resonance arteriography (MRA) provide detail of large vessel disease to the level of the wrist. Catheter-based arteriography is reserved for nondiagnostic CTA/MRA or if small vessel disease is suspected. Unilateral arm or hand ischemia in an athlete is suggestive of subclavian or axillary artery aneurysmal disease, and multiple imaging views should focus on this area. Bilateral digital ischemia warrants bilateral upper extremity arteriography as well as blood testing for systemic disease. Studies for unilateral hand or finger ischemia include duplex ultrasonography, echocardiography, bilateral arteriography, and blood test screening. Blood test screening for autoimmune disease entails erythrocyte sedimentation rate, C-reactive protein, antiphospholipid antibodies, antinuclear antibody titer, and rheumatoid factor. There should be a low threshold for rheumatology consultation if blood screening tests are positive in the setting if digital ischemia.

Management

Surgical As opposed to most lower-extremity revascularizations being completed endovascularly, upper-extremity therapy for acute ischemia has stayed predominately with an open surgical approach, likely because of the infrequency of interventions and the underlying arterial causes. Most of the literature describes treatments of occlusions in the axillary, brachial, radial, and ulnar arteries with surgical bypass or embolectomy.[29,30] Brachial artery embolectomy is the most common upper-extremity embolectomy. Exposure of the distal brachial artery is recommended as well as exposure of both the forearm artery origins to assure embolectomy catheter (2 or 3 French) passage down each artery. Upper-extremity bypasses have excellent patency rates compared with lower extremity. Autogenous vein conduits with greater saphenous vein or upper-extremity vein (basilic, cephalic) are recommended for bypass with anatomic tunneling along the axillary or brachial artery axis.[31] Arterial thoracic outlet syndrome is most commonly treated with a hybrid approach requiring thrombolysis of the affected extremity followed by cervical/first rib resection and possible subclavian artery aneurysm repair. Because of the infrequency of the pathologic condition (least common of all thoracic outlet pathologic condition, 1%), arterial thoracic outlet should be treated at centers with up-to-date endovascular technology and experience in open decompression of the thoracic outlet.

Endovascular The main exceptions to open therapy with large vessel arterial endovascular interventions have been described with proximal subclavian artery and axillary artery angioplasty and stent placement. There are increasing reports of covered stents for subclavian and axillary injury.[32] Numerous other endovascular case reports are reported in the literature with low case numbers and minimal follow-up.

Medical For patients presenting with acute digital ischemia with normal results on physical examination, screening blood tests and noninvasive vascular laboratory tests but a history of vasospasm, Raynaud phenomenon is diagnosed. Raynaud phenomenon diagnosis is one of exclusion after other causes are ruled out. Medical management is the mainstay of therapy. Two medications have proven beneficial in randomized, double-blinded control trials: nifedipine (30 mg daily) and losartan (50 mg twice daily).[33,34]

POSTOPERATIVE COMPLICATIONS

Myoglobinuria

Myoglobinuria is common after treatment of acute limb ischemia. Myoglobinuria exerts its nephrotoxic effects by inducing renal vasoconstriction, tubular cast formation, and direct heme protein–induced cytotoxicity.[35] Preexisting renal insufficiency, large volumes of iodinated contrast (>150 mL) delivery, and hemoglobinuria are all risk factors for myoglobinuria and subsequent acute kidney injury. Hemoglobinuria is commonly seen after percutaneous mechanical thrombectomy, which causes lysis of red blood cells. Treatment mandates maintaining a urine output more than 100 mL/h and alkalinization of the urine with sodium bicarbonate added to IV fluids. Acute renal failure due to myoglobinuria may require temporary dialysis until the kidney function improves.

Compartment Syndrome

Compartment syndrome, regardless of cause or anatomic location, is caused by an increase in intracompartmental pressure (ICP) within an unyielding fascial envelope that impairs tissue perfusion.[36] The most common vascular causes for compartment syndrome are ischemia-reperfusion injury associated with acute ischemia, arterial and venous traumatic injuries, crush injuries, phlegmasia cerulea dolens, and hemorrhage within a compartment. Compartment syndrome may complicate up to 21% of case of acute limb ischemia.[24,37] Risk factors for compartment syndrome after acute arterial ischemia include prolonged ischemia time (>6 hours), young age, insufficient arterial collaterals, acute time course for arterial occlusion, hypotension, and poor back-bleeding from the distal arterial tree at embolectomy.[24]

The diagnosis of compartment syndrome relies on a high index of suspicion. Pain disproportionate to the injury and paresthesias in the distal extremity are the key symptoms of compartment syndrome.[38] On examination, the most common finding is a tense, swollen compartment with pain on passive movement of the muscles in that compartment. ICP measurements are not required for a diagnosis but can be useful in equivocal cases, unconscious patients, and pediatric patients. Normal compartment pressures measure less than 10 to 12 mm Hg. Fasciotomy is recommended if the difference between ICP and mean arterial pressure decreases to less than 40 mm Hg or the difference in ICP and diastolic pressure is less than 10 mm Hg.[39]

Compartment syndrome is a surgical emergency, and once clinically diagnosed, fasciotomy of the affected compartment is indicated. Several fasciotomy techniques (lower extremity, thigh, and forearm) will be described below with accompanied operative diagrams.

- Lower-extremity fasciotomy is carried out most commonly through the double-incision technique (**Fig. 3**) (single-incision fasciotomy is an accepted technique but not described here). A longitudinal incision in made on the lateral aspect of the lower leg between the fibula and crest of the tibia (approximately 4 cm lateral to the tibia crest). The intermuscular septum is identified, and the anterior and lateral compartments are decompressed with attention to avoid injury to the common superficial and deep peroneal nerves near the fibula head. The second incision is made on the medial lower leg 2 cm posterior to the tibia to decompress the 2 posterior compartments. Deep posterior compartment decompression requires dividing the attachments of the soleus muscle to the tibia.[40]
- The thigh contains 3 compartments: anterior, posterior, and medial. Thigh decompression is accomplished most commonly through a single lateral incision to decompress the posterior and anterior compartments (**Fig. 4**). Medial compartment decompression is rarely required. A lateral thigh incision is placed just distal to the intertrochanteric line and extends distally to the lateral

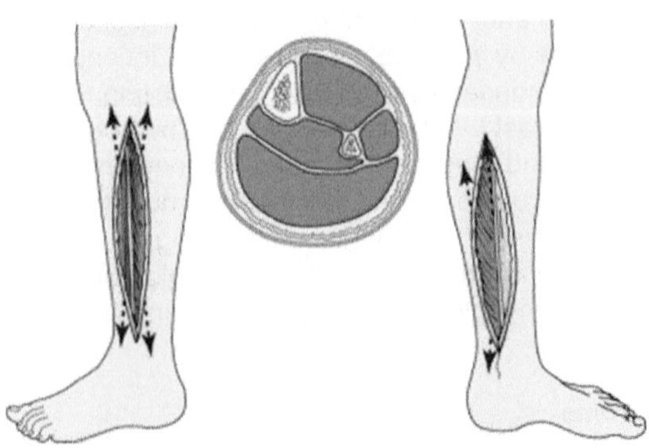

Fig. 3. Fasciotomy technique: lower-extremity double-incision technique. (*From* Janzing H, Broos P, Rommens P. Compartment syndrome as a complication of skin traction in children with femoral fractures. J Trauma 1996;41:156; with permission.)

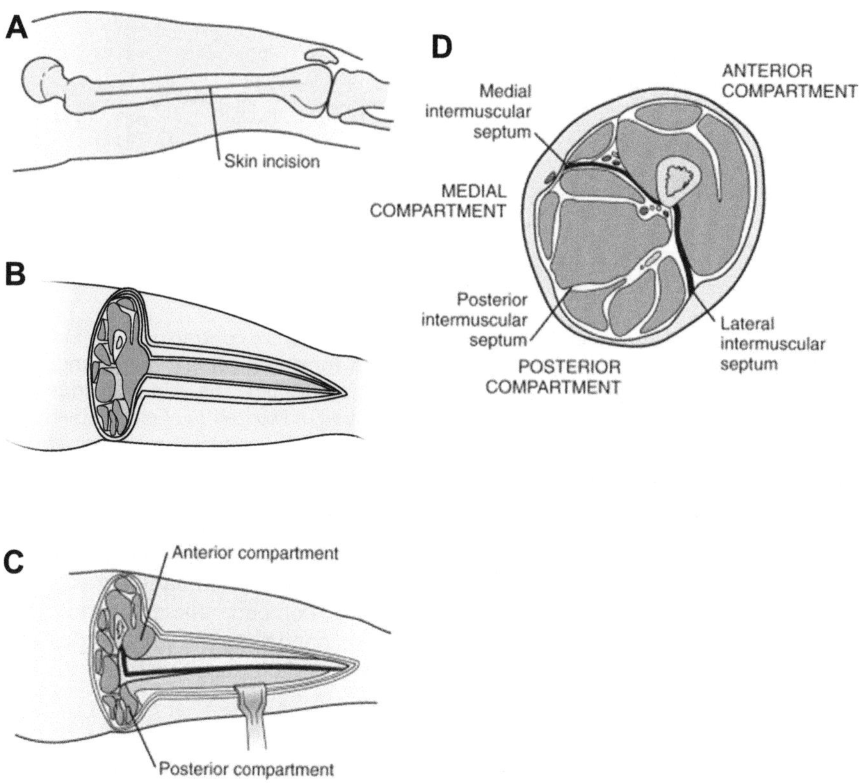

Fig. 4. Fasciotomy of the thigh. (*A*) The incision extends from the intertrochanteric line to the lateral epicondyle. (*B*) Skin incision with anterior and posterior muscle compartments visualized in transverse plane. (*C*) The anterior compartment is opened by incising the fascia lata. The vastus lateralis is retracted medially to expose the lateral intermuscular septum, which is incised to decompress the posterior compartment. (*D*) Thigh compartments and appropriate incision. (*From* Chung J, Modrall JG. Compartment syndrome. In: Cronenwett JL, Johnston KW, eds. Rutherford's vascular surgery. 8th ed. Philadelphia, PA: Elsevier; 2014: 2544–54; with permission and Tarlow SD, Achterman CA, Hayhurst J, et al. Acute compartment syndrome in the thigh complicating fracture of the femur: a report of three cases. J Bone Joint Surg Am 1986;68:1439; with permission.)

epicondyle. The iliotibial band is exposed and incised longitudinally to decompress the anterior compartment. The vastus lateralis is reflected medially to expose the lateral intermuscular septum, which is then incised for posterior compartment decompression. If necessary, a separate incision over the adductor muscle group in the medial thigh will decompress the medial compartment.[41]

- Upper-extremity compartment syndrome is seen most frequently in the forearm. The forearm compartments consist of the volar (flexor, superficial, deep), lateral (mobile wad), and extensor (dorsal, superficial, deep) compartments. The volar approach decompresses the lateral and volar compartments with a single incision (**Fig. 5**). A curvilinear incision begins proximal to the antecubital fossa and medial to the biceps tendon, crosses the antecubital crease, and extends to the radial side of the forearm, where it extends distally along the medial border of the brachioradialis muscle. From the distal forearm, the incision extends

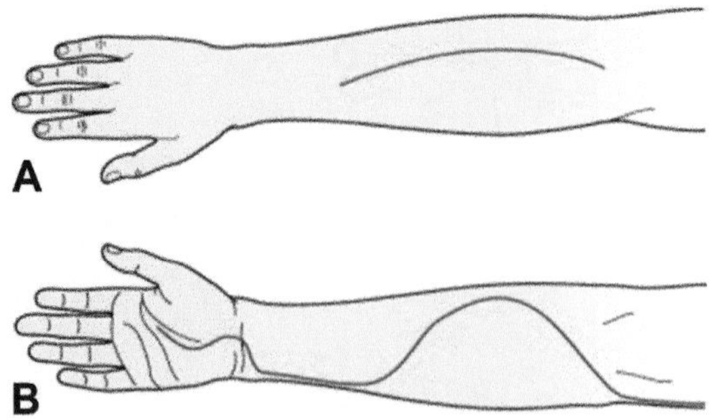

Fig. 5. Fasciotomy of the volar forearm for severe Volkmann's contracture. (*A*) Extensive opening of the fascia of the dorsum of the forearm for dorsal compartment syndromes. (*B*) Incision used for anterior forearm compartment syndromes. The skin and underlying fascia are released completely throughout. (*From* Chung J, Modrall JG. Compartment syndrome. In: Cronenwett JL, Johnston KW, editors. Rutherford's vascular surgery. 8th edition. Philadelphia: Elsevier; 2014. p. 2544–54; with permission.)

across the carpal tunnel along the thenar crease. The fascia overlying the superficial flexor compartment is incised along the entire length of skin incision. The fascia overlying each of the muscles of the deep flexor compartment is incised to complete the volar fasciotomy. The extensor compartment is decompressed through a separate incision from the lateral epicondyle to the wrist between the extensor carpi radialis brevis and the extensor digitorum communis.[42]

REFERENCES

1. Norgren L, Hiatt WR, Dormandy JA, et al. Inter-Society consensus for the management of peripheral arterial disease (TASC II). J Vasc Surg 2007;45(Suppl S):S5–67.
2. Suggested standards for reports dealing with lower extremity ischemia. Prepared by the Ad Hoc Committee on Reporting Standards, Society for Vascular Surgery/North American Chapter, International Society for Cardiovascular Surgery. J Vasc Surg 1986;4:80–94.
3. Rutherford RB, Baker JD, Ernst C, et al. Recommended standards for reports dealing with lower extremity ischemia: revised version. J Vasc Surg 1997;26:517–38.
4. Ouriel K, Veith FJ, Sasahara AA, et al. A comparison of thrombolytic therapy with operative revascularization in the initial treatment of acute peripheral arterial ischemia. J Vasc Surg 1994;19:1021–30.
5. Tawes RL Jr, Harris EJ, Brown WH, et al. Peripheral arterial embolism: a 20-year perspective. Arch Surg 1985;120:595–9.
6. Javid M, Magee TR, Galland RB. Arterial thrombosis associated with malignant disease. Eur J Vasc Endovasc Surg 2008;35:84–7.
7. Abbott WM, Maloney RD, McCabe CC, et al. Arterial embolism: a 44 year perspective. Am J Surg 1982;143:460–4.
8. Jivegärd L, Wingren U. When is urgent revascularization unnecessary for acute lower limb ischaemia? Eur J Vasc Endovasc Surg 1995;9:448–53.
9. Mackman N. Triggers, targets and treatments for thrombosis. Nature 2008;451:914–8.
10. Campbell WB, Ridler BM, Szymanska TH. Two year follow-up after acute thromboembolic limb ischaemia: the importance of anticoagulation. Eur J Vasc Endovasc Surg 2000;19:169–73.

11. Ouriel K, Veith FJ, Sasahara AA. A comparison of recombinant urokinase with vascular surgery as initial treatment for acute arterial occlusion of the legs. Thrombolysis or Peripheral Arterial Surgery (TOPAS) Investigators. N Engl J Med 1998;338:1105–11.
12. Suwanabol PA, Tefera G, Schwarze ML. Syndromes associated with the deep veins: phlegmasia cerulea dolens, May-Thurner syndrome, and nutcracker syndrome. Perspect Vasc Surg Endovasc Ther 2010;22(4):223–30.
13. Oguzkurt L, Ozkan U, Demirturk OS, et al. Endovascular treatment of phlegmasia cerulea dolens with impending venous gangrene: manual aspiration thrombectomy as the first-line thrombus removal method. Cardiovasc Intervent Radiol 2011;34(6):1214–21.
14. Sarwar S, Narra S, Munir A. Phlegmasia cerulea dolens. Tex Heart Inst J 2009;36:76–7.
15. Mumoli N, Invernizzi C, Luschi R, et al. Phlegmasia cerulea dolens. Circulation 2012;125(8):1056–7.
16. Kearon C, Julian JA, Newman TE, et al. Noninvasive diagnosis of deep venous thrombosis. McMaster diagnostic imaging practice guidelines initiative. Ann Intern Med 1998;128:663–77.
17. Thomas SM, Goodacre SW, Sampson FC, et al. Diagnostic value of CT for deep vein thrombosis: results of a systematic review and meta-analysis. Clin Radiol 2008;63:299–304.
18. Carpenter JP, Holland GA, Baum RA, et al. Magnetic resonance venography for the detection of deep venous thrombosis: comparison with contrast venography and duplex Doppler ultrasonography. J Vasc Surg 1993;18:734–41.
19. Casey ET, Murad MH, Zumaeta-Garcia M, et al. Treatment of acute iliofemoral deep vein thrombosis. J Vasc Surg 2012;55(5):1463–73.
20. Nagarsheth KH, Sticco C, Aparajita R, et al. Catheter-directed therapy is safe and effective for the management of acute inferior vena cava thrombosis. Ann Vasc Surg 2015;29(7):1373–9.
21. Comerota AJ, Gale SS. Technique of contemporary iliofemoral and infrainguinal venous thrombectomy. J Vasc Surg 2006;43:185–91.
22. Frykberg ER, Dennis JW, Bishop K, et al. The reliability of physical examination in the evaluation of penetrating extremity trauma for vascular injury: results at one year. J Trauma 1991;31:502–11.
23. Cox MW, Whittaker DR, Martinez C, et al. Traumatic pseudoaneurysms of the head and neck: early endovascular intervention. J Vasc Surg 2007;46:1227–33.
24. Papalambros EL, Panayiotopoulos YP, Bastounis E, et al. Prophylactic fasciotomy of the legs following acute arterial occlusion procedures. Int Angiol 1989;8:120–4.
25. Kauvar DS, Sarfati MR, Kraiss LW. National trauma databank analysis of mortality and limb loss in isolated lower extremity vascular trauma. J Vasc Surg 2011;53:1598–603.
26. Casey RG, Richards S, O'Donohoe M, et al. Vascular surgery of the upper limb: the first year of a new vascular service. Ir Med J 2002;95:104–5.
27. Stonebridge PA, Clason AE, Duncan AJ, et al. Acute ischaemia of the upper limb compared with acute lower limb ischaemia; a 5-year review. Br J Surg 1989;76:515–6.
28. McLafferty RB, Edwards JM, Taylor LM, et al. Diagnosis and long-term clinical outcome in patients presenting with hand ischemia. J Vasc Surg 1995;22:361–93.
29. Roddy SP, Darling RC, Chang BB, et al. Brachial artery reconstruction for occlusive disease: a 12-year experience. J Vasc Surg 2001;33:802–5.

30. Hughes K, Hamdan A, Schermerhorn M, et al. Bypass for chronic ischemia of the upper extremity: results in 20 patients. J Vasc Surg 2007;46:303–7.
31. Brunkwall J, Berggvist D, Bergentz SE. Long-term results of arterial reconstruction of the upper extremity. Eur J Vasc Surg 1994;8:47–51.
32. DuBose JJ, Rajani R, Gilani R, et al, Endovascular Skills for Trauma and Resuscitative Surgery Working Group. Endovascular management of axillo-subclavian arterial injury: a review of published experience. Injury 2012;43:1785–92.
33. Kiowski W, Erne P, Bühler FR. Use of nifedipine in hypertension and Raynaud's phenomenon. Cardiovasc Drugs Ther 1994;4(Suppl 5):935–40.
34. Dziadzio M, Denton CP, Smith R, et al. Losartan therapy for Raynaud's phenomenon and scleroderma: clinical and biochemical findings in a fifteen-week, randomized, parallel-group, controlled trial. Arthritis Rheum 1999;42:2646–55.
35. Ward MM. Factors predictive of acute renal failure in rhabdomyolysis. Arch Intern Med 1988;148:1553–7.
36. Matsen FA III. Compartment syndrome: a unified concept. Clin Orthop 1975;113: 8–14.
37. Bates GJ, Askew AR. Arterial embolectomy: a review of 100 cases. Aust N Z J Surg 1984;4:137–40.
38. Jensen SL, Sandermann J. Compartment syndrome and fasciotomy in vascular surgery. A review of 57 cases. Eur J Vasc Endovasc Surg 1997;13:48–53.
39. McQueen MM, Court-Brown CM. Compartment monitoring in tibial fractures. The pressure threshold for decompression. J Bone Joint Surg Br 1996;78:99–104.
40. Murbarak SJ, Owen CA. Double-incision fasciotomy of the leg for decompression in compartment syndromes. J Bone Joint Surg Am 1977;59:184–7.
41. Tarlow SD, Achterman CA, Hayhurst J. Acute compartment syndrome in the thigh complicating fracture of the femur. J Bone Joint Surg Am 1986;68A:1439–623.
42. Gelberman RH, Garfin SR, Hergenroeder PT, et al. Compartment syndromes of the forearm: diagnosis and treatment. Clin Orthop 1981;161:252–61.

Aggressive Soft Tissue Infections

Nicole M. Garcia, MD*, Jenny Cai, MD

KEYWORDS

• Necrotizing fasciitis • Soft tissue infection • Sepsis • Gas gangrene

KEY POINTS

- Necrotizing soft tissue infections (NSTIs) are rapidly progressive and lead to sepsis, multisystem organ failure, and sometimes death.
- The diagnosis of NSTI is based on clinical findings with the aid of certain laboratory values and imaging.
- Prompt diagnosis and immediate surgical debridement are necessary for the management of NSTIs.
- Surgical debridement should involve complete excision of all tissues that were involved in the disease. Multiple operations may be required.
- Broad-spectrum empiric antibiotics should be given once the diagnosis is suspected, but should not be a substitute for surgical management. Antibiotics can then be tailored to cultures obtained from debridement.

BACKGROUND

Necrotizing soft tissue infections (NSTI) are relatively rare but potentially fatal diseases that are caused by virulent, toxin-producing bacteria. Necrotizing fasciitis has been originally used to describe these infections, but now the term necrotizing soft tissue infection is used to include infections wherein the necrosis extends beyond the fascia. Incidence is varied, about 3800 to 5800 cases yearly, but this is likely underreported because of different reporting practices.[1] Mortality has been reported to range from 21% to 43%,[2,3] but recently, there has been decline in mortality to 10% to 12%.[4] Proposed explanations include increased awareness and early diagnosis, improvements in intensive care and resuscitation, better wound care options, and improved antibiotic coverage.

PATHOPHYSIOLOGY

The hallmark of NSTI is the progressive infection, toxin production, activation of cytokines, thrombosis, ischemia, tissue destruction, and death, which all differentiate it

Disclosure Statement: The authors have nothing to disclose.
Department of Surgery, Division of Trauma and Acute Care Surgery, East Carolina University, Brody School of Medicine, 600 Moye Boulevard, Greenville, NC 27858, USA
* Corresponding author.
E-mail address: Garcian16@ecu.edu

Surg Clin N Am 98 (2018) 1097–1108
https://doi.org/10.1016/j.suc.2018.05.001
0039-6109/18/

from uncomplicated skin and soft tissue infections. Any infection that is left untreated can progress to local necrosis. The pathophysiology depends on the specific bacterium involved in the infection. Necrosis can be secondary to toxins that cause vascular occlusion and necrosis. Bacteria can also produce toxins that lead to progressive systemic inflammation, sepsis, and death. NSTI has been originally described by 2 distinct microbiological profiles, but the classification has evolved over time with additional pathogen classes.

TYPE I INFECTIONS

Type I infections are the most common type of NSTI (55%–80%). These type I infections involve mixed infections, including aerobic and anaerobic bacteria. Streptococcus is the most common aerobic bacteria (and overall), and bacteroides is the most common anaerobe.[5] Diabetes mellitus, obesity, immunosuppression, chronic kidney disease, cirrhosis, malignancy, and alcohol abuse are common risk factors and contribute to the underlying failure of host immune system that leads to these infections.[6]

Some NSTIs are named based on their anatomic location. Fournier gangrene involves the perineum or genital areas.[7] Ludwig angina involves the submandibular space that can spread into the neck and mediastinum, causing a cervical necrotizing fasciitis.[8]

TYPE II INFECTIONS

Type II infections involve either beta-hemolytic *Streptococcus* or *Staphylococcus aureus* (10%–15%).[9] Typically there is a history of trauma to the area, including surgery and intravenous drug use, which supplies the initial inoculation.[10] The bacteria involved in these infections produce exotoxins, and their specific features contribute to their virulence. M proteins on the surface bind directly to T-cell receptors, causing rapid proliferation and a resultant immense proinflammatory cytokine release that produces the septic shock associated with NSTI.[11,12] The inflammatory response then causes widespread thrombosis of blood vessels, preventing host's immune system from attacking the infection as well as necrosis of the tissues.[13] Varied exotoxins produced by the bacteria cause neutrophil damage, break down connective tissue structural components, and decrease viscosity of the purulent fluid so that it transmits along fascial planes.[14,15]

TYPE III INFECTIONS

Infections caused by *Clostridium* spp and *Vibrio vulnificus* (from warm coastal seawater or consumption of raw oysters) are classified as type III infections. These infections are more common in Asia. Water that is contaminated can penetrate the smallest of wounds and spread rapidly. The mortality is high, ranging around 30% to 40%.[16,17]

TYPE IV INFECTIONS

Aeromonas hydrophila and fungi are found in these infections. *Candida* spp are typically found in immunocompromised patients and zygomycetes in immunocompetent patients. Frequently these fungal infections are a result of penetrating traumatic injury. Type IV infections are rare, but aggressive, with rapid extension, and the associated mortality is high, especially when immunocompromised.[18]

PRESENTATION

The initial symptom of NSTI is pain. Typically this pain is out of proportion to examination findings, and it is the most consistent clinical finding.[19,20] The initial appearance of the skin can be deceiving. Commonly, there is minimal erythema and edema. The skin contains a rich vascular network of collaterals, so the skin may be spared in those with deep NSTI. Once the infection progresses, there can be blistering, crepitus, bullae, hemorrhagic blebs, and obvious necrosis that develops (**Fig. 1**). These signs are the typical "hard signs" of infection and should prompt immediate debridement and antibiotics. Patients can also present with signs and symptoms of systemic inflammatory response, sepsis, and profound shock. Multisystem organ failure is a common sequela of the overwhelming infection; thus an NSTI should be suspected in those with a soft tissue infection who rapidly deteriorate.[21]

DIAGNOSIS

The gold standard for diagnosis of NSTI is a clinical diagnosis confirmed by operative exploration. The diagnosis is confirmed when there is either pasty gray necrotic tissue, thin purulent fluid ("dishwater"), lack of resistance to digital pressure against fascial planes, lack of bleeding, thrombosed vessels, and/or muscles that do not contract to electrocautery stimulation.[22,23] Some have proposed a limited operative incision when the diagnosis is equivocal by using a 2-cm incision down to the superficial fascia at the bedside under local anesthesia. If the findings are suspicious, then the patient is brought to the operating room for debridement under general anesthesia. The diagnosis is obvious when there are signs of necrosis.[24] The challenge lies in those without the pathognomonic signs and differentiating necrotizing infections from the more common nonnecrotizing skin infections, especially when early in the course.

Laboratory Values

No specific laboratory values have been proven as diagnostic. However, there have been a few studies to help aid surgeons in earlier diagnosis or increased suspicion. Wall and colleagues[25,26] have demonstrated a negative predictive value of 99% in patients who have a white blood cell (WBC) count less than 15,400/uL or serum sodium greater than 135 mEq/L on admission and 90% sensitivity for NSTI detection using the same parameters.

The Laboratory Risk Indicator for Necrotizing fasciitis (LRINEC) score has been proposed as an adjunct for clinically detecting early cases of NSTI. The score includes total WBC count, hemoglobin, sodium, glucose, serum creatinine, and C-reactive

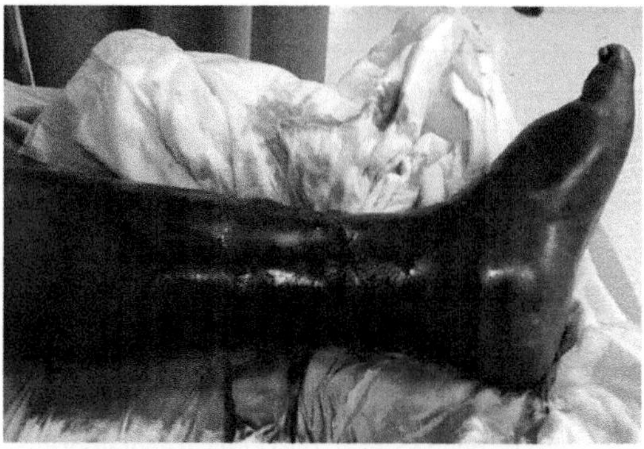

Fig. 1. Left lower extremity with edema, hemorrhagic bullae, and skin necrosis with foul-smelling discharge.

protein. Scores are given to each value, and a total score of 6 or above is highly suspicious for NSTI (**Table 1**). The score corresponds to a positive predictive value of 92% and negative predictive value of 96%.[27] A recent multicenter prospective study on the LRINEC score has shown that a score less than 6 failed to distinguish those with or without evidence of septic shock, high cytokine levels, and death. Thus, the scoring system should not be solely relied on for the diagnosis or exclusion of NSTI.[28]

IMAGING

Plain radiographs can be helpful when gas is demonstrated in the soft tissues. However, subcutaneous emphysema is only seen in 17% to 30% of NSTIs.[13] Computed tomography (CT) often demonstrates nonspecific inflammatory changes, which make it nondiagnostic. In addition, the fascial thickening and edema without asymmetry are nonspecific. Identifying gas on CT images has a high specificity but low sensitivity for NSTI (**Fig. 2**).[29,30]

MRI has a low sensitivity (80%–90%) and lower specificity (50%) in aiding with the diagnosis. It can demonstrate hyperintense signal on T2-weighted images. However, the time typically required to obtain and complete can delay diagnosis and increase mortality; thus, its role in diagnosis is very limited.[31,32]

Point-of-care ultrasound is becoming more ubiquitous given its portability and rapidity, especially in the field of emergency medicine. It is readily available but relies heavily on operator experience. There have been limited case series using point-of-care ultrasound

Table 1
The laboratory risk indicator for necrotizing fasciitis

Variable	Score
C-reactive protein	
<15	0
≥15	4
Total WBC (1000s per mm^3)	
<15	0
15–25	1
>25	2
Hemoglobin (g/dL)	
>13.5	0
11–13.5	1
<11	2
Sodium (mmol/L)	
≥135	0
<135	2
Creatinine (mg/dL)	
≤1.59	0
>1.59	2
Glucose (mg/dL)	
<180	0
≥180	1

Adapted from Wong CH, Khin LW, Heng KS, et al. The LRINEC (Laboratory Risk Indicator for Necrotising Fasciitis) score: a tool for distinguishing necrotizing fasciitis from other soft tissue infections. Crit Care Med 2004;32(7):1536; with permission.

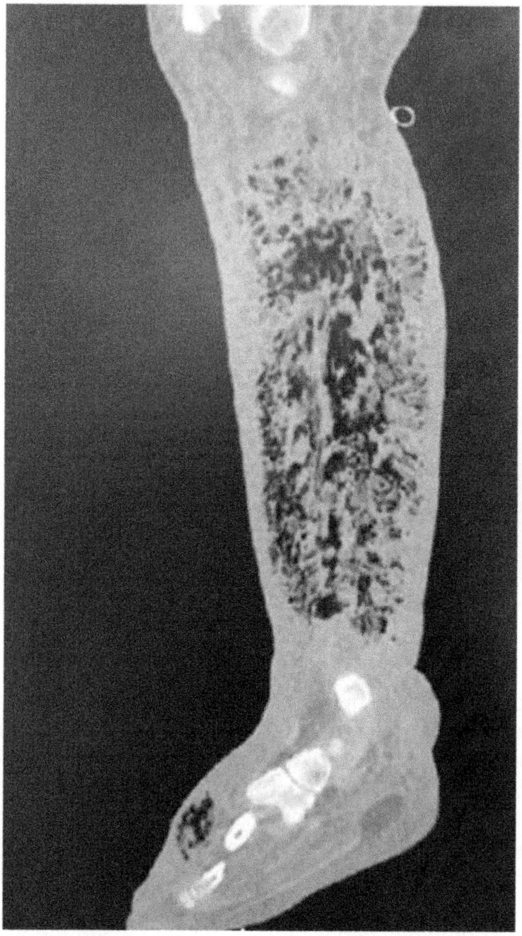

Fig. 2. Evidence of air tracking along the leg on coronal CT images of the right lower extremity.

to assess soft tissue infections.[33,34] There is no compelling evidence for their routine use because the literature is limited to sporadic reports, and additional data are needed before it can be considered a mainstream diagnostic modality.

SURGICAL MANAGEMENT

The single most important determinant of survival is immediate surgical debridement.[35–37] Surgical debridement involves excision of all necrotic skin, subcutaneous tissue, fascia, and muscle within the first operation (**Fig. 3**). Complete excision helps prevent further progression of the disease.[37] Inadequate or more than 24-hour delay in debridement is associated with a 9-fold increase in death.[19,37] The excision and debridement can be debilitating and disfiguring, but essential to halt the disease and maximize survival. Necrotic tissue should be aggressively debrided back to healthy, viable, bleeding tissue (**Fig. 4**). After debridement, the area should be covered with saline-soaked gauze and absorbent pads. The resuscitation is completed, and the wound is monitored for progression of the infection.

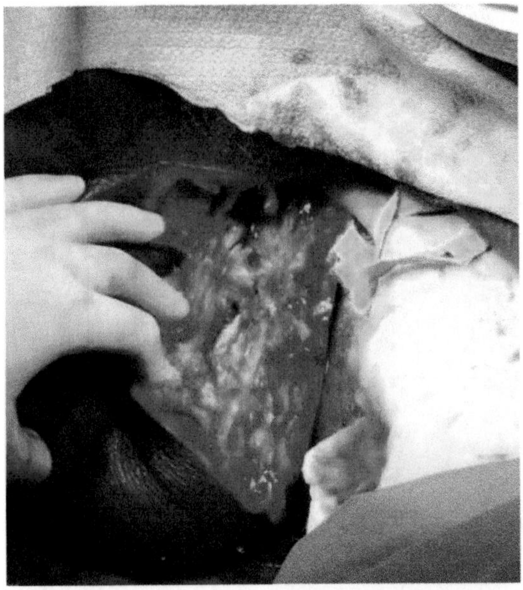

Fig. 3. Intraoperative debridement of a perineal NSTI with evidence of necrosis of subcutaneous tissue and muscle.

These patients typically require multiple operations. It is very common to have additional areas of necrosis that will require additional debridement, so it is recommended that the patient be taken back to the operating room for a thorough exploration after initial resuscitation after 12 to 24 hours.[21,35] Serial explorations and debridement are usually necessary until no infection remains (**Fig. 5**). Once the necrosis and infection are controlled, a vacuum-assisted closure system can accelerate wound healing, and eventually, the defect can be covered with skin grafts or rotational flaps.[38,39]

Amputations are sometimes necessary for patients when the affected limb is not viable or not expected to be functional after debridement. Those with extensive limb involvement may need an amputation to control the infection. Typically, a

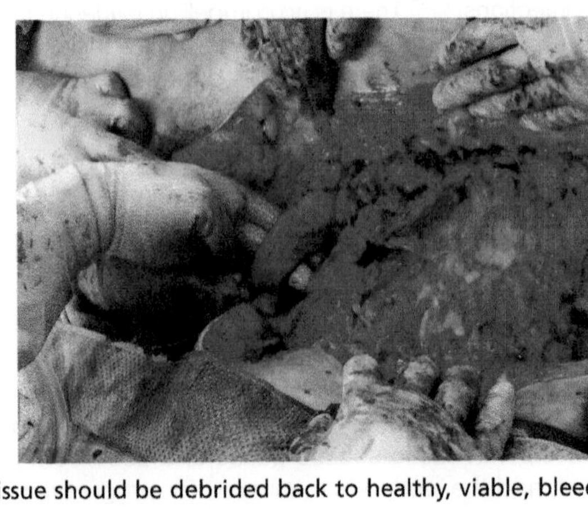

Fig. 4. Necrotic tissue should be debrided back to healthy, viable, bleeding tissue.

guillotine amputation is the initial procedure of choice, especially in those in extremis, in order to perform serial evaluations to ascertain that the infection does not spread more proximally.[40] In those patients with perineal infections, a diverting colostomy may be needed to control soilage of the wound. These patients usually have involvement of their perianal area and become incontinent of stool. Orchiectomy is rarely needed for Fournier because the blood supply to the testicles is usually preserved.[41]

ANTIBIOTICS

Initiation of antimicrobial therapy is an important component for the management of NSTIs. Antibiotics aid in the systemic manifestations of the infection, but they are not effective on necrotic tissue. Thus, antibiotics are not a replacement for an operation. Initial antibiotic regimen should be broad spectrum, including coverage of gram-negative, gram-positive, and anaerobic bacteria, and later deescalated based on culture results and clinical response[23] (**Table 2**). Because of the increased prevalence of

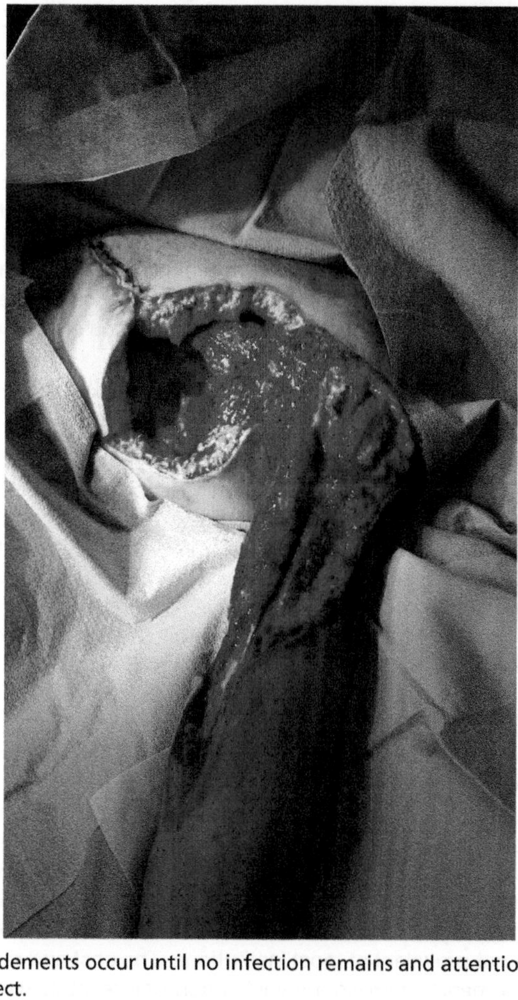

Fig. 5. Serial debridements occur until no infection remains and attention can be turned to closure of the defect.

Table 2
Types of necrotizing soft tissue infections, common patient populations, most common pathogens, and initial antibiotic choices

Type of Infection	Patient Population	Most Common Pathogen	Antibiotic Choices
Type I	DM, CKD, cirrhosis, obesity	Mixed aerobic (streptococcus) and anerobic (bacteroides)	Gram negative, gram positive, including MRSA + anaerobic
Type II	Trauma, postoperative, IVDA	Beta-hemolytic streptococcus, *S aureus*	Gram negative, gram positive, including MRSA + anaerobic + clindamycin
Type III	Marine organisms	*Clostridium* spp, *V vulnificus*	Gram negative, gram positive, including MRSA + anaerobic + tetracycline
Type IV	Immunocompromised, penetrating trauma	*A hydrophila*, *Candida* spp, zygomycetes	Gram negative, gram positive, including MRSA + anaerobic + antifungal

Abbreviations: CKD, chronic kidney disease; DM, diabetes mellitus; IVDA, intravenous drug abuse; MRSA, methicillin-resistant *S aureus*.

methicillin-resistant *S aureus* in the community and hospital, it is mandatory to include empiric treatment of these strains. Clindamycin is unique in that it attenuates the toxins produced by *S aureus*, hemolytic streptococci, and clostridia. If infection with *Vibrio* or *aeromonas* is suspected, doxycycline or another tetracycline should be added to the regimen.[42,43] There are no clinical trials that have evaluated the duration of antibiotic therapy for NSTI; however, guidelines suggest continuing antibiotics for at least 48 to 72 hours after resolution of systemic signs of infection and completion of source control.[23]

ADJUVANT THERAPIES

Intravenous Immunoglobulin

Immunoglobulins have been studied in streptococcal infections that cause toxic shock syndrome.[44,45] Because streptococcus is known to cause many NSTIs, it is reasonable to hypothesize that it may aid in the treatment of NSTIs. The intravenous immunoglobulin (IVIG) binds and inactivates the circulating superantigens, therefore blunting the cytokine cascade. Case reports and observational studies involving IVIG in NSTI show no survival benefit to therapy.[46] The most recent INSTINCT study, which is a Danish multicenter randomized controlled trial, evaluating the effect of 3 days of IVIG therapy found no benefit on survival at 6 months.[47]

Hyperbaric Oxygen

The fascia is a relatively hypoxic environment; it has been proposed that by increasing the plasma dissolved oxygen concentration, hyperbaric oxygen can enhance oxygen delivery and be used as a direct toxin to fight anaerobic bacteria. There are some small studies, mostly observational, that show a shorter length of treatment and increased overall survival with hyperbaric oxygen, whereas other studies show no effect.[48–50] These studies are flawed in that this disease process is relatively uncommon, making adequate statistical analysis difficult with low-powered studies. Also, hyperbaric oxygen chambers are not prevalent at most institutions. The cost and relative unavailability of this treatment mandate broader investigation before implementation.

SPECIAL PATIENT POPULATIONS

Obesity

Obesity is a growing issue in the United States. Obesity is associated with many medical diseases as well as poor outcomes in multiple disease processes. However, the "obesity paradox" has been recognized, in which a high body mass index can have a protective effect across several disease states.[27,51] One study has demonstrated a protective effect of obesity on in-hospital mortality in NSTI.[52] The mechanism behind the obesity paradox is still being investigated, and theories include increased cardiopulmonary reserve and malnutrition inflammation syndrome.

Pediatrics

NSTI has been documented in the pediatric population. Predisposing factors have consistently included varicella lesions as well as intramuscular injections. Rapid diagnosis and surgical management remain the mainstays of treatment in this population. The pathogen is more likely monomicrobial secondary to streptococcus pyogenes.[53]

SUMMARY

NSTI continues to be a disease fraught with high morbidity and mortality. Early diagnosis is essential to improving outcomes. The diagnosis can be challenging in that it is difficult to distinguish between common superficial cellulitis and NSTIs. Patient presentation can range from subtle physical examination findings to multisystem organ failure. There are some diagnostic tools that can be used as an adjunct, but nothing has been found to be very sensitive and specific. Imaging can be used to aid in the diagnosis, but should not delay treatment. Prompt aggressive wide surgical debridement is the mainstay of treatment and is the single most important factor in controlling the disease process. Broad spectrum antibiotics should also be administered as soon as possible and can be refined based on results of cultures obtained during debridement. Other therapies such as IVIG and hyperbaric oxygen have been explored, but they have been found to be ineffective and not routinely recommended. Early recognition and diagnosis, expeditious treatment and debridement, and support with the best available critical care significantly improve the burden of this disease.

REFERENCES

1. Psoinos CM, Flahive JM, Shaw JJ, et al. Contemporary trends in necrotizing soft-tissue infections in the United States. Surgery 2013;153:819–27.
2. Ward RG, Walsh MS. Necrotizing fasciitis: 10 years' experience in a district general hospital. Br J Surg 1991;78:488–9.
3. Wong CH, Chang HC, Pasupathy S, et al. Necrotizing fasciitis: clinical presentation, microbiology, and determinants of mortality. J Bone Joint Surg Am 2003;85-A:1454–60.
4. Mills MK, Faraklas I, Davis C, et al. Outcomes from treatment of necrotizing soft-tissue infections: results from the National Surgical Quality Improvement Program database. Am J Surg 2010;200:790–6.
5. Elliot DC, Kufera JA, Myers RA. The microbiology of necrotizing soft tissue infections. Am J Surg 2000;179:361–6.
6. Henry S, Scalea T. Soft tissue infections. Acute care surgery. New York: McGraw Hill Medical; 2009.
7. Eke N. Fournier's gangrene: a review of 1726 cases. Br J Surg 2000;87:718–28.

8. Boscolo-Rizzo P, Da Mosto MC. Submandibular space infection: a potentially lethal infection. Int J Infect Dis 2009;13:327–33.
9. Center for Disease Control and Prevention (CDC). Invasive group A streptococcal infections-United Kingdom. MMWR Morb Mortal Wkly Rep 1994;43:401–2.
10. Chen JL, Fullerton KE, Flynn NM. Necrotizing fasciitis associated with injection drug use. Clin Infect Dis 2001;33(1):6–15.
11. Schrager HM, Alberti S, Cywes C, et al. Hyaluronic acid capsule modulates M protein-mediated adherence and acts as a ligand for attachment of group A Streptococcus to CD44 on human keratinocytes. J Clin Invest 1998;101:1708–16.
12. Lancefield RC. Current knowledge of type-specific M antigens of group A streptococci. J Immunol 1962;89:307–13.
13. Sarani B, Strong M, Pascual J, et al. Necrotizing fasciitis: current concepts and review of the literature. J Am Coll Surg 2009;208(2):279–88.
14. Salcido RS. Necrotizing fasciitis: reviewing the causes and treatment strategies. Adv Skin Wound Care 2007;20(5):288–93.
15. Cainzos M, Gonzales-Rodriguez FJ. Necrotizing soft tissue infections. Curr Opin Crit Care 2007;13(4):433–9.
16. Goodell KH, Jordan MR, Graham R, et al. Rapidly advancing necrotizing fasciitis caused by Phytobacterium (vibrio) damsela: a hyperaggressive variant. Crit Care Med 2004;32(1):278–81.
17. Present DA, Meislin R, Shaffer B. Gas gangrene: a review. Orthop Rev 1990;19:333–41.
18. Morgan MS. Diagnosis and management of necrotising fasciitis: a multiparametric approach. J Hosp Infect 2010;75:249–57.
19. Childers BJ, Potyondy LD, Nachreiner R, et al. Necrotizing fasciitis: a fourteen-year retropsective study of 163 consecutive patients. Am Surg 2002;68(2):109–16.
20. Stevens DL, Bisno AL, Chambers HF, et al. Practice guidelines for the diagnosis and management of skin and soft-tissue infections. Clin Infect Dis 2005;41:1373–406.
21. Elliot DC, Kufera JA, Myers RA. Necrotizing soft tissue infections: risk factors for mortality and strategies for management. Ann Surg 1996;224:672–83.
22. Green RJ, Dafoe DC, Raffin TA. Necrotizing fasciitis. Chest 1996;110:219–29.
23. Stevens DL, Bisno AL, Chambers HF, et al. Practice guidelines for the diagnosis and management of skin and soft tissue infections: 2014 update by the Infectious Diseases Society of America. Clin Infect Dis 2014;59:147–59.
24. Andreasen TJ, Green SD, Childers BJ. Massive infectious soft-tissue injury: diagnosis and management of necrotizing fasciitis and purpura fulminans. Past Reconstr Surg 2001;107(4):1025–35.
25. Wall DB, Kleain SR, Black S, et al. A simple model to help distinguish necrotizing from non-necrotizing soft tissue infection. J Am Coll Surg 2000;191(3):227–31.
26. Wall DB, de Virgilio C, Black S. Objective criteria may assist in distinguishing necrotizing fasciitis from non-necrotizing soft tissue infection. Am J Surg 2000;179(1):17–21.
27. Wong CH, Khin LW, Heng KS, et al. The LRINEC (Laboratory Risk Indicator for Necrotising Fasciitis) score: a tool for distinguishing necrotizing fasciitis from other soft tissue infections. Crit Care Med 2004;32(7):1535–41.
28. Hansen MB, Rasmussen LS, Svensson M, et al. Association between cytokine response, the LRINEC score and outcome in patients with necrotizing soft tissue infection: a multicentre, prospective study. Sci Rep 2017;7:42179.
29. Wysoki MG, Santora TA, Shah RM, et al. Necrotizing fasciitis: CT characteristics. Radiology 1997;203(3):859–63.

30. Becker M, Zbaren P, Hermans R, et al. Necrotizing fasciitis of the head and neck: role of CT in diagnosis and management. Radiology 1997;202(2):471–6.
31. Schmid MR, Kossman T, Duewell S. Differentiation of necrotizing fasciitis and cellulitis using MR imaging. AJR Am J Roentgenol 1998;170(3):615–20.
32. Hopkins KL, Li KC, Bergman G. Gadolinium-DTPA enhanced magnetic resonance imaging of musculoskeletal infectious processes. Skeletal Radiol 1995; 24(5):325–30.
33. Castleberg E, Jenson N, Dinh VA. Diagnosis of necrotizing faciitis with bedside ultrasound: thhe STAFF Exam. West J Emerg Med 2014;15(1):111–3.
34. Yen ZS, Wang HP, Ma HM, et al. Ultrasonographic screening of clinically suspected necrotizing fasciitis. Acad Emerg Med 2002;9:1448–51.
35. McHenry CR, Piotrowski JJ, Petrinic D, et al. Determinants of mortality for necrotizing soft-tissue infections. Ann Surg 1995;221:558–63.
36. Sudarsky LA, Laschinger JC, Coppa GF, et al. Improved results from a standardized approach in treating patients with necrotizing fasciitis. Ann Surg 1987;206: 661–5.
37. Bilton BD, Zibari GB, McMillan RW, et al. Aggressive surgical management of necrotizing fasciitis serves to decrease mortality: a retrospective study. Am Surg 1998;64:397–400.
38. Kiyokawa K, Takahashi N, Rikimaru H, et al. New continuous negative-pressure and irrgation treatment for infected wounds and intractable ulcers. Plast Reconstr Surg 2007;120(5):1257–76.
39. Lee JY, Jung H, Kwon H, et al. Extended negative pressure wound therapy assisted dermatotraction for the closure of large open fasciotomy wounds in necrotizing faciitis patients. World J Emerg Surg 2014;9:29–39.
40. Anaya DA, McMahon K, Nathens AB, et al. Predictors of mortality and limb loss in necrotizing soft tissue infections. Arch Surg 2005;140:151–8.
41. Kilic A, Aksoy Y, Kilic L. Fournier's gangrene: etiology, treatment, and complications. Ann Plast Surg 2001;47:523–7.
42. Zanetti S, Spanu T, Deriu A, et al. In vitro susceptibility of Vibrio spp. Isolated from the environment. Int J Antimicrob Agents 2001;17:407–9.
43. Aravena-Roman M, Inglis TJ, Henderson B, et al. Antimicrobial susceptibilities of Aeromonas strains isolated from clinical and environmental sources to 26 antimicrobial agents. Antimicrob Agents Chemother 2012;56(2):1110–2.
44. Linner A, Darenberg J, Sjölin J, et al. Clinical efficacy of polyspecific intravenous immunoglobulin therapy in patients with streptococcal toxic shock syndrome: a comparative observational study. Clin Infect Dis 2014;59(6):851–7.
45. Darenberg J, Söderquist B, Normark BH, et al. Differences in potency of intravenous polyspecific immunoglobulin G against streptococcal and staphylococcal superantigens: implications for therapy of toxic shock syndrome. Clin Infect Dis 2004;38(6):836–42.
46. Kadri SS, Swihart BJ, Bonne SL, et al. Impact of intravenous immunoglobulin on survival in necrotizing fasciitis with vasopressor-dependent shock: a propensity-score matched analysis from 130 US hospitals. Clin Infect Dis 2016;64(7):877–85.
47. Madsen MB, Hjortrup PB, Hansen MB, et al. Immunoglobulin G for patients with necrotizing soft tissue infection (INSTINCT): a randomized, blinded, placebo-controlled trial. Intensive Care Med 2017;43(11):1585–93.
48. Shupack A, Shoshani O, Goldenberg I, et al. Necrotizing fasciitis: an indication for hyperbaric oxygenation therapy? Surgery 1995;118:873–8.
49. Jallali N, Withey S, Butler PE. Hyperbaric oxygen as adjuvant therapy in the management of necrotizing fasciitis. Am J Surg 2005;189:462–6.

50. Riseman JA, Zamboni WA, Curtis A. Hyperbaric oxygen therapy for necrotizing fasciitis reduces mortality and the need for debridements. Surgery 1990;108: 847–50.
51. Ahmadi SF, Streja E, Zahmatkesh G, et al. Reverse epidemiology of traditional cardiovascular risk factors in the geriatric population. J Am Med Dir Assoc 2015;16(11):933–9.
52. Rios-Diaz AJ, Lin E, Williams K, et al. Obesity paradox in patient with severe soft tissue infection. Am J Surg 2013;214:385–9.
53. Bingol-Kologlu M, Yildiz RV, Alper B, et al. Necrotizing fasciitis in children: Diagnostic and therapeutic aspects. J Pediatr Surg 2007;42(11):1892–7.